Doing Right

Fourth Edition

Doing Right

A Practical Guide to Ethics
for Medical Trainees
and Physicians

Philip C. Hébert
Wayne Rosen

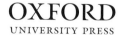

OXFORD
UNIVERSITY PRESS

OXFORD
UNIVERSITY PRESS

Oxford University Press is a department of the University of Oxford.
It furthers the University's objective of excellence in research, scholarship,
and education by publishing worldwide. Oxford is a registered trade mark of
Oxford University Press in the UK and in certain other countries.

Published in Canada by
Oxford University Press
8 Sampson Mews, Suite 204,
Don Mills, Ontario M3C 0H5 Canada

www.oupcanada.com

Copyright © Oxford University Press Canada 2020

The moral rights of the author have been asserted

Database right Oxford University Press (maker)

First Edition published in 1996
Second Edition published in 2009
Third Edition published in 2014

Library and Archives Canada Cataloguing in Publication

Title: Doing right : a practical guide to ethics for medical trainees and physicians / Philip C.
Hébert and Wayne Rosen.
Names: Hébert, Philip C., author. | Rosen, Wayne, 1961- author.
Description: Fourth edition. | Includes bibliographical references and index.
Identifiers: Canadiana (print) 20190051833 | Canadiana (ebook) 20190062037 |
ISBN 9780199031337(softcover) | ISBN 9780199034734 (loose-leaf) |
ISBN 9780199031344 (EPUB)
Subjects: LCSH: Medical ethics.
Classification: LCC R724 .H39 2019 | DDC 174.2—dc23

Cover image: Caiaimage/Robert Daly/OJO+/Getty Images
Cover design: Laurie McGregor
Interior design: Sherill Chapman

Oxford University Press is committed to our environment.
This book is printed on Forest Stewardship Council® certified paper
and comes from responsible sources.

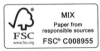

MIX
Paper from
responsible sources
FSC® C008955

Printed and bound in the United States of America

1 2 3 4 — 22 21 20 19

Contents

Cases   ix
Preface   xii
Acknowledgements   xiv
Introduction: A Revolution in Learning   xvi

1   **Ethics Matters   1**
    I. Great Expectations: Healthcare Professionals and Ethics   1
    II. Four Ethical Principles and Questions   2
    III. The Principles and Ethical Reasoning in Medicine   5
    IV. Beyond Principles   9
    V. The Hidden Curriculum   10
    VI. Overcoming Obstacles to Ethics   12

2   **Broadening the Horizon: What Law and Ethics Say   15**
    I. What the Law Says   16
    II. What Ethics Says: Virtues, Rules, and Consequences in Medicine   17
    III. Expanding the Horizons of Ethics   23
    IV. Professional Ethics   28

3   **Managing Medical Morality   33**
    I. Managing Ethical Dilemmas   33
    II. Really Hard Choices Are Not Always about Ethics   34
    III. "Doing Right": A Process for Managing Ethical Choice   37
    IV. The Ethics Process in a Little More Detail   38
    V. Applying the Ethics Process   43

4   **The Times are Changing: Autonomy and Patient-Based Care   50**
    I. The Autonomy Principle   51
    II. Autonomy as the Patient's Preference   54
    III. The Case of Ms Malette and Dr Shulman   56
    IV. Choices: The Good, the Bad, and the Ugly   58

5   **Reasonable Persons: The Legal Roots of Informed Consent   69**
    I. Medical Consent   69
    II. Informed Consent: A Brief Legal History   71
    III. Informed Consent: The Canadian Context   74
    IV. Significance of *Reibl v Hughes*: The Modified Objective Standard   79

6 Informed Choice and Truthtelling: The Centrality of Truth and Trust 85
I. Disclosure and Truthtelling 85
II. The Elements of Informed Choice 89
III. Consent as Trust 95
IV. Other Special Circumstances 97
V. Special Circumstances and Limits on Truthtelling 101

7 Keeping Secrets: Confidentiality and Privacy in the Electronic Age 108
I. Confidentiality and Privacy 108
II. Privacy, confidentiality, and Trust 110
III. New Risks to Privacy 115
IV. Limits to Confidentiality 121
V. To Warn and Protect 128

8 The Waning and Waxing Self: Capacity and Incapacity in Medical Care 131
I. Incapacity and Its Discontents 131
II. Assessing Capacity 134
III. Capacity and Consent 136
IV. Treating and Protecting the Vulnerable 137
V. Substitute and Assisted Decision-Making 139
VI. Mental Illness and the Right to Refuse 142
VII. Children's Right to Refuse 145

9 Helping and Not Harming: Beneficence and Nonmaleficence 151
I. The Principles of Beneficence and Nonmaleficence 151
II. A Duty to Attend? 156
III. Risks to the Professional 158
IV. Endangering One's Self 160
V. Parental Refusals of Treatment 165
VI. Parental Requests for Treatment 169

10 Conduct Becoming: Medical Professionalism 175
I. Maintaining the Connection 175
II. A New Professionalism 177
III. Conflicts of Interest 181
IV. Professionals and Industry 183
V. Boundaries Large and Small 186
VI. Fitness to Practise Medicine 191

11   The End of Forgetting: Ethical and Professional Issues with Social Media   197

I. Friends, Boundaries, and Privacy in the Age of Social Media   197
II. The Personal and the Private   201
III. Patients Using Social Media   204
IV. Photographs and Patient Privacy   206
V. Internet Etiquette and Telling Others' Stories   209

12   The Error of Our Ways: Managing Medical Error   214

I. Medical Error   214
II. Error and Being Responsive to Patients   222
III. How to Disclose Error   223
IV. Apologies   224
V. Large-Scale Adverse Events   225

13   Beyond the Patient: Doing Justice to Justice   230

I. Justice in Everyday Medicine   230
II. A System of Mutual Recognition   234
III. Distributive Justice   239
IV. Squeezing the Balloon   242
V. Guidelines and Rationing   245
VI. Justice for All?   247

14   Labour Pains: Ethics and New Life   254

I. Birthing and Reproductive Choice   254
II. Termination and Choice   260
III. The New Age of Reproduction   262
IV. Desperately Seeking Stem Cells   272

15   A Dark Wood: End-of-Life Decisions   276

I. Allowing Death: Refusals by Patients   276
II. Competent Decisions, Living Wills, and Advance Directives   281
III. Decisions to Withhold or Withdraw Life-Sustaining Treatment   284
IV. Persistent Vegetative States and Prognostic Error   287
V. Unilateral Decisions Regarding Life-Sustaining Treatment   289
VI. Palliative Sedation   292

16   Medical Assistance in Dying: The Triumph of Autonomy   296

I. Assisted Death: Terminology and Other Jurisdictions   298
II. Medically Assisted Death in Canada: A Brief History   300
III. Legislating Medical Assistance in Dying: Bill C-14   302

IV. MAID: Minors, Advance Requests, and Mental Illness   304
V. MAID and Issues of Conscience   313

17   Nature and Culture: Of Genes and Memes   319
I. All in the Genome?   319
II. Cultural Connections   327
III. Worlds Apart?   331
IV. Culture and Defying Death   332
V. Transcending Culture   335

18   The Ethical Regulation of Research   340
I. Medicine's Legacy   340
II. The Purpose of Research   341
III. Consent for Research   344
IV. The Tissue Issue   347
V. Some Questions and Answers Regarding Research   350

Conclusion: Setting our Sights   358
Notes   362
Index   406

Cases

1.1 To Prescribe or Not to Prescribe (resource allocation, justice, professionalism) 2
1.2 "I'm Not Ready to Die!" (resource allocation, respect for autonomy) 8
1.3 A Risky Teaching Tool (professionalism, moral distress) 11
2.1 "You Have No Right to Touch Me!" (capacity, autonomy) 16
2.2 Silent Witness (confidentiality, beneficence, nonmaleficence) 19
2.3 The Worrier (beneficence, truthtelling, medical error, autonomy) 22
2.4 "Don't Tell!" (confidentiality, truthtelling) 27
3.1 Hidden Trauma (confidentiality, truthtelling, cultural issues) 33
3.2 To Feed or Not to Feed? (autonomy, capacity, end of life, consent) 43
4.1 More Surgery Wanted! (autonomy, beneficence, cultural issues) 51
4.2 A Man Who Would Live on Eggs Alone (autonomy, beneficence) 54
4.3 Ligation Litigation (autonomy, consent, reproductive ethics) 58
4.4 "Don't Touch My Arm!" (autonomy, consent, beneficence) 60
4.5 Tranquillizer Trap (autonomy, beneficence) 62
4.6 This Lady's Not for Turning (autonomy, nonmaleficence) 64
5.1 A Simple Question (consent) 70
5.2 New Grads and Small Centres (consent, truthtelling) 74
5.3 How Not to Get Informed Consent (consent, autonomy) 77
5.4 "You'll Be Back to Work in No Time!" (consent, autonomy) 80
5.5 What You Don't Know Won't Hurt You (consent, truthtelling) 81
6.1 A Dark Secret (truthtelling, consent) 87
6.2 "If I Had Only Understood" (consent, autonomy) 89
6.3 "Thanks but No Thanks!" (consent, capacity) 92
6.4 Ratcheting up the Rhetoric (consent, coercion) 94
6.5 "I Trust Ya, Doc" (consent, disclosure, autonomy) 98
6.6 "Stop the Test!" (consent, capacity, autonomy) 100
6.7 A Reflex Response (truthtelling, nonmaleficence) 105
7.1 The Shame of It All! (confidentiality, privacy) 108
7.2 Mum's the Word (confidentiality, privacy, minors, autonomy) 110
7.3 A Favour, Please (confidentiality, privacy, professionalism) 112
7.4 "Just Email Me, Doc" (confidentiality, privacy) 115
7.5 For the Record (confidentiality, privacy) 118
7.6 A Pain in the Butt (confidentiality, privacy, limits of confidentiality) 125
8.1 "Talk to Me, Not My Daughter!" (autonomy, capacity) 131
8.2 A Questionable Consent (autonomy, capacity) 134
8.3 Whose Life Is It Anyway? (autonomy, capacity, withdrawal of care, SDM) 140
8.4 An Odiferous Condition (autonomy, capacity, consent) 142
9.1 No Surgery Wanted (autonomy, beneficence, consent) 152
9.2 A Rush of Blood to the Head (autonomy, beneficence, consent) 154
9.3 Is There a Doctor in the House? (beneficence, professionalism) 157

9.4   No Fools Allowed (autonomy, beneficence)   160
9.5   An Acceptable Request? (autonomy, beneficence, consent, capacity)   162
9.6   The Pillow Angel (autonomy, beneficence, consent, capacity, minor)   171
10.1   An Unexpected Death (beneficence, professionalism)   175
10.2   Show a Little Respect! (professionalism)   179
10.3   Who's Helping Whom? (professionalism, conflict of interest, boundaries)   182
10.4   Supping with the Devil (professionalism, conflict of interest)   183
10.5   Drug Redux (professionalism, conflict of interest)   185
10.6   An Uncomfortable Revelation (professionalism, boundaries)   188
10.7   Too Far from Away (professionalism, boundaries)   189
10.8   An Unfair Rating (professionalism)   191
11.1   To Friend or Not to Friend (professionalism, boundaries)   197
11.2   More Than Just a Friend (professionalism, boundaries, confidentiality)   200
11.3   My Personal Life Is My Business! (professionalism, boundaries, privacy)   201
11.4   A Google Dilemma (professionalism, boundaries, privacy)   204
11.5   Whose Wound Is It Anyway? (professionalism, boundaries, privacy)   206
11.6   A Soldier's Story (professionalism, confidentiality, privacy)   209
12.1   "I'm Just So Tired!" (medical error, truthtelling)   214
12.2   A Lapse in Care (medical error, truthtelling)   219
12.3   The Newfoundland Breast Hormone Assay Inquiry (medical error, truthtelling)   225
13.1   Time Well Spent? (justice, beneficence)   230
13.2   Misfortune Begetting Injustice (justice, advocacy)   232
13.3   Should He Wait or Should He Go? (justice, resource allocation, beneficence)   237
13.4   Terms of Entitlement (justice, resource allocation, autonomy)   240
13.5   A Transplant Tourist (justice, resource allocation, beneficence)   249
14.1   A Trivial Matter? (reproductive, abortion, autonomy)   254
14.2   A Right to Be Tested? (reproductive, abortion, professionalism)   255
14.3   Whose Baby Is It Anyway? (reproductive, beneficence)   270
14.4   The Saviour Child (reproductive, minors, genetics)   273
15.1   The Story of Nancy B (autonomy, end of life, withdrawal/withholding)   277
15.2   No Crap, No CPR (autonomy, end of life, withdrawal/withholding)   280
15.3   Don't Leave Home without It! (autonomy, end of life, withdrawal/withholding)   282
15.4   "She's Not Dying!" (autonomy, end of life, withdrawal/withholding)   284
16.1   An End Foretold (MAID, autonomy)   297
16.2   A Minor Problem (MAID, minor, autonomy)   305
16.3   Advance Notice (MAID, autonomy)   307
16.4   A Depressing Condition (MAID, autonomy)   310

16.5   A Conscientious Objection (MAID, autonomy, professionalism)   314

17.1   A CRISPR View (consent, genetics)   319

17.2   All in the Family? (genetics, consent)   323

17.3   A Cultural Gap (culture)   327

17.4   A Dispute over Death (culture, end of life, withdrawal/withholding)   333

17.5   A Wound Too Terrible (culture, end of life, withdrawal/withholding)   335

18.1   A Reversal of Fortune (research ethics)   341

18.2   Poles Apart (research ethics)   344

18.3   An Unexpected Association (research ethics, genetics)   347

18.4   Are You Coming Home Soon, Dad? (research ethics, privacy)   353

18.5   An Unfair Trial (research ethics, justice)   354

Preface

The future ain't what it used to be.

Colloquialism, but attributed to New York Yankees'
catcher and manager Yogi Berra [1]

Why is there a need for a new edition of a textbook on ethics? Isn't ethics constant and enduring? The answer to this is, simply, no. Our attitudes to numerous practices common in the past—such as slavery, racism, the sexual harassment of women, 100-hour work weeks for medical interns, discrimination against gay and transgender people, the untreated suffering of the terminally ill—have changed dramatically [2].

In the 20 years since the first edition of *Doing Right*, medical ethics has continued to change and many questionable practices have withered away [3]. This book is intended to contribute in a small way to the ongoing evolution towards more ethical medical practice.

Doing Right has been updated to include recent developments in bioethics and jurisprudence. It represents the most comprehensive revision of the book to date. In addition to new chapters on topics such as assisted dying and social media, there have been substantial revisions made to other chapters as well.

All who work in healthcare must face difficult ethical issues, so we have included cases affecting not only physicians but also other healthcare professionals such as nurse practitioners, nurses, social workers, and trainees. Interprofessional practice has become the new norm for healthcare. With that in mind, this text has been written from the perspective of the well-intentioned healthcare professional, the good clinician, regardless of their focus. Although different healthcare professionals will have different degrees of agency and responsibility for handling dilemmas in clinical practice, the "right way" of doing so should reflect a common professional point of view, as seen from those with an abiding commitment to the healing enterprise. This is best arrived at by consensus and through critical interprofessional discussion.

When a troublesome issue must be addressed, consider following three simple steps:

- *Look to the wisdom of others.* Don't try to make hard decisions alone.
- *Be humble and admit you don't know when you don't know.* Consider your limitations and be open about them. No one can do or know everything.
- *Turn to your best resource, the patient beside you.* They may know more than you realize.

Remember that medicine, although a difficult enterprise, need not be a lonely one.

Dialogue and progress in ethical matters, as in medicine and society generally, may not require a common language. However, they do require allegiance to the core and pre-eminent values requisite for all professions: a respect for human dignity and a dedication to critical thought. Thus, the work to abolish—within and *across* cultures—human bondage, female degradation, and child labour, as well as the achievement of medical milestones, such as the eradication of smallpox and soon polio and other viral plagues, are definitive indicators of progress. They also result from recognition of our shared humanity and our ability to change. This book will explore the commitment to these values and their implications for medicine and society.

Ethics taps into the human penchant for regulation to transform and increasingly moralize aspects of social life, such as healthcare. "*Ethical rules are 'advantage-reducing' rules*"[4], claims the less powerful can make against those with more authority. They can reduce unfair advantages of the more powerful. At the same time, they can enhance the position of the less well-situated, such as patients and the public generally, giving voice to those heard less often and speaking truth to power.

Ethical rules are well suited to challenging existing hierarchical or authoritarian systems. Rules and attitudes of showing respect for others, seeking consent, abiding by confidentiality, and being honest attempt to level out what is an uneven playing field. Together, ethics and the new information technologies, with their emphasis on patient self-determination, transcend the secretive and paternalistic Hippocratic ethos. They also give rise to new expectations of healthcare when the old institutions are revealed to be inadequate to the tasks at hand. The point is not to build an exceptionless ethical system—all ethical systems have fault lines and limitations—but to better understand and more fully respond to the new and emerging capacities made possible by healthcare. Advances in ethics, as in medicine, are achieved by seeing the miscalculations and errors in our ways.

A final word about words. We shy away from thinking of "patients" as "consumers," "customers," or "clients" of healthcare and instead think of them as "partners" or "participants" in care. In our view, these "p-words" better capture what healthcare is all about. Those we serve and try to help are unwell and vulnerable. They deserve protection as well as promotion. When travelling through the unfamiliar country of illness, people do not want or need to feel boondoggled and cajoled as if in a commercial marketplace. On the contrary, they need to feel respected, cared for, and heard, not treated as a commodity.

Finally, *morality* is used interchangeably with *ethics*, although many would use morality to refer to the local custom and ethos and ethics to refer to the critical reflection on diverse practices. Medicine is used interchangeably with healthcare, although the latter implies a broader scope of care.

Acknowledgements

Unlike the previous editions, the fourth edition of *Doing Right* is the result of a rich and fruitful collaboration between the original author (PCH) and Wayne Rosen, a surgeon based at the University of Calgary. Both of us had our starts in Philosophy at Queen's University, clearly a department with a propensity for turning out medically minded philosophers (or philosophically minded physicians)! Philip would like to express his gratitude to Wayne for his wisdom, hard work, and patience. This edition would never have been completed without him. Wayne would similarly like to express his gratitude to Philip. It has been an honour to work with him on this project.

We both would like to express our extra special thanks to our editors at OUP (Canada) and to Nancy Carroll of WordReach whose excellent editing hands helped us navigate treacherous waters.

Insightful feedback and help came from a tremendous number of knowledgeable and supportive family, friends, colleagues, and students who read and commented on portions of *Doing Right*. Thanks must go to Erika Abner, Priscilla Alderson, Lisa Alexander, Peter Allatt, Sharone Bar-David, Cécile Bensimon, Lenny Berlin, Carrie Bernard, Anne Berndl, Wendell Block, Ivy Cheng, Sara Cohen, Eoin Connolly, Kristine Connidis, Chip Doig, Neda Ghiam, Rocco Gerace, Mona Gupta, Janice Hébert, Paul Hébert, Jonathan Hellmann, Yiwei Hu, Ian Jarvie, Hanna Jones-Eriksson, Kelly Jordan, Michael Kaufman, John Kingdom, Eva Knifed, Peter Landstreet, Winnie Lem, Mary Rose MacDonald, Maria McDonald, Martin McKneally, Chryssa McAlister, Sue MacRae, Cliodhna McMullin, Eric Meyer, Brian Murray, David Naimark, Florin Padeanu, Kathy Pritchard, Daryl Pullman, Melanie Randall, Deb Selby, Norman Siebrasse, Laura Sky, Gavin Smith, Robert Storey, Frank Wagner, Dick Wells, Shawn Winsor, Hilary Young, and Rhonda Zwingerman. The errors and limitations of this book remain ours.

Wayne would like to also express his sincere appreciation to a number of people at the University of Calgary who made his work on this project possible. Sean Grondin and Elijah Dixon of the Department of Surgery supported and enabled a somewhat atypical sabbatical for a surgeon. Ron Bridges and the University of Calgary Medical Group provided much-appreciated financial support for Wayne's sabbatical. Wayne could also not have carried out this work without the generous support of his surgical colleagues at the Peter Lougheed Centre in Calgary, who took care of his patients and picked up the extra work while he was away. It is a privilege to work with this special group of surgeons.

Not surprisingly, the biggest debts of gratitude we owe are to our spouses—Victoria (herself a tireless editor and fierce grammarian) and Laurie—and to our children—Neil and Raven, Ben and Sam. You have instructed us in more ways than you can know and we can count. To paraphrase Marx, the educators must themselves be educated[1], and we have been re-educated by your welcome critical reflections and by your lessons from life. This has been not just an education of the intellect, but also an education of our emotions—or our "sentiments," as they were once known[2]. Without your unwavering support, forbearance, and suggestions, this edition of *Doing Right* would not have been possible. We are indeed blessed and fortunate to have you in our lives.

Philip C. Hébert, MD, PhD, FCFPC

Professor Emeritus
Department of Family and Community Medicine
University of Toronto
Toronto, Ontario, Canada
philip.hebert@sunnybrook.ca

Wayne Rosen, MD, MSc, FRCS(C)

Clinical Assistant Professor
Department of Surgery
University of Calgary
Calgary, Alberta, Canada
wrosen@ucalgary.ca

Winter 2019

Introduction
A Revolution in Learning

You talk and I'll listen.

Inscription on a park bench, 2017

A new medical curriculum

Beside a peaceful pond in San Francisco's Golden Gate Botanical Garden can be found a bench with the following inscription: "You talk and I'll listen." Although it's not entirely clear what this really means, two doctors had dedicated it, so we'd like to think it was meant for patients and doctors together: *You [the patient] talk and I [the doctor] will listen.*

This is the starting point for the new journey any healthcare professional is expected to take with patients. It begins with making the effort to understand the patient's world, an important instruction, given the number of studies suggesting how time-constrained modern physicians are. At the bedside and in the office, patients are given as little as 12 seconds to tell their story before physicians start interrupting them [1]. And then they keep on interrupting them . . . . No wonder patients often feel they can't get a word in edgewise (with the physician, anyway). Traditionally, communication with nurses and other healthcare professionals has, by contrast, been considered superior, but this may be changing—and not for the better. Nurses too can be swamped with charting and computer work that can erode their time with patients [2].

Our hurriedness undoubtedly contributes not only to the epidemic of error but also to the dissatisfaction with modern medical care on the part of patients *and* practitioners. (Of this, more later; see Chapter 10.) A partial remedy to this problem has been suggested by one family doctor: "If there is one thing to learn, to do really well as a physician, it is to listen. In the midst of the intensity of medicine, the crises, the sadness and the everyday, and the wall of computer screens, always listen to your patient. The patient will give you a better history if they see you are listening" [3].

Good healthcare professionals have always known they need to learn a lot more about their patients and their circumstances—their hopes, fears, dreams, and nightmares—in order to most effectively help them. What has changed in medical education is the more explicit emphasis on encouraging our ability to elicit and respond to unique patient factors. In the midst of the hustle and bustle of modern medical life, there is much to be said for paying attention—as well as for self-reflection and for critical thought.

As a response to the unbalanced world of communication between doctors and patients, the traditional curriculum of medical schools has undergone, and continues to undergo, dramatic changes[4]. Although medical trainees continue to study traditional subjects such as anatomy and physiology, pharmacology and cardiology, they are also taught communication skills, organizational aspects of medicine, the social determinants of health and illness, and the full meaning of respect for others: empathy, honesty, altruism, and trustworthiness. In place of long days full of tedious lectures, students participate in subject-integrated, problem-based cases of the week teaching appreciation of the many-sided—the physical, psychological, and cultural—aspects of the illnesses and the needs of patients.

Medical trainees are taught that the patient in Room 1102 is not just any old aging patient admitted to the hospital with cognitive decline and poor self-care. She is Ms B, who decades ago, as an education consultant, devised new classrooms for children throughout the country. They learn that in Room 613 is not simply an "interesting myeloma patient with a fractured femur" but a former Olympian, Mr Y, who is eager to know as much as possible about his condition, while also feeling terrified about its implications for his future and for his young family.

The best of the new pedagogies stress critical reflection and lifelong learning, rather than rote memorization and regurgitation of facts. Trainees must learn *how* to learn and how to keep up to date as part of an occupation that will last for decades—far longer than most medical fads and fancies. This is a sea change in medical pedagogy. The nature of learning and information exchange in general is changing dramatically. With the advent of the Internet and the digital revolution, information (if not always expertise) is at the fingertips of not only health professionals but also patients and families. Democratic in its implications, this revolution in teaching and learning resists attempts to return to the era of medical paternalism. In a digital world, excluding patients from decision-making will be impossible[5].

A contemporary philosopher of science, Sam Harris, has written that "the most important facts... are bound to transcend culture"[6]. Democratic values and practices are among the "transcendent facts" that stand above individual cultures, helping throughout the world to unite patients with healthcare providers. In the new era of scientific medicine, the humanities—among them ethics, great art, and literature—provide crucial balance to a humane universal education[7]. Becoming a better medical practitioner may be achieved not only by learning the biochemistry of the Krebs cycle or how to recognize geriatric depression but also by reading books such as Miriam Toews' *All My Puny Sorrows*[8] or Tolstoy's *Anna Karenina*[9] or watching a classic film such as Kurosawa's *Red Beard*[10]. Exposure to the humanities not only enriches the lives of practitioners, making them better, more compassionate, citizens of the world, but also increases the likelihood they will understand and empathize with the worlds of patients and their families[11].

One key focus of this new edition of *Doing Right* is the impact of digital technologies on medical practice and the resulting ethical dilemmas. Since the last edition, the digital revolution has continued to profoundly transform how physicians practise medicine. Patients' charts are now electronic, their radiographs digital, hospital orders typed into computer terminals, and communication between patients and health professionals almost instantaneous. Patient safety has been improved with automated alerts of drug incompatibilities or allergies. Many of the minimally invasive interventions that have dramatically improved patient care, whether radiological or surgical, are a result of digital technologies. And now most medical information is no longer hidden away in arcane textbooks and journals, accessible only through expensive subscriptions or by experts in musty libraries, but is more easily retrieved at home by the lay public through Open Access[12]. This has had a lasting impact on democratizing medical knowledge, allowing patients, if they so wish, a greater role in their healthcare[13].

Rather than pining for the old days prior to the advent of the computer and e-communication, the twenty-first-century physician must become an expert in the new technologies of information in order to keep up with what patients are reading and be able to use these to better understand and help their patients. (For more on the impact of social media on medicine, see Chapter 11.) The dramatic explosion of medical information goes far beyond what any one healthcare practitioner can master. The ever-burgeoning amount of information from research and practice can only be managed by learning how to utilize the tremendous gain in cognitive capabilities offered by computerization.

Box I.1

"Medical thinking has become vastly more complex, mirroring changes in our patients, our health care system, and medical science. The complexity of medicine now exceeds the capacity of the human mind."[14]

These changes in medical teaching and learning have been generally all to the good, although seen as a threat by some and a distraction by others. "Computers," Obermeyer and Lee write, "far from being the problem, are the solution"[14]. Well, not entirely. An uncritical infatuation with new technology can also be bad for your health and the health of your patients. The new teaching and learning can enhance healthcare professionals' expertise *only if* they are more willing *to listen to patients and to each other*. Although the learning curve is long and treacherous, computerization should make this task easier and more robust.

"You talk and I, the doctor, will listen."

What is ethics?

Ethics is fundamentally about the virtues and principles necessary for good medical practice (respect for persons being the most basic) and the critical reflection exercised by healthcare professionals to try to do the right thing. It is about acting in ways consistent with what we have the overall "best (moral) reasons" to do [15]. Ethics is also about critically examining these reasons, looking at what we do every day, and trying to do it better. Having a process for considering and managing ethical dilemmas is helpful, we believe, as a structured approach to the ethical quandaries certain to arise for all healthcare practitioners.

For example, should practitioners always inform patients fully about their condition? Is it ever appropriate to disclose confidential information about a patient to a third party? To what extent should the odd views of an eccentric patient be respected? May desperate patients be allowed to take part in medically risky research? Do parents have the right to refuse medically indicated treatment for their children? Are religious objections to accepting that a loved one is dead ever valid? To how much of society's healthcare resources is a patient entitled? Should there be limits to the allocation of scarce resources for procedures such as artificial reproduction or genetic manipulation? How far ought clinicians to go in helping their patients die? Can suicide ever be a rational choice?

The unavoidable uncertainty of practical judgment in medicine—the so-called "grey zone" of practice [16]—is characteristic of most of medicine. Faced with a clinical problem, the healthcare professional asks: "What are we going to do?" But there is a huge gap for most areas of practice between knowing and doing. Medical practice is not simply detective work with clear-cut answers and error-free methods for finding solutions to puzzles [17]. It can never be value free and is rarely simple.

The goal of ethics is not to get the "right" answer to ethical issues. It is to recognize dilemmas, to worry about them, and to do so in ways sensitive to and respectful of the views and practices of others, seeking where possible a broader, more comprehensive perspective. Ethics works towards an unblinkered point of view, unhampered by inappropriate bias; it does not necessarily call for, or result in, easy or singular resolutions.

What can ethics offer to the tentative or reflective practitioner?

What ethics can offer

Ethical dilemmas arise out of perceived conflicts between our basic values and beliefs and the resulting ill-at-ease feelings, sometimes a sense of moral distress or a worry, that some rule or norm of proper behaviour has been violated or transgressed. *They arise when there are good reasons for, and/or strong sentiments regarding, different ways of proceeding. Ethical issues can thus stir our innermost feelings.* The resolution of the issues at stake sometimes requires choices involving mixed emotions, better and worse solutions, optimal and less-than-optimal ways of proceeding.

What medical ethics can offer is an expanded set of critical considerations—ethical values, virtues, moral principles—to take into account when making a difficult decision. The choice in hard circumstances is not between following simple rules versus exercising individual moral judgment, or between an algorithmic versus an intuitive approach to managing moral problems. Virtues and principles need not routinize decision-making; they can, however, aid us in making deeper, less reflexive, more informed, and more heartfelt decisions. In a world of distractions and chaos, ethical deliberation should help to *clarify* and to *remind* us when we ought to be concerned, why we ought to be concerned, who else should be involved, and what we should do about it. Ethics cannot replace all the other important elements, such as discernment, sensitivity, compassion, common sense, prudence, and critical appraisal, factoring into a wise and right medical decision, the decision that seems to be the optimal one for the individual patient and/or practitioner to make.

Ethical responses are, or should be, tentative and uncertain. Thoughtful clinicians understand the importance of seeking support for their decisions by obtaining input from various sources, communicating with other involved healthcare professionals but also, most importantly, engaging in ongoing dialogue with patients and their networks of support. Here lies one of the virtues of interprofessional cooperation and patient-based medicine: to ensure that contentious decisions, if later called into question, have had the benefit of more than one opinion and incorporate patient preferences. This thereby can avoid charges of unilateral, high-handed, ham-fisted, or paternalistic decision-making.

Ethical practice entails a commitment to patient-based and value-infused medicine. The components of patient-based care—for example, respecting patients, focusing on their needs and values, and providing timely care—are not always complex, often requiring only a few extra minutes of being present at the patient's bedside. The good clinician welcomes input from patients, families, and indeed any healthcare professional, as this will improve the quality of care the patient receives. Speaking up, when faced with concerns over patient safety is, for example, an important skill to be taught and learned in the new climate of striving for less error-prone medicine. Patient-based medicine is simply what good medicine strives to be[18, 19].

Diversity

One challenge may seem to be the diversity of bioethics across cultures and throughout history. Diversity is not necessarily an obstacle to a transnational practice of biomedical ethics—differences of opinion can encourage critical thinking, open discussion, and forge new ideas[20]. The idea of a global approach to healthcare

---

Box I.2

....

Patient-based medicine

- identifies and respects patient feelings and values,
- provides high-quality information,
- addresses physical and emotional needs,
- involves the patient and significant others,
- offers coordinated care,
- provides access to appropriate care, and
- ensures continuity of care.

---

ethics may seem a long way off in a world rife with assassinations, brutal wars, mass starvation, parochial nationalisms, and widespread denials of basic human rights. The shift away from culturally based or idiosyncratic medical practices is hastened by ready access to information everywhere and the democratic forms of communication this enhances. Steps in the right direction can be seen in, for example, agreements on an international code of medical rights for patients, the ongoing updates to the Declaration of Helsinki regarding Principles for Medical Research Involving Human Subjects [21] and in the widespread opposition to physicians participating in torture [22] and in state executions, no matter how "humane" [23]. Nonetheless, in the present-day world complexities abound. Tremendous gaps still exist between how things are and how they should be [24].

Aim of book

Given the movement towards patient-based medicine, a reflective and practical understanding of medical ethics and how to approach decision-making has never been more relevant—or more necessary. This book aims to provide a readable and practical introduction to modern professional medical ethics appropriate for the new pedagogies and curricula of healthcare. We hope to make the complex topic of ethics more accessible to, and usable for, medical trainees and practitioners. The twentieth-century Austrian philosopher of science Karl Popper [25] held that anything important could and should be said clearly without obfuscation or technical language. Ethics needn't be obscure and cannot be now, if it ever was, the sole domain of an expert ethicist. When it comes to moral action, all those involved in healthcare—the patient, the public, and health professionals alike—have legitimate views deserving consideration.

Our hope is that by the end of this book you will have acquired the skills and confidence to analyze and manage ethical problems and conflicts of values in medicine in a reasonable way. Although there can be no guarantees you will have made the "right" choice in responding to an ethical issue, you should be satisfied you have tried to solve it in a comprehensive and careful fashion.

Throughout this book we provide cases followed by a focused discussion of each. Many of the cases are real-life dilemmas encountered in clinical practice with details altered significantly to protect privacy. Other cases are taken from the public domain and reflect important principles of medical jurisprudence. This is not a source book on the law and so cannot serve as a comprehensive guide to the ever-changing world of jurisprudence. We are physicians, not lawyers or judges. Nevertheless, we have tried to discuss important legal cases—often from Canadian law, but also from American and British law—with which the clinician needs to be familiar, as they impact medical care. None of the case discussions should in any way be taken as legal advice. Nor should our opinions be taken as the "right answers." In the ethical problems of real life, as in medicine generally, decisions are fraught with uncertainty and even the seemingly best choice may have reasonable alternatives. In each of the cases, we encourage you to develop your own opinions and to listen to your emotions. You will also have the opportunity to apply what you've learned in the cases presented at the end of each chapter.

Book outline

The plan of the book is as follows. In Chapter 1 we discuss some basic ethical principles but also argue that no one ethical theory or set of principles will apply to every situation. Chapter 2 distinguishes law from ethics and provides a brief examination of various accounts of ethics as a discipline. Chapter 3 examines an ethical management tool in some detail and looks at a more complex case. Chapter 4 presents the crucial principle of contemporary medicine, patient autonomy. Chapters 5 and 6 look at informed consent, truthtelling, and trust, other concepts closely bound up with autonomy. Duties as regards confidentiality and privacy are presented next in Chapter 7. Chapter 8 considers the ethical problems involved in incapacity and substitute decision-making. Chapter 9 examines another fundamental principle of medicine, beneficence. Chapter 10 discusses the new professionalism. Chapter 11 focuses on the professional and ethical issues arising out of the advent of the new digital media in medicine. Chapter 12 examines the issue of medical error—when medicine goes astray. Justice, a principle recognized by Aristotle and Hippocrates and now of increasing concern in everyday healthcare, is the topic of Chapter 13. Chapter 14 looks at ethical issues at the onset of life and issues arising out of the new reproductive technologies. Chapter 15 concerns the care of the dying, and Chapter 16, new developments regarding medical assistance in dying (MAID). Then in Chapter 17 we consider the influence of culture and genetic knowledge ("memes and genes") and finally, in Chapter 18, ethical issues in medical research. The Conclusion contains some cautions about the future of medicine and provides suggestions for further reading.

Medicine is a challenging job. Trainees and mentors can suffer under the weight of information and decision-making [26], but better and more satisfying experiences in learning and practising medicine are possible when we use ethical, patient-based decision-making and address the inefficiencies in care by working in new ways with other healthcare professionals [27, 28]. The advantages are many: a sense of humility, shared decision-making, lightened responsibilities, and more realistic expectations by all.

◆ 1 ◆

Ethics Matters

The foundations of moral motivations are not the procedural rules or a kind of discourse, but the feelings to which we can rise. As Confucius saw long ago, benevolence or concern for humanity is the indispensable root of it all.

Simon Blackburn, 2001 [1]

I. Great Expectations: Healthcare Professionals and Ethics

In a lecture to senior level medical students in 1967, Dr Reg Perkin, one of the founders of the College of Family Physicians of Canada, alerted them they would, throughout their careers as physicians, have their ethical conduct continually examined—by their patients, their peers, and society. His views about the duties of the physician continue to be widely held today (see Box 1.1).

Box 1.1

"Physicians are . . . recognized as being in a class set apart . . . . The practice of medicine asks more morally of the practitioner than the community as a whole asks of its members . . . . The professional . . . is expected to go the second mile [for the patient]." [2]

Dr Perkin's words were prescriptive, not simply descriptive. Addressed to doctors in training, they could apply to members of any regulated healthcare profession. These professionals' primary duty is a moral one: to serve the best interests of their patients, to go that extra mile if that's what it takes to do so. Whether physicians or any other healthcare practitioners have a special obligation to counter society's bigger social and political ills was left open by Dr Perkin. For many practitioners, it seems hard enough just to do their job and to see the next patient.

For other practitioners, however, being a healthcare professional, whether an MD, a nurse, or other first responder, means to have special obligations of service and commitment that may entail going many miles. There are numerous accounts of doctors and nurses who have devoted themselves to patients in distant places like rural China[3] or war-ravaged Sudan[4] or to those with desperate needs such as the inner-city poor[5]. These are outstanding exemplars for us all, but it is behaviour and action most of us can only hope to emulate in small, everyday ways. We can't all be heroes—in any case the real heroes are our patients—but we can all practise exemplary ethical care close to home.

II. Four Ethical Principles and Questions

Let's start where ethics begins in medicine: out of the special connections between people, between care providers and patients. Medical care is fundamentally about offering a helping hand to those in need. The medical encounter often begins with a simple facilitative question, such as "How are you doing?" or "What can I do for you?" These questions immediately put the clinician at the service of the patient. Here is a commonly encountered scenario.

Case 1.1   To Prescribe or Not to Prescribe

You are a primary care practitioner in the downtown core of a large city. A 32-year-old factory worker, Mr M, attends your clinic as a new patient.

You start by asking him the usual accommodating questions. Mr M tells you he has been unwell for 24 hours with a runny nose, aching muscles, a dry cough, and hoarseness. Apart from some tender neck muscles, however, his physical examination is entirely normal; indeed, he barely seems ill. You say by way of conclusion that he has got a simple viral illness. "We can get to the moon, but we can't cure the common cold. It will get better on its own."

Unconvinced, Mr M requests an antibiotic because he "always got one from the clinic down the road." He then, rather loudly, voices concern you do not really have the experience or skills to make the proper diagnosis.

"I felt so under the weather today I couldn't go to work! How do you know I don't have one of those new superbugs I heard about? One of my buddies at work picked something up. He went to see his doctor, who said it was nothing, and the next thing you know he was almost dead in the ICU."

Is there an ethical issue here?
Would you do what the patient requests?

Discussion of Case 1.1

There is one obvious ethical issue here: the conflict between what you, a trained health professional, believe is the right treatment for the patient and what the patient wants or believes he needs. The choice is either to prescribe the antibiotics the patient requests or not to do so.

In this case there are some pros for prescribing antibiotics:

- you may be mistaken about the nature of the patient's illness,
- the patient may benefit because of a placebo effect,
- the drugs can be prescribed quickly, and
- the patient will not go away disappointed.

However, there are many cons to prescribing unnecessary antibiotics:

- they waste medical resources,
- they may cause side effects,
- they may encourage the growth of resistant organisms in the community, and
- they perpetuate the idea of a quick cure for every illness.

Rather than a blanket refusal, you should take some time to talk with Mr M. Perhaps he felt your initial response to his request was dismissive of his concerns. Inquire about his expectations, find out more about his background, and spend a little time explaining the reasoning behind your reluctance to prescribe the antibiotic. Although time is at a premium in modern-day healthcare practices, time spent listening to the patient—often only a few minutes—can be time well spent. If Mr M remains unconvinced, you *might* propose a compromise: you could offer to call his pharmacy in a day or two with a prescription if he is not improving.

However, even *this* degree of compromise may be inappropriate. Some physicians have noted that with "the casual attitude towards antibiotics . . . resistance

continued

[to them] has increased worldwide over the past few decades." [6] Therapies in medicine, as we shall see in future chapters, all come at some cost to the wider community.

Another important feature of this case is Mr M's criticism of your expertise as a clinician. The patient may have viewed you as uncaring, which does not augur well for a therapeutic alliance. Rather than openly addressing the patient's criticism, the practitioner might be tempted to write him off as difficult and demanding and ignore what are, from the patient's perspective, legitimate concerns.

Listening to a patient does require humility and openness. As a general rule, practitioners should provide only care likely to help their patients. Of course, the line between helpful and useless care may not always be clear (and can be quite contentious as we will see in this and in future chapters), but the overuse of drugs, especially antibiotics, is an all too common occurrence in medicine. Each time clinicians give in to inappropriate demands for tests or treatment, their ethical fibre is weakened, making it less likely they will act properly in other situations and "hold the line."

How can you prepare yourself, as a healthcare professional, to provide effective and appropriate medical care? In considering what should be done, the practitioner or trainee needs to step back from the situation at hand. A simple reflective exercise can help you ensure that you have acted properly. Consider the following simple questions corresponding to the fundamental ethical principles of healthcare (see Box 1.2).

Box 1.2

These core questions correspond to fundamental ethical principles of healthcare:

1. What are the patient's wishes and values? (Autonomy)
2. What can be done for the patient? What are the harms and benefits of the options? (Beneficence/Nonmaleficence)
3. Is the patient being treated fairly? Given the competing claims of others, how can the needs of all be best satisfied? (Justice)

Reflecting on ethics goes back thousands of years, but the most influential modern theorizing about ethics began in the 1960s, the era of modern transformative medicine. A number of high-level reports from American Presidential

Commissions on research[7], end-of-life care[8], and consent[9] were released in the late 1970s and early 1980s. The reports rest on four basic principles of bioethics to be used in good decision-making in medicine—patient autonomy, justice, beneficence, and nonmaleficence. They have been extremely influential, leading to their widespread adoption by physicians, philosophers, and medical educators in and outside North America[10]. The use of these principles has become *the* standard paradigm for the practice of modern medical ethics.

In Case 1.1, if it is clear that a drug is not going to help Mr M, it is better for everyone, as well as more honest and more professional, to refuse his request. Although saying no to patients can be difficult, there are concrete strategies on how to do so (see Box 1.3) [11], [12]. It does require fortitude on the part of the healthcare professional.

Box 1.3

How to say "no" to a patient[12]:

- Just say no: don't be vague.
- Be kind and not dismissive: explain why you are saying no.
- Offer alternatives: for example, offer to see the patient again if there is no improvement.
- Don't argue: be empathetic and allow the patient room to vent.
- Be consistent.
- Understand why a patient is making a request so you can better address the underlying reason.

Behind the ability to refuse inappropriate demands lies the world of principles, the foundation of excellent, high-quality ethical medical care.

III. The Principles and Ethical Reasoning in Medicine

There is no simple algorithm providing the "right answer" to many moral dilemmas in medicine. (The easy ones, such as whether one needs to get consent from capable adults before a medical intervention—for example, for doing an HIV blood test before surgery—can be readily resolved by pointing to established law or precedent.) Complex cases often arise from competing ethical principles, for example, between a patient's privacy interests involving security and autonomy of the person and the safety and best interests of other people. Guidelines may emphasize one principle or another but do not eliminate the need for moral evaluation and discretion when it comes to deciding on the best course of action in particular circumstances. The lack of consensus as to how best to proceed—and the presence of ethical issues and dilemmas—is not unusual in nursing[13] and medical practice[14, 15].

The principle of autonomy

The importance of the patient's point of view should be the cornerstone when deciding what to do in medicine. What are the patient's concerns, wishes, and values? Consider, for example, the competent patient's wishes for treatment. So long as these are informed wishes not contravening any other important moral principles, the patient's wishes should guide decisions about their treatment.

While the patient's agenda sets the tone for a meeting, it does not always rule the roost. Patient-based medicine is a collaborative enterprise. To understand the issues as the patient sees them, a good clinician will listen to, but also question, the patient. Asking patients to tell you about themselves is a good beginning.

The principle of beneficence

Having (at least initially) established the patient's main concerns, skilful clinicians will carefully attend to their professional agenda. The appropriate dialogue with the patient begins by initiating a conversation and following a set of focused questions in order to better establish what troubles the patient and how they see themselves.

Problems can arise when healthcare professionals make assumptions about what their patients believe, value, or should do, or what resources, financial and social, patients have at their disposal. Instead, they need to appreciate *what life is like* for their patients[16]. This can be accomplished only through conversation, listening, examination, and careful observation.

The principle of justice

This principle includes fairness: is a patient's care reflective of their fair share of what are often scarce healthcare resources? A patient's wishes and concerns are rarely considered in isolation from the needs of others. For example, will other persons, such as the family, other patients, or professional staff, be unduly burdened by the treatment chosen? The clinician's job is to try to access appropriate, not inordinate, care and time for patients and to attempt to give priority of focus to the needs of their patients, all the while not ignoring the impact of the recommendations on the interests of others—not an easy task. Nevertheless, fairness should play a significant part in our decision-making.

Nonmaleficence: "Above all, do no harm"

This is the Hippocratic principle of *primum non nocere* ("above all, do no harm"), the oldest and seemingly least controversial moral rule in medicine. This principle could be incorporated (and some do include it) in the principle of beneficence. All things being equal, the wise practitioner would, of course, recommend the intervention leading to the least possibility of harm to the patient [17].

Truly nonmaleficent interventions are rare in medicine. Simple interventions, such as taking a venous blood sample or discussing a diagnosis with a patient, involve some small risk of harm, even when done well. Most surgical interventions, for example, involve considerable harm initially, with the hope of eventual good, but sometimes that good never materializes. While many healthcare professionals refer to the nonmaleficence principle [18], it cannot serve as the guiding principle for medical practice—otherwise, "therapeutic nihilism" (the view that *all* medical treatment is worse than the disease) may ensue. Such thinking is behind the radical view that "the medical establishment has become a major threat to health" [19].

Scepticism about medical interventions is frequently appropriate, as much of what practitioners do—such as overprescribing dangerous drugs—is not helpful or can actually harm patients [20] (see Chapter 12). At times a wait-and-see attitude, rather than intervening with risky or uncertain measures, is the better route to take.

Think of *do no harm* as an ideal limit to, and a regulative guideline for, the principle of beneficence—something you will always strive to do. The best choice is the option where the potential benefits outweigh the risk of harms. Although evil physicians do exist (such as the British doctor in the late twentieth century who succeeded in killing several hundred patients before his arrest [21]), most doctors do not go to work with the explicit intent to harm their patients. They can act maleficently, however, as a result of ignorance, conflict of interest, incompetence, dishonesty, mental illness, or a lack of fortitude when faced with the "reality" of rationing (see Chapter 13). They can also do harm to patients through overaggressive prescribing of unproven or ineffective therapies [22].

Empathy and ethics

In general, harm and benefit cannot be understood as purely objective notions. They must be defined with input from the patient and tailored to that patient's situation. What might be a great harm to one patient could be relatively harmless to another. Lack of awareness of, or interest in, a patient's illness experience is one factor that can lead practitioners to act in a less than ethically optimal manner.

Case 1.2 "I'm Not Ready to Die!"

A 46-year-old man, Mr H, dying of multiple myeloma, has fought the disease every step of the way with a remarkable determination to live. He has undergone every known treatment—bone marrow transplantation, experimental therapies, naturopathic remedies. Thin and wasted, Mr H is now on dialysis. The disease has, it seems, finally reached its terminal stages. He has but a few weeks to live. Although Mr H recognizes he is dying, he refuses to agree to a "palliative care only" order. To him this would mean giving up. There is still so much he wants to do. He wants any extra moment of life that aggressive interventions might give him. Mr H's treating team wants to transfer him to a palliative care ward, which, they feel, could better serve his needs. The patient refuses this.

"I'm not ready to die!" Mr H states categorically.

What would be the next best step to take with Mr H?

Discussion of Case 1.2

Mr H seems to be asking his caregivers—his nurses, his physicians—to break the *primum non nocere* rule: he is asking them to do something (staying in acute care) that will almost certainly cause him more harm than good. If we strictly followed the nonmaleficence principle, we would not agree to a dying man's request to continue to receive aggressive care. On balance, however, it is Mr H's life and his death. By his values it would be better to try likely futile gestures than none at all. The physician or nurse clinician needs to understand how Mr H views and experiences his circumstances, and what life is like for him at his life's end.

The next best step would be to try to understand the gap between the differing perspectives held by Mr H and his care providers. This is where empathic communication comes into play[23]. Mr H may believe accepting palliative care means others will give up on him. He needs reassurance his care providers will not abandon him on the doorstep of death or be indifferent to his needs (see Chapter 15). This is not a job for doctors alone.

The "right" response, the ethical response, to this patient is to exercise compassion—to make sure he knows you intend to be with him, to be present with him, through his suffering by saying in effect, "Here I am. I am ready to help, ready to witness, ready to respond to suffering. Here for you"[24]. This is the definition of empathy: identifying what the patient feels and needs. Requiring listening and imagination[25], it starts with trying to understand the situation from the patient's perspective—the reality for them of their world of serious illness (see Chapter 2).

The best resolution of the case depends very much on the clinician taking time for a patient for whom ostensibly "nothing more" can be done. Sometimes holding on, rather than letting go, is the right thing to do [26]. It seemed to be so for Mr H. A virtuous experienced clinician from any of the health professions will know when and how to encourage hope and acceptance in a dying patient.

Central to the exercise of empathy is understanding the stories behind our patients' illnesses. This story-based approach, narrative medicine, allows us to connect with our patients and gain a better understanding of their needs by eliciting their concerns and their personal experience of illness (see Chapter 2). So it went for Mr H. Understanding his perspective—the depth of his wish for any intervention that might prolong his life, his worries that others would give up on him and would not do everything to help him—allowed him to die in the acute care setting.

Box 1.4

To increase empathic communication, ask patients, [23]

- What do you understand about your situation now?
- What are you hoping for?
- How do you want things to be when you die?
- How do you feel about all of this?

IV. Beyond Principles

Knowing when and how to follow the principles, as well as when and how we may bend or break them, requires some practical and pragmatic knowledge of medical practice, ethics, and the law. Recent scholarship in ethics emphasizes the importance of other factors in medicine. Adhering to ethical principles will not resolve every real-world dilemma. Contemporary philosopher Harry Frankfurt argues there are other concerns and values—familial, aesthetic, cultural, or religious—an individual may consider more important than strictly ethical considerations in making a decision [27]. Martha Nussbaum stresses the centrality of the emotions to proper decision-making [28]. Emotions can lead to moral action by encouraging "people to think larger thoughts and recommit themselves to a larger common good" [29].

Another late-twentieth-century philosopher, Bernard Williams, held that we sometimes *ought* to be swayed by other factors when making a serious moral choice— such as deciding to rescue a family member first when other people are also at risk and not everyone can be rescued. To ignore the instinct to rescue loved ones, based on the belief one should respond impersonally to moral dilemmas (as some moral theories would have us believe), would be to have, Williams said, "one thought too many" [30].

In difficult situations, doing right and achieving good ends cannot rest with a purely reflexive or emotional response. Faced with a hard choice, don't overthink it; do what feels right, but be prepared to defend it later on.

V. The Hidden Curriculum

The tension of ethics versus "non-moral" factors in medical decision-making applies particularly to healthcare trainees and allied healthcare professionals in subordinate positions who may be uncertain of their rights [31]. Moral agents may be swayed from doing the right thing by emotions such as fear, by discriminatory attitudes or intimidation, or by local mores or habits (not mutually exclusive factors).

In hospitals, power and prestige have traditionally held sway over sense and reason [32]. Doctors have traditionally been at the top of the hierarchy (with specialists above generalists), other health professionals next, and trainees usually last. One followed "doctors' orders," right or wrong, fearing for one's professional survival otherwise.

Healthcare trainees especially may be smothered by the organization of medicine. Medical students, for example, may be intimidated into undertaking tasks or performing procedures they know to be wrong [33], such as pelvic examinations on anaesthetized patients just prior to surgery [34]. Why do students feel compelled to comply? They may not want to lose a learning opportunity or may feel they cannot speak up without being ridiculed or worse. Ethical infractions are common and not unique to one country or one medical school [35, 36].

Box 1.5

Ethical erosion:
"Under the pressure to conform in order to succeed and not imperil a career, even a virtuous student will need extra courage to resist." [37]

Unfortunately, studies [38, 39] have revealed students still face considerable abuse, despite attempts to resist and to improve the curriculum [40].

Box 1.6

Medical students [39, 40]

- are not simply overly sensitive—the abuse they experience is real;
- most commonly encounter humiliation and being "dressed down" publicly;
- may experience even gentle criticism as abusive if not given properly;
- if female, may worry more about their competence and are more likely to be distressed if judged incompetent by an attending doctor; and
- if male, are more likely to experience physical mistreatment.

That hierarchically induced unethical practices still exist in many places is a measure of the degree to which various professions and institutions within medicine remain uninformed by moral practices ("under-moralized"). In rigid hierarchies there is often a power imbalance, without a culture of respect—resulting in unhappy trainees, disgruntled patients, and dissatisfied staff (see Chapter 10). We could do better in medicine and many places are trying to do better [41]. Unethical practices in professional schools and institutions are threats to their reliability. They create the conditions for what has been called a "hidden curriculum," tolerating and encouraging a poor learning environment [42, 43].

Here is one such case.

Case 1.3 A Risky Teaching Tool

A fourth-year medical student, Michael, on a two-week elective in anaesthesia, is observing a patient being intubated in preparation for surgery. Suddenly, the staff anaesthetist, Dr B, removes the patient's endotracheal tube, asking Michael to demonstrate how he would re-intubate the patient. Not surprisingly, the student, having no prior experience with the procedure, cannot do so. Dr B must eventually and hurriedly do the re-intubation himself. He angrily dresses Michael down in front of others in the OR. Humiliated about his failure, the student does not mention the episode to anyone until much later.

What could Michael have done at the time?

continued

Discussion of Case 1.3

It is hard to say why Dr B acted the way he did. Was he simply mistaken about the trainee's abilities? Or was Dr B in the habit of similarly challenging other novice learners—the old school "sink or swim" philosophy ("If I learned this way, so can you . . .")? Such pedagogic practices are liabilities that should be left in the past, whether or not this particular patient suffered any harm related to the delayed intubation. The not-so-hidden message is that it is acceptable to treat patients in this fashion. The behind-the-scenes learning environment is the hidden curriculum—the perfect medium for breeding unethical practices and attitudes.

The situation and the actions of Dr B are unacceptable for many reasons. First of all, Michael was unprepared and the patient's well-being was endangered. Such action was an assault upon the patient, unless prior consent to this teaching lesson had been given. Ongoing trends in medical education remind everyone the patient's interests must come first[44].

Secondly, Dr B's behaviour towards Michael was abusive. The student felt overwhelmed and unable to see past his own embarrassment to do anything about it at the time. Although it was, no doubt, an intimidating situation, Michael could have let Dr B know how difficult the situation was for him. This may not have been a realistic option, however. A clinician teaching in this manner is not likely to take kindly to a trainee who questions his pedagogic technique! If fearful of Dr B's response, Michael should consider seeking direction from a student advocacy office or ombudsman, where trainee and patient concerns should be (but are not always, quite frankly) taken seriously.

Box 1.7

"Neophytes cannot perform high-stakes procedures at an acceptable level of proficiency . . . [We must] develop approaches to skills training that do not put our patients at risk in service to education."[44]

VI. Overcoming obstacles to ethics

The hidden curriculum and the tangled web of fear and power imbalances create roadblocks to proper moral decision-making. There is no easy way to overcome such obstacles to acting ethically in practice. If you encounter them, you should not ignore your feelings of outrage, disappointment, and sadness. You could start by seeking support from your peers. Then, if the ethical infraction is serious, consider having a second, tactful, conversation with other clinicians, sympathetic teachers, or members of the healthcare institution's administration. It is critical to act and to raise your concerns in some venue; it is only by the voiced opinions of many people that institutions and unethical routines change. This is the value of virtue (and the "danger" of critical thinking): it may question the established order of things and invite reprisal. We hope that clinicians who are teachers can accept critical feedback as an opportunity for learning ("Help me to understand why you . . .").

The risk of *not* speaking up is far greater in our estimation. It's important to be aware that one can become inured to unethical practices, negative work environments, and toxic supervisors. These practices and attitudes can affect not only the welfare of the patient but also one's own sense of integrity and well-being as a trainee or healthcare professional. Not doing something about such negative practices and mindsets is one of the sources of moral distress for healthcare trainees and can contribute to cynicism, burnout[45], and student self-harm[46].

Conclusion

Situations of ethical challenge hardly end with training. Most practitioners experience situations of far greater ethical difficulty when practising in the real world of looking after patients and their families. The good news is that institutions of medicine *are* changing. In the recent past, there were few, if any, resources for addressing ethical infractions within institutions. Many hospitals and medical schools have resources to help trainees troubled by the medical hierarchy to raise issues without fear of reprisal. There are now complaints processes, patient advocates, patient safety offices, bioethics departments, and so on—all of which can lend a sympathetic ear to disenchanted staff and learners.

In the next chapter, various approaches to bioethical issues in medicine will be briefly examined. The reader less interested in theory may wish to skim over that chapter.

Cases for Discussion

Case 1: "What's Up, Doc?"

You are a healthcare trainee on a multidisciplinary team looking after a previously well 66-year-old married Armenian patient, Mr I, admitted recently due to a two-week history of vomiting and dramatic weight loss. Tests done two

continued

days ago revealed he has advanced metastatic gastric cancer. The internist responsible for this patient tells you Mr I is unaware he is dying of cancer. "It was the family's wish not to tell him and I went along with it. He doesn't speak much English and the family said in their culture the family is always told first," she says. "He thinks he has a bad infection in his colon, so don't say anything."

One evening, when everyone else has left for the day and you are on call, the patient asks to see you. He tells you he has been gradually feeling worse since admission. "Why am I still vomiting? Is there nothing you can do for me?" His English seems perfectly fine to you.

He then adds, "Tell me, Doc, it isn't just an infection, is it?" [47]

Questions for Discussion

1. How should you respond?
2. What if you were not a "doc" but a medical student or another member of the healthcare team?

Case 2: Use of Force

Dr G works for a medical NGO (Non-Governmental Organization) in rural Ethiopia, an impoverished region of the developing world. There is a wave of diphtheria sweeping through the countryside as the recent vaccine campaign did not reach many of the smaller villages. Several children died of the illness, something quite preventable had there been early diagnosis and prompt treatment.

A poor family asks Dr G to come their house in an affected small town. The youngest child in this family, 5-year-old Liya, has developed a fever and refuses to swallow. She defiantly refuses to open her mouth. No amount of arguing, bribing or cajoling by Dr G or her parents will budge her.

Dr G decides, with the parents' consent, to hold Liya down and force her mouth open. She is fierce in her resistance. Dr G is finally able to see a grey web in her posterior pharynx, typical of diphtheria. Exhausted and sweaty from the struggle, she falls back into a chair. Liya stares at her in anger. Dr G thinks to herself, "What did I just do? What kind of person am I?" [48]

Questions for Discussion

1. What makes this scenario so distressing?
2. How could Dr G's actions be justified?
3. What other options could have been explored?

✦ 2 ✦

Broadening the Horizon
What Law and Ethics Say

These people are climbing the same mountain on different sides.

Derek Parfit, 2011 [1]

How should healthcare professionals assess what is right in situations of ethical difficulty? For whom is it right? The patient? The patient's family? Ourselves? The profession? Society at large? This chapter will briefly examine the direction some legal and philosophical approaches to medical morality provide. As we shall see, the ethical principles discussed in Chapter 1 will not provide satisfactory or complete answers in all situations.

Although it matters why we do what we do, the differences between the various approaches to ethics are not as great as some believe them to be. Moreover, it is our view that one overarching theory of ethics is not needed to explain every moral issue in medicine.

Traditionally, people relied—and many still rely—on religion for the answers to moral issues. Indeed, devout religious practice has been and can be an important fount of moral belief and action. There are problems with a theological approach, however: religious mores can vary with ethnicity and culture; they also change slowly, if at all. This can be a good thing—to be rock steady in a seemingly rootless world—or less than helpful—to be inflexible and unresponsive in a rapidly changing world. Ethics, while similarly aiming at something less temporally based, looks for common values that are less culturally specific but upon which different religions can agree [2]. This may not be easy to do.

Case 2.1 "You Have No Right to Touch Me!"

You are a healthcare trainee doing your rotation in a community health centre. An 80-year-old widow, Ms B, is brought by her son for her annual influenza vaccine. In explaining its risks and benefits, you realize the patient is not following your explanation. An inspection of her chart reveals she has a five-year history of progressive dementia with a decline in many aspects of daily functioning.

A brief examination reveals Ms B to be very confused, having difficulty understanding what is being asked of her. She blankly looks at her son and asks, "Who is that person and what does she want?" The son gives you permission to give his mother the injection, saying she always wanted it in the past. However, normally quite docile and quiet, she vociferously refuses.

"What do you want my arm for? You have no right to touch me there!"

Do you have a right to touch her?
What would you do?

I. What the Law Says

When faced with an ethical quandary, many healthcare practitioners ask: "What does the law say?"[3] Defining what is right and wrong on the basis of laws and regulations is an understandable response when confronted by challenging moral or ethical dilemmas. Legal rulings are almost always relevant as to what healthcare professionals ought to do (they are part of the professional's moral landscape). Yet concern about the legal and political basis for one's actions may be overly cautious. This may be quite prudent, given the daily attacks on the safety and well-being of medical personnel taking place throughout the world[4]. However, following the law too assiduously can lead to an unhealthy kind of defensive medicine.

This in turn can lead to unethical or unprofessional practices or events—such as the needless death in 2012 of Dr Savita Halappanavar, a pregnant dentist in Ireland. Imperilled by a threatened miscarriage at 17 weeks' gestation, she made repeated requests for a therapeutic abortion. Her doctors refused this because a fetal heartbeat could still be detected, circumstances under which Irish law at the time prohibited terminating a pregnancy. They waited instead for the fetus to die *in utero* before extracting it. By then it was too late to save Dr Halappanavar. Her death from septicemia motivated Irish society to change its law[5].

Physicians are usually not lawyers. Where a law seems to stand in the way of what obviously should be done to help a patient, clinicians ought to carefully examine their professional judgment—first ask themselves what is needed to save the patient, and worry about fallout from the law later. It is problematic to uncritically accept the law as a gold standard for ethically exemplary practice. Laws that interfere with offering proper care to patients or that cause needless suffering are ethically questionable from a medical perspective. For instance, recognizing the negative impact on the well-being of individuals, healthcare professionals should call into question the requirement in many countries to report illegal immigrants (who, even if critically ill, may be subject to summary deportation)[6, 7, 8]. This moral foundation for medicine does not create an ethical requirement for doctors to break unjust laws or to sacrifice their own well-being for the sake of others (see Chapter 10), but it does suggest there is a critical advocacy role for doctors.

The law and medical ethics, while often in agreement, can diverge[9]—especially if the law is spiritlessly applied[10]. As well, the law often does not address, let alone resolve, many challenging moral issues. Established legal precedent—the kind of law that healthcare professionals like to know—may come many years after a moral issue arises, too late to help the practising clinician. Practically speaking, when a dispute comes to court, the legal resolution *can* seem to have the last word about what to do. Medicine's boundaries are for the profession itself to determine, but "within the framework of . . . law"[11]. In many places the spirit of the law allows for professional discretion—the exercise of clinical judgment—as to what to do, especially, for example, if a patient's life is at stake and the clinician is acting in "good faith"[12].

Discussion of Case 2.1

You have every right to touch Ms B—her son has the authority to make decisions on her behalf (see Chapters 6 and 8)—and to act in her best interests. Her strenuous refusal ought to be met by a calm, deliberate approach on your part. In circumstances such as this case—the refusal of appropriate care by a patient with impaired capacity—it is the clinician's job to know how and when to proceed. Being a trainee should not mean one cannot act within one's graded responsibility. On this point, ethics and the law would agree.

How, then, should we think in general about the actions of a good clinician?

II. What Ethics Says: Virtues, Rules, and Consequences in Medicine

The virtues

Pellegrino and Thomasma talk about the necessity for virtues to be exhibited by the good clinician[13]. Deeds that abide by or arise from virtues are typically considered good actions[14]. A person motivated by the opposite of virtue—vice, such as dishonesty, avarice, or prejudice—is simply less trustworthy.

In the ancient philosophy of Aristotle, one came to know the "good" by *doing* good deeds[15]. The virtuous agent is not born with virtues but provided "by nature" with the capacity to receive them and then to act on them. The more one practises doing right, the more likely one will learn how to act properly.

Box 2.1

Aristotle on virtue:
"Moral virtue . . . is formed by habit, ethos . . . . Whether one habit or another habit is inculcated in us from an early age makes all the difference."[15]

The theory of virtue ethics is prominent historically. This school of thought focuses on the requisite personal character of the healthcare provider. Virtues are those morally upright tendencies to be emulated by others and are taken to provide more surefooted guides to right action. One trains in medicine by apprenticing oneself to a mentor and one learns, not just the *what* of being a doctor, but the *how* of being a good one.

Box 2.2

A Typology of Some Ethical Theories:

1. Consequentialism
   a. Utilitarianism
2. Deontology
   a. Kantian theory
   b. Contractualism
3. Virtue Ethics
   a. Aristotelian ethics
   b. Virtue theory
4. Hybrid theories
   a. "Principlism"
   b. Narrative ethics
   c. Feminist bioethics
   d. Casuistry
   e. Capability theories

Case 2.2 Silent Witness

Sam E is in the first month of his training to be a healthcare professional. Recently learning about the dangers of suntanning, he has taken to cautioning his friends about melanoma, the most serious form of skin cancer. He's seen pictures of some nasty-looking lesions in his Dermatology atlas. One hot summer's day, standing in a crowded bus going to school, he happens to notice a small but ominous-looking lesion on the posterior shoulder of a fellow passenger wearing a halter top. He has never seen her before.

Is this an ethical dilemma?
What should Sam say, if anything, to the stranger?

It is impossible to imagine a good clinician without conceiving of them acting on the basis of the core virtues of clinical practice. The prime virtues this book recommends to healthcare practitioners are

- *compassion*, the feeling of concern inclining one to empathize with and to desire to relieve the suffering of others;
- *prudence*, taking due care and exhibiting due diligence in one's deliberations and actions;
- *altruism*, putting the interests of others before one's own;
- *trustworthiness, demonstrating a consistent commitment to patients;* and
- *humility*, having the ability to admit one might be wrong ("fallible").

It is important that healthcare professionals not just praise good character (or censure bad character) but also be able to state *why* certain actions or values are viewed as good or bad. This is useful during times of medical change when "new" virtues are called for or when old values need to be overthrown, as, for example, in the cases of medical assistance in dying (see Chapter 16) and the new technologies of assisted reproduction (see Chapter 14). Do the basic virtues of healthcare ever change? And, if they do, how ought we to think about morality? What distinguishes a virtue from a vice? Are good acts in medicine possible if the clinician is motivated solely by self-interest or by malignant narcissism?

Discussion of Case 2.2

The ethical dilemma in this case is the conflict between the principle of respecting a person's privacy and the principle that one ought to act to prevent harm.

continued

For someone so early in his training, Sam should be careful how he approaches the stranger with the nasty-looking lesion. While motivated only by good intentions, he should be wary of being too intrusive. That said, where he sees a potential serious harm, he also should not ignore his desire to prevent that harm. Sam could approach the woman with a caution about his own inexperience and offer to give his opinion. He could say something such as, "I have just begun my medical training. May I offer you a concern I have about your health?" If she agrees, Sam could go on to say, "I don't want to alarm you, but are you aware . . . ?"

Virtue theory asks people to reflect on who they are and what they do: "What kind of person do I want to be? What would a virtuous person—your role model, your mentor—do in this situation?" [16] Sam is faced with this dilemma: he knows he won't sleep well at night if he does not try to warn the stranger. Just weeks into his medical training, he is already thinking and acting as a good doctor would.

Deontology and morality

One account of what makes something a virtue or a vice is deontology. Deontology views duties and/or rights to be fundamental to any account of morality. What makes an action suitable or a trait virtuous is determined by its compatibility with a duty or a universal rule.

This duty-based account of morality is most notoriously exemplified in the dense writings of the eighteenth-century Prussian philosopher Immanuel Kant. He viewed ethics as arising out of universal laws (maxims) of reason, of which one formulation is his "categorical imperative"—an action is right only if everyone could do it; if that is impossible, then that act is wrong or unacceptable. Kant's test is this: "Can you will that your maxim should become a universal law?" [17] Only rules passing this uncompromising test are acceptable (see Box 2.3). Lies and deceptions are, for example, always wrong as they undermine the duties of promise keeping and truthtelling. Thus, for Kant a clinician must always give the patient the unvarnished truth, no matter how harmful the consequences [18].

Kant's commitment to truthtelling was an important moment for philosophy, countering the tendency in society to treat the truth in a purely instrumental way. However, he could not imagine circumstances where this duty could conflict with other compelling professional responsibilities, such as prudence and compassion. His equally famous associated maxim—that one is never to treat oneself or another "merely as a means to an end, but always at the same time as an end" [19]—embodies the principle of respect for humans, quite progressive for the time. (This should have led him to oppose institutions such as slavery that utilize humans as mere tools for the ends of others. Kant did not, however, oppose slavery or colonialism [20].)

John Rawls' "contractualism" updates Kant [21, 22]. His idea of justice asks: what type of, and how much, inequalities would individuals be prepared to accept if they did not know in advance (behind a "veil of ignorance") where they would end up in the social hierarchy?

Consequentialism and ethics

A contrasting major theory of ethics is consequentialism, of which utilitarianism is the best-known example. Duties or Kantian maxims of actions are judged by the impact they have upon human welfare. As one of this philosophy's greatest exponents, John Stuart Mill, explained in his book *Utilitarianism*, "actions are right in so far as they tend to promote happiness, wrong as they tend to produce the reverse of happiness. By happiness is intended pleasure, and the absence of pain; by unhappiness, pain, and the privation of pleasure" [23]. Thus, certain consequences or outcomes, such as increasing pleasure or happiness, are to be preferred and other states of affairs, such as pain or suffering, to be avoided. Conflicts of duties—for example, between compassion and honesty—are resolved by examining their impact upon humans. No duties are sacrosanct.

Crudely speaking, in contrast to deontology, utilitarianism is a philosophy whereby the "end justifies the means." It is an attitude permeating medicine, an activity weighing good outcomes against the risk of causing (or threatening to cause) harm and suffering (think needles, surgery). Taking an instrumental view of truthtelling, this philosophy has been used to withhold the truth from patients, if, on the doctor's view, the truth would cause more harm than good for the patient.

Utilitarianism has been criticized for its view that all that matters is the total improvements in outcomes. This supposes that it is possible to measure outcomes—such as welfare, pleasure, satisfaction of desires, and happiness—in one way and in one dimension. Others have argued this philosophy, in being concerned with overall good outcomes, fails to care who performs an action and for what reason, so long as the preferred outcomes are maximized in the long run [24].

A crude form of utilitarianism has been used in medicine to support deceiving patients, where, sometimes and in some cultures, the truth has been taken as too brutal to reveal. (It has also been seen as tolerating tyrannies of majorities over minorities. Mill was himself a staunch opponent of all forms of tyrannies and a vigorous proponent of liberty and individual worth [25].)

Utilitarianism does seem to capture the common-sense ideal that some outcomes do matter (for example, in treating patients, is pleasure not better than pain? Or, if two groups of desperate refugees are awash at sea, in danger of drowning, is it not better to devote your efforts to saving the larger group first?). Utilitarianism has its defenders today[26, 27]. The Australian philosopher Peter Singer, for example, is well known for his very practical defence of a utilitarian ethics championing assisted death and terminating the lives of severely disabled infants and patients in a persistent vegetative state—all in the name of minimizing suffering and against the deontological view that all human life is equally sacred[28]. (For a *very* simplified way of looking at these ethical theories, see Box 2.3.)

Box 2.3

Traditional tests of ethical judgment, simplified:

1. Aristotle's test: What would a good person do?
2. Kant's test: Could you imagine everyone acting as you recommended?
3. Mill's test: Does your choice maximize pleasure or happiness?

Case 2.3   The Worrier

A married, 72-year-old retired construction worker, Mr G, has a history of severe coronary artery disease (CAD), Type 2 diabetes, and recurrent depression. Perpetually in a gloomy state of mind, he worries considerably about his health. His family doctor, Dr Y, receives a letter from the local hospital informing her Mr G may have had his prostate biopsy done last year with improperly sterilized equipment. A patient on whom it had been used just prior to Mr G was recently diagnosed with Creutzfeldt-Jakob disease (CJD).

Dr Y had read of CJD being transmitted by surgical instruments, but the risk was, she thought, "incredibly low." She has seen no evidence for this disorder in this patient. She also recalls Mr G reacting almost hysterically when she asked him several years ago about testing for hepatitis C ("What's this? You want to give me another illness to worry about? I'm sick enough already."); it took her an hour to calm him down, but eventually Mr G took the test (which was negative).

Dr Y decides, on grounds of compassion, not to tell Mr G about his possible exposure to CJD.

Was Dr Y's response the right course of action?
What are the arguments you could make for and against warning Mr G?

> **Box 2.4**
>
> ....
>
> Three practical tests of moral acceptability of an action.
>
> In all cases ask,
>
> 1. What if everyone knew? (Publicity test—a utilitarian view)
> 2. Is this how you would want to be treated or those closest to you treated? (Golden Rule test—a Kantian view)
> 3. Can you sleep at night with your choice? (Good conscience test—an Aristotelian view)

III. Expanding the Horizons of Ethics

Four hybrid theories

The ethics procedure adopted in this book (see Chapter 3) incorporates, and in some ways goes beyond, the perspectives of virtue theory, deontology, and consequentialism. In a situation of ethical difficulty, we think it is always worth considering what one should do from the perspectives of the law and various ethical theories. In this book we advocate use of a version of "principlism" (see Chapter 1). The advantage of principlism is its opposition to "moral monism," the theory that all moral judgments must be justified by, and subsumed under, one principle or one account of ethics[29]. Instead, we espouse a pluralistic view that tolerates and utilizes different norms and values depending on the circumstances. We also believe that acceptable solutions to ethical problems in medicine need not, in general, be complex. Sometimes better answers can come from responding to very simple questions (see Box 2.4).

The question is this: does the use of the four principles (principlism) make for the best account of medical morality? Although there exist many theories and approaches to ethics that combine, modify, and even claim to overthrow these basic principles, no one theory predominates. Capability theories, narrative ethics, virtue theory, feminist bioethics, and casuistry are chief among ethical approaches rivalling or completing the dominant ethical paradigms of duty-based deontology and outcome-based consequentialism. The accounts we provide here are but brief summaries and cannot, quite frankly, do justice to them.

Capability theory and ethics

The capability theories of Martha Nussbaum[30] and Amartya Sen[31] have a different focus as to the proper aim of moral action. Ethical acts should maximize the realization in the real world of human capabilities (such as living a life of normal length, enjoying good health, being secure against violent assault, thinking and reasoning, experiencing emotions such as love, justified anger, and so on [32]) in order to contribute to human flourishing. "A society that does not guarantee these to all its citizens," Nussbaum writes, "falls short of being a fully just society" [33]. Using elements taken from consequentialism and virtue ethics, a unitary global ethics perspective transcending cultural differences is sought. Still quite abstract, these theories are currently being operationalized [34]. However, from this perspective, it is clear how far we are today from realizing these very practical requirements for human well-being.

Nussbaum argues emotions have been given a bad rap. She emphasizes the central role emotions play in developing the list of human capabilities and the possibility of making proper ethical decisions. "Part and parcel of the system of ethical reasoning" [35], emotional evaluations can help us focus on what is important and ignore the rest. Without an emotional underpinning to our beliefs and actions—such as being grounded in compassion—our principles and norms of action would be "lifeless and calculating" [36].

Narrative theory and ethics

Narrative ethics calls for rich descriptions of cases encouraging greater input from the patient and the care provider. (See Chapter 1, Box 1.6, for questions to elicit the patient's story.) This approach is readily familiar to clinicians used to writing up detailed case studies. Narrative ethics focuses its attention on making coherent sense of the stories behind the lives of our patients: "[i]llness itself unfolds as a narrative" [37]. Understanding the patient's story should be the goal in any good clinical encounter, but eliciting such stories does require time, compassion, and having a "receptive ear" [38].

Narrative ethics, in treating the patient's story as a text to be interpreted, is less interested in applying ethical rules than in understanding the patient's story *from the inside*: what is life really like for the patient, the family, the practitioner? The goal is to find the hidden treasure, the empathic lesson that will help a story make sense. "I can only answer the question 'What am I to do?' if I can answer the prior question 'Of what stories do I find myself a part?'" [16].

Box 2.5

Strategies for narrative-based medicine [39]:

- Ask patients, "What would you like me to know about you?"
- Listen and don't interrupt.
- Elicit the patients' views of their condition.

- Ask patients about the impact of the illness on their lives.
- Assess the distress and suffering of the patient.
- Examine your assumptions and stereotypes about patients and their culture.
- See noncompliance as the patient's hidden story—one that you need to understand.

Vigilant listeners and readers are encouraged by good literature to put themselves in the place of another. This helps develop in us the urge to assist others—altruism—and the aptitude for an insightful—an empathic—reflection into the lives of others. One comes to see that other ways of being and responding are possible and perhaps even necessary. This skill of reflection is so important for healthcare professionals in order to understand and appreciate the suffering of patients and fellow practitioners. Some of the most gifted writers of modern medicine are physicians—Oliver Sacks, Richard Selzer, and Atul Gawande, for example—who can enthrall us with compelling narratives. They help us appreciate the ethical aspects of medicine in deeper and more intimate and empathic ways.

Box 2.6

Less traditional tests of moral reasoning:

- Capability theory: Do your actions reflect those a compassionate person would take to maximize the capabilities of others?
- Narrative ethics: Do your actions make sense once you know the details of the person's story?
- Feminist bioethics: What action would those closest to you recommend?
- Casuistry: Does your action follow from a set of similar cases?

Discussion of Case 2.3

Our response to this case will be brief: Dr Y, in not warning Mr G of his possible exposure to CJD, takes the responsibility upon herself should he suffer some ill outcomes on account of not knowing this. She has taken a narrow

continued

consequentialist view of the truth in deciding that telling Mr G would do him more harm than good. This could be backed up by a compassionate, protective view of Mr G's life story. But, the alternate, more modern, view is to see this as his life story and not to assume he cannot handle the truth. The view that he has a "right" to the truth is, of course, a deontological position.

Feminist bioethics

Feminist theory considers how men and women may approach ethical issues differently. It emphasizes caring relationships and responsibilities rather than more abstract rights and duties of moral agents. Feminist bioethics is not one approach but a complexity of many strands, including cultural critiques and studies of inequalities between the sexes. One core theme is the emphasis on an "ethics of care" over the use of abstract ethical principles, such as rights-based individualism. Feminist bioethics reminds us of the importance of relations with others and of social structures that can limit the choices people—especially women and minorities—face. Restrictions on the choice and freedom of women are "advantage-increasing" rules for men ("patriarchal" rules) discriminating against women.

Feminist bioethics also tends to look at less-examined topics such as reproductive ethics, disability ethics, women in research, and hierarchies of power in medicine. It considers moral issues from the perspectives of the disadvantaged and marginalized, rather than from the viewpoint of those presently in power[40]. It is not one theory of ethics but pushes the boundaries of ethics into a more inclusive field. It reminds us of the importance of relational ethics: "persons are, inevitably, connected with other persons and with social institutions"[41]. The notion of "relational autonomy" focuses on the critical contribution of the context and of other individuals to how and what decisions we make[42]. Feminist bioethics tries to render visible hidden interests and voices of the disadvantaged and the powerless[43].

Modern casuistry and ethics

Casuistry or case-based ethics regards each case or situation as a starting point for ethical deliberation. This approach to ethics uses analysis of practical cases to arrive at an appropriate response to ethical dilemmas. It avoids overarching moral theories, such as deontology or consequentialism, and grounds its decisions in the particular details of actual cases[44].

Casuistry, for example, would look at a case where promise-breaking is wrong (for example, a father has promised to take his daughter out for her birthday but does not turn up because he has decided to go out with his friends instead) and then find changed circumstances that might justify this behaviour (perhaps, in the example, the father is a health professional and was called away for an emergency). What justifies an action is, then, not a general rule but local circumstances[45].

Case 2.4 "Don't Tell!"

You are seeing Ms R, a 34-year-old woman, and her partner, Mr P, for the first time. They have been trying unsuccessfully for the last five years to have their first child. As part of the workup for infertility, you need to examine each of them. After spending time talking to the couple, you ask Ms R to disrobe in the next room so you can conduct your physical examination of her. As you enter the room, she appears nervous and hesitant. Finally, she says, "I have to be really honest with you, I had an STD when I was 19 and then again when I was 25. I have never told my partner. Please don't tell him now."

This information is important in your workup of the couple's infertility.

What is the ethical issue here?

Discussion of Case 2.4

The central issue is the duty of physicians to respect patients' privacy and the expectation by patients they will do so. What is the ethical rationale for patients such as Ms R to have control over their personal health information and what are its limits? An adherent to Kantianism might say granting the patient the right to control her own information is no different than the promise of privacy made by clinicians and the healthcare system in general to patients. Kant would say promises, once made, are to be kept ("irrespective of consequences").

But there is also a consequentialist ("dependent-on-outcomes") view on the right to privacy. Breaching Ms R's privacy would threaten the trust on which healthcare depends. This, in turn, might lead to negative outcomes such as avoidance of care by patients and disciplinary proceedings against healthcare professionals. It is to avoid such negative outcomes—rather than the obedience to any abstract rule—that would favour non-disclosure of Ms R's past. All this seems rather straightforward.

But suppose the circumstances were different. What if the workup of the couple revealed one of them had an active sexually transmitted disease that could only have come from an outside affair? Suppose that patient asked for confidentiality. Would that change the doctor's duty to respect the patient's privacy?

A Kantian might maintain it would not—the right to privacy of the patient would eclipse any duty to warn an unsuspecting partner. However, if the danger were life-threatening, even the most ardent Kantian would, these days, place the obligation to prevent serious harm above the duty to protect confidences.

continued

A utilitarian would say protection of another person's well-being would favour warning that person even if that person was not your patient (although one ill-consequence of too hastily breaching privacy might mean that at-risk individuals would not come in for care, thus increasing the risk of harm to all).

A capability theorist might say the individual at risk of getting an STD from the infected partner would be wronged if not warned of the dangers of transmission. They are wronged and their dignity as humans is denied because they are treated as the object of someone else's means. The question might be asked: who is responsible for preventing this[46]? Is the would-be malefactor responsible for not warning the other? Ought there to be a law?

Or would we say everyone is responsible for their own well-being in sexual encounters and ought to take precautions to protect themselves under any circumstance? Thus, a casuist might say the paradigmatic case to follow is that of a surgeon preparing to operate on a patient—any surgeon ought to take appropriate precautionary measures, no matter what they have been told of a patient's serological disease status. Their working idea should be to *always* assume another person harbours the agent of a serious transmissible disease. This paradigmatic case recommends protection rather than disclosure as the best way to prevent infection.

A feminist bioethics perspective might in this case invoke a duty of care to prevent harm to others that would outweigh any abstract commitment to privacy. Feminist ethics would be particularly concerned with how badly treated women historically have been by men whose seropositive STD status had been hidden from them by doctors, under the guise of protecting a man's right to privacy.

IV. Professional Ethics

Principles and doing what is best overall

From our perspective, it is interesting how the various theories of ethics consider the moral dilemma of Case 2.4 from different angles, yet also overlap. Almost any ethical issue can be seen in this way—not that the theories arrive at the same conclusion in the same way or at the same time.

All these approaches to ethics seem fruitful and could be usefully elaborated. It is unlikely the differences between them will ever be eliminated. Each offers a unique and important perspective on ethics and right action. Moreover, the disputes between them do not have to be resolved for ethics to be clinically useful or to be taught. It is notable, for example, that two authors, who diverged on the level of grand ethical theory (deontology versus consequentialism), could still agree on concrete, everyday ethical issues and write the most well-known textbook on bio-ethics, *Principles of Biomedical Ethics*[47.] The principles of ethics they espouse can encompass or be completed by the competing accounts of ethics—narrative ethics can fill in details of the stories behind the dilemmas and so provide a richer account of the dilemmas patients and physicians face. Feminist bioethics and capability theories also deepen our understanding of caring and justice in cases where people are owed duties of confidentiality and protection from harm. Thus, the principles of ethics seem consistent with a variety of accounts of ethical issues in medicine.

This does not, in our view, entail a collapse into incoherence or arbitrariness. Most importantly, the conclusions can be reasoned and coherent, open to discussion, refinement, and reflection, "even if," as the anthropologist Gellner wrote, "no absolute point of view is possible"[48.] The requirement for modern medical ethics need not be "universalism" (what has been called the moral "monist" perspective) in ethical theory but pragmatism, thoughtfulness, and reflection.

Prior to his premature death in 2017, the prominent British philosopher Derek Parfit argued that, while the perspectives of contractualism, utilitarianism, and deontology differ, they are (in his interpretations) ultimately concerned with the same end—the search for a "single true morality"[49.] What matters most, in the end, is that "all things go well." They may if we always strive to do what is "best overall." This does not end the controversy, of course. The philosopher John Kekes has argued, for example, that taking all the relevant factors into account will exclude some options as unacceptable but not necessarily all competing answers. "We are all encumbered by conflicts and ambivalence, which perhaps we can ameliorate but not eliminate"[50.]

Fallibilism and the underlying requirements for ethics

Healthcare professionals frequently must make fateful decisions with and for patients armed only with uncertain and incomplete evidence. The important questions to ask oneself in such situations are self-reflective ones: *Could I be wrong? What would it take for me to be mistaken about my diagnosis? What else could this be?*[51] In philosophy this is known as "fallibilism" or "critical rationalism"[52.]

> **Box 2.7**
>
> "To be a fallibilist at the bedside is to exercise the understanding [that] the very 'facts of the case' of the patient presenting in front of you may indeed be wrong. It means always being open to the possibility that you are wrong about the way you are interpreting the patient's presentation and the treatments they need."[52]

Fallibilism is not an ethical theory. Rather, it is an approach at the heart of medical reasoning generally, forming the basis for the art of the "differential diagnosis" —the trial-and-error process of recommending tests and consultations that would help favour one diagnosis over another.

When it comes to difficult moral decisions, rather than espousing one theory of ethics (no one theory can encompass all judgments in medicine), we prefer the use of a toolbox of mid-level ethical principles that do not derive from one ethical theory. Instead, we promote a critical examination and management, a "resolution" if you will, of cases. The two cardinal features required for good clinical practice are self-awareness and openness to criticism.

This admittedly eclectic ethics toolbox is what the great twentieth-century anthropologist Lévi-Strauss might have called a *bricolage*—a hodgepodge of different elements that in this case is nevertheless insightful and effective in having an impact on the everyday world of medical professionals[53].

Box 2.8

The toolbox approach to ethics in our view is best served by acknowledging two basic commitments:

1. the principle of "respect for humans" (or "respect for human dignity") and
2. a fidelity to reason and to critical appraisal.

These two commitments constitute the underpinnings of all professional medical practice, required in everything we, as healthcare providers, do. Without respect for others and a commitment to reason, it is hard to see how medicine and society could advance. Our use of mid-level principles in ethics is not meant to imply that other perspectives are not possible or useful. We will return to and at times utilize these other views throughout the book. Whether an outcome or decision is the right answer to any particular moral situation discussed in the cases in this book will depend upon the reader's considered moral judgment.

Conclusion

In its original form from ancient Greece, the Hippocratic oath saw trust as possible only if the doctor kept his professional training, his apprenticeship, a secret— as perhaps befitted a tradition that had few truly helpful interventions. Today, trust in medicine requires informational transparency and patient involvement. The old, narrow guild mentality and the monetary self-interest of some modern healthcare professionals are ongoing threats to the public's trust in the profession. So, too, is the view of medicine as a corporate enterprise. These issues will be discussed more fully in Chapters 10 and 13.

In the next chapter we will turn to a complex and sad case to illustrate in greater depth the application of one way of managing ethical dilemmas in medicine.

Cases for Discussion

Case 1: "I've Seen Worse!"

You are the attending physician at a chronic care facility. One of the residents, Mr T, an 84-year-old war veteran with no living relatives, unable to look after himself owing to physical frailty and mild cognitive decline, develops gangrene in his foot due to poor circulation; it does not respond to medical treatment. Advised to have the foot amputated, Mr T refuses, saying, "My foot will get better on its own. I've seen lots worse during the war!"

Question for Discussion
1.   Should you accept his refusal of treatment?

Case 2: "It's My Life!"

Ms R is a 46-year-old single woman from the Dominican Republic with a 10-year history of rheumatoid arthritis. It has become very disabling; her small hand and finger joints are barely usable despite numerous corrective surgeries. Pain control has also been a significant issue. Ms R is taking 300 mg of morphine a day and complains bitterly that she is still in pain. Your colleagues are appalled at the dose of opiates you have prescribed for her.

Ms R comes to see you today as she needs more painkillers and to talk about methotrexate, the only drug she has found at all helpful in remitting her symptoms. She has been taking the drug much longer than recommended; there are changes in her lab tests suggesting damage to her liver. There are some new biologic agents, but she is skeptical about whether they will help her. In any case, these new drugs are far too expensive for Ms R to afford.

continued

You have advised her several times to stop the methotrexate, but Ms R refuses. "It's the only thing that helps me! Damn the liver, I just want some relief!"

Questions for Discussion

1. As Ms R's physician, what should you do?
2. What are the pros and cons of following Ms R's request?

✦ **3** ✦

·······································

Managing Medical Morality

Morality, therefore, is more properly felt than judged of.

David Hume, 1739 [1]

I. Managing Ethical Dilemmas

Various formal techniques of resolving ethical dilemmas were developed some time ago by, among others, Lo [2], Thomasma [3], and Jonsen, Siegler, and Winslade [4]. All presume an organized approach is useful in arriving at the most appropriate management of such quandaries. To make the process seem familiar to medical students, Thomasma described this organized approach as an ethics "workup." However, the idea that we can "resolve" ethical issues is problematic. Rather, healthcare providers are encouraged to be careful in what they do and to consider their views and practices critically. Ethical issues and dilemmas are not to be readily solved and then forgotten. Sometimes these are best opened up to the light of day with alternative solutions examined. Admittedly, this may leave involved healthcare professionals more perplexed and worried than they were before. This is why we now consider it more appropriate to recommend an ethical *management* process.

Case 3.1   Hidden Trauma

·······································

You are the primary care provider for Ms T, a 45-year-old woman admitted with syncope and a possible seizure disorder. This is her second such admission. During a similar hospitalization three months ago, a complete neurological workup, including a brain scan, failed to reveal a cause for

continued

---

these symptoms. The attending physician on this admission orders the same tests to be repeated.

Informed of the admission, you come to visit Ms T in the hospital. You are extremely worried. Two days previously, the patient had come to see you and had confided the real cause of her last admission was a beating, one of many she had suffered at the hands of her abusive husband. Ms T had never disclosed this to anyone before and asked you to keep the matter a secret. In their culture, she explained, men are allowed to beat their wives for actions such as going out without the husband's approval. Ms T does not disagree with this cultural allowance. She does not even regard this as "abuse"—it's "just how things are." It's what she learned growing up.

You are pretty sure that the husband's actions are again the cause for Ms T's admission. After reviewing the admission notes, you realize this has not been considered by the attending physician.

Should you reveal the patient's secret to her admitting doctor?

The importance of circumstances

In ethical matters, as in other matters, the right people must be involved for good decision-making. It is not surprising to find great variance in this. The people involved, the specific circumstances of the case, and the milieu will help to determine the best thing to do. People make decisions in a particular context and in concert with (or against) other people[5]. The complexity of the context and the circumstances are reasons why the "correct" answer to real-world dilemmas cannot be deduced from a recitation of the case.

II. Really Hard Choices Are Not Always about Ethics

Cultural factors in particular may seem overwhelming in some circumstances (see Chapter 17). Issues such as race, gender, income, housing, literacy, and education—of the healthcare practitioner and of the patient and the similarities or gaps between the two—have an obvious impact on the care patients may request and practitioners can provide[6]. Add to this the emotional reactions, as well as the cultural norms and practices in the communities where practitioners and their patients reside, and you have fertile grounds for a sense of futility. Ethics cannot treat patients as abstract entities but must be able to recognize their individuality. We are "diversely diverse," as the economist Amartya Sen has written[7].

Box 3.1

Doing right for a particular patient will mean being aware of such circumstances as

- institutional regulations,
- local laws,
- the attitudes of your fellow healthcare professionals,
- your emotions,
- the patient's cultural background,
- the patient's significant others, and
- other upstream issues that may impact on the patient (such as poverty, homelessness, illiteracy).

Discussion of Case 3.1

This is a typical ethical dilemma: the patient's well-being is at odds with her autonomous wishes. Involved in this case as well are the issues of confidentiality, trust and privacy, social justice, cross-cultural issues, and the social determinants of illness. This is a challenging, complex assortment of issues but we will focus on one: the safety of the patient (the principle of beneficence) versus her expressed wishes (the principle of autonomy).

Spousal abuse is underreported and often not suspected by healthcare professionals [8]. Cultural factors and norms can play a role in its occurrence and in its continuance. This does not make it acceptable as just another cultural custom. There are important screening questions to identify domestic violence that the clinician should initiate in private (such as, Does your partner ever physically hurt you? Insult or talk down to you? Threaten you with harm? Scream or curse at you? How often does this happen?) [9].

It is remarkable Ms T has been able to confide this much to you. (If she does not share a common language with you, this is where reliance on a professional interpreter, as opposed to a family member such as the husband, is critical.) Abused women sometimes resist help even when the problem is identified; this reluctance to seek help must be of concern to healthcare professionals. But, unless a patient is in "imminent" or serious danger (see Chapter 7), you cannot breach her confidentiality until she is ready to have her secret revealed.

In most jurisdictions, a patient's consent for medical information to be shared among members of the "circle of care" (those healthcare professionals

continued

and entities such as pharmacies, laboratories, and hospitals providing or assisting in providing healthcare to a specific patient) is implied (see Chapter 6). However, this patient's explicit refusal of such information-sharing must be respected. Premature disclosure could undermine the patient's trust in you and make it harder for her to ask for the help she needs. Although Ms T may be given unnecessary medical tests if you do not reveal her secret, this is not a strong enough reason to override the duty of confidentiality. You should try to reassure her that all involved in her care must respect her privacy.

The greater worry would be the consequences of Ms T returning to her husband. You could try to ensure her physical safety by referring her to culturally sensitive services and shelters. The unacceptable cultural mores that tolerate domestic violence need to be addressed as well.

In the end, Ms T is persuaded that she can safely disclose the true cause of her injuries to the admitting medical team and seeks help for her troubled home situation.

Box 3.2

....

The hidden lesson: "We cannot avoid secrets, disconcerting or otherwise. They come to us unsolicited and by surprise, and, once heard, they change forever the way we feel about a patient." [10]

There are many lessons to be taken from Case 3.1: the importance of listening to the patient, of thinking outside the box, of taking background ("upstream") issues into account, and of considering patient safety in a cultural context. The secret story of a patient can change everything, utterly.

An ethical dilemma may involve hard choices and risk very real sacrifices. It is important always to ask yourself: "Is this what a ('reasonably') good person/ clinician would do?" If you cannot in good faith answer this question, you may not be ready to address or resolve the dilemma. You may need more information. The best resolution of an ethical dilemma, of course, depends on healthcare professionals possessing the most up-to-date facts and having good colleagues to consult.

The decision process outlined here is not a moral algorithm that will churn out right answers to any dilemma like a sausage-making machine. As well, not all dilemmas are simply *ethical* dilemmas; many difficult decisions concern matters of living as well—so-called "existential" dilemmas. A heartbreaking example occurs in the movie *Sophie's Choice*, based on the book by William Styron [11], in which a mother is forced to decide which one of her two children she must give up to the Nazis and certain death. A similar choice had to be made in the real world by millions of parents of twins in Mao's China as to which twin would be "sent down" from urban areas for rural re-education ("rustication") [12]. These terrible choices are being repeated around the world today as refugees, fleeing murderous regimes, wars, and famines, are treated as criminals and face the forcible separation of children from their parents. This completely unnecessary human suffering due, in part, to the inaction by most well-off counties must be of concern to the professions of healthcare (see Chapter 13).

There is nothing philosophy can say to ever make such situations right in any way. The question medicine has to ask is what it can do to make things right again. Managing ethical issues may help open them up to proper analysis and scrutiny, but it is vigilant and caring healthcare professionals acting as advocates for patients who can ensure situations of ethical difficulty are not forgotten.

III. "Doing Right": A Process for Managing Ethical Choice

The process for analyzing ethical problems in medicine cannot help health professionals escape the emotional consequences of their decisions. If anything, the process of ethical deliberation will intensify the emotional consequences and import of the decisions healthcare professionals have to make. Working through a difficult situation can be helpful for identifying what the issues and options are and for offering resolutions.

In the workup we use, there are eight steps (see Box 3.3). Keep in mind you do not have to follow all of the steps in every case. In some instances, it will be obvious how to proceed after a few moments' reflection because you just know the right thing to do or because an ethical consideration suggests the best way to proceed. The full procedure is most helpful for decisions concerning difficult cases or when you wish to ensure your decision is backed up by critical reflection.

Box 3.3

An Ethics Management Process

1. Outline the case simply but with pertinent facts and circumstances.
2. What is the dilemma? What decisions need to be made?
3. What are the alternatives?

continued

4. How do the key considerations apply?
   (a) Autonomy: what are the patient's wishes and values?
      - Consider the patient's mental capacity, wishes, beliefs, goals, hopes, and fears. If capacity is lacking, look to local laws when considering substitute decision-makers.
   (b) Beneficence: what can be done for the patient?
      - Consider the benefits and burdens of the various alternatives from the perspective of the clinician, the patient, and possibly the family, and the probable result of each one.
   (c) Nonmaleficence: which option poses the least risk of harm?
      - Consider that any intervention involves some chance of harm.
   (d) Justice: is the patient being treated fairly?
      - Consider the patient's fundamental right to their fair share of medical resources as well as the interests and claims of the family, other patients, and healthcare staff.

5. Consider involving others and consider context: what emotions and situational factors are important? Consider others who ought to be involved. Be familiar with cultural and local practices, institutional policies and guidelines, professional norms, and legal precedents.

6. Propose a resolution: weigh these factors for each alternative; then say what you would do or recommend. Consider, in the circumstances, what your role would be—what would a "good doctor/person" do?

7. Consider your choice critically: under what circumstances would you be prepared to alter it? Consider the opinions of your peers, your conscience, and your emotional reactions. Know your resources. Formulate your choice as a general maxim and see how far it might extend; suggest cases where it would not apply; decide if you—and others—are comfortable with the choice made. If not, reconsider key considerations and consider consultations with specialists in ethics, law, or in the local culture.

8. Do the right thing—"all things considered."

IV. The Ethics Process in a Little More Detail

The ethics consideration process can be truncated or made more detailed depending on the complexity of the issues being examined and how familiar the situation is to those involved.

Step 1. Recognize that a case raises an important ethical problem.

Ethical problems arise when there is a genuine conflict of values or ethical princi-ples leading to different possible paths of action. For example, the relatives of an elderly woman with dementia wish to have her placed in a nursing home, some-thing she refuses to consider (safety versus autonomy); a patient does not want his sexual partner to know he carries a herpes virus (confidentiality versus nonmalefi-cence); a 15-year-old girl, 16 weeks pregnant, is resisting the abortion her parents insist she have (autonomy versus beneficence); a patient, now floridly psychotic, re-fuses drug treatment that he, when well, had said he would take (autonomy versus nonmaleficence). In all these cases, clinicians must make difficult decisions about what to do or to recommend; in many cases there are more than two choices.

It is important, of course, to be as knowledgeable as possible about the situation. You should know the most relevant aspects of the patient's life story and family context, the patient's medical condition, the working diagnosis, and the various treatment options as well as the associated burdens and benefits of each. A true ethics consultation for a case will usually not rest content with the kind of "thin" case studies (due to space limitations) used in this book. The devil, they say, lies in the details, but sometimes in the details is the angel, the best solu-tion to the case. This is where narrative medicine is so important to the ethical management of patient issues.

Step 2. What is the problem that has to be solved?

State what you take to be the central problem. This is often the most important step. Should the woman with dementia be institutionalized without her consent? Should the partner of the patient with herpes be informed of his condition? Should the parents have a say in their daughter's decision? Should the patient with psych-osis, now refusing the antipsychotic drugs he previously said he would take if psy-chotic, be treated against his will according to his prior wish?

Always be clear on what needs to be resolved. Ethical problems can seem intractable when the participants are not asking the same question. For example, a family resists for some time the transfer of their cognitively impaired father to another ward. Consultation reveals the problem is not that the family wants some-thing inappropriate; the problem is a disagreement among the siblings. What they need is help as a family in resolving their differences. When this is achieved, a solution to the ward problem is found. Sometimes an ethical dilemma turns out to be a communication problem or a cultural factor or an issue for Psychiatry. Once the problem is precisely identified, you will be better able to decide what resources are needed to resolve it. (For example, miscommunication or misunderstanding frequently occurs in discussions around discontinuing life-sustaining care. It is important to convey that the patient will be cared for just as much, but in a different way, with the focus directed towards the patient's comfort. See Chapter 15.)

Step 3. Determine reasonable alternative courses of action.

Asking what is the right thing to do for a patient presupposes that alternative procedures—usually two or three—exist for this patient. The list of options need not be exhaustive, but clear alternatives should be given. They may be quite simple: for example, either the woman with dementia should be placed or not; the partner should be told or not; the parents should have a say in their daughter's decision or not. They can also be quite complex. For example, should the psychotic patient be treated, following his prior wish, or not, following his current wish? How clear was his prior wish and how determined is he with his current wish? Is he now resisting all manner of treatment or just certain antipsychotics? Perhaps the patient with dementia can be gradually introduced to a long-term care institution; perhaps there are untapped resources to support her at home; perhaps she has funds to be used to make her environment safer. The final resolution of the case may be one of these options or some other previously unconsidered choice. Use your imagination!

Step 4. Consider each option in relation to the four fundamental ethical principles.

This is a critical and difficult step. The ethical healthcare practitioner or trainee is expected to utilize and consider the four fundamental ethical principles of autonomy, beneficence, nonmaleficence, and justice. Knowing just how to interpret the principles in light of circumstances and the agents involved can be problematic. What to do when the principles seemingly conflict is another, not infrequent, problem. Broadly speaking, the patient's wishes come first, but the acceptability of these wishes will sometimes depend upon the medically possible, socially available, and culturally plausible options. As conflicts between principles can never be entirely eliminated, healthcare professionals may have to make judgment calls in particular circumstances. The principles can help eliminate some options as unacceptable but cannot always be counted on to unequivocally favour one option.

You obviously need not agree to fulfill a patient's wishes if what the patient suggests is illegal, immoral (even if locally accepted), or unusually burdensome to others. For example, for the woman with dementia who refuses to leave her home, you will want to weigh the significance of her wish against its effect on her well-being and the safety of others. Does she pose a risk serious enough to outweigh her wish? What if she smokes in bed? What if she is prone to leaving the stove on? Or wanders in the snow shoeless? Complicating all this is that patients can change their minds: if the patient who had previously said, "Don't listen to me when I'm psychotic," now says, "Listen to me even though I'm psychotic," which self should you heed?

Step 5. Consider who should be involved and other circumstances.

You will want to ensure, insofar as is possible, that the right people—those in the patient's circle of care: the family (if the patient has no objection) and other healthcare providers—are consulted. If the patient is not capable or is acting out of character and putting others in harm's way, you should attempt to contact the patient's significant others or, where appropriate, a substitute decision-maker. You may also need to involve others, such as a public guardian or, if culturally appropriate, a local sage or healer, who may be appointed, or may be expected, to "look after" an incapable person in their community.

You should also consider other circumstances, such as institutional policies, professional guidelines, cultural norms, and personal or emotional factors. Are there upstream issues that are at the root of the dilemma? In deciding what to do for the woman with dementia, for example, you will have to take into account specific factors such as legislation that might (or might not) allow an incapable person to be removed from her home. You may also wish to reflect on practical matters such as what resources might be made available to allow the patient to stay in her home or how strenuously the patient would resist being "placed" without her consent. These factors can help you to choose between the various options.

Step 6. Decide on a resolution to the problem.

Sounds like a lot, doesn't it? It can be. This is why you may need to seek advice from others, such an ethicist, a peer, or another colleague, who can help you sort out the various complexities. At the end of the day, you must take a stand as to what you think is the right course of action. Try to follow your best guess as to the right thing to do, all things reasonably considered. Some scenarios will test your patience— for example, patients who are suffering and could be treated were it not for their prior wishes not to be—and your ability to empathize with the patient. Your conclusion may be disputed, so you should be able to justify your choice as the best one, if not the only one. Be flexible: if the evidence changes, be prepared to change.

Step 7. Consider your position critically.

Before and after the decision, keep an open mind and consider what could be done differently. The reflective practitioner will ask, *under what circumstances would one advocate a different course of action*? It may help to formulate your position as a general "maxim" or principle. For example, if you decide the woman with dementia should be allowed to stay at home, you might generalize this into a statement such as, "Persons with dementia may stay at home, providing they are not putting others in danger."

The next step would be to consider the limits of such a principle. What if the impaired person refused any help or monitoring of their condition? What if they didn't smoke but had weak legs, which could result in a high risk of falling down the stairs? What if the community has no home-support resources for patients with dementia?

At the end of the day, ask yourself: What is your role in the resolution of the problem? Are you prepared to be an advocate for the patient? Will you be able to sleep soundly given your decision? Would you be comfortable if your decision were to be made public? Will your colleagues stand behind you? If they will not step forward to support you, this may be telling you something you should not ignore.

If you or others feel ill at ease with the decision, carefully reconsider the main features of the case. Take into account the emotional, cultural, and ethnic factors that may result in differing views. Where no option seems satisfying, compromises may have to be made. Not all moral disagreements can be readily settled, however. Indeed, some may never be. In the end, people in disagreement have to learn to work with one another or agree to disagree.

In considering what *your* role would be in achieving what you take to be the right choice, do not be pushed by abstract ethical principles to do things your conscience or emotions tell you are wrong[13]. Sentiments can be a helpful corrective to reason[14]. Your conscience, emotional reactions, and, yes, intuition in response to a case can provide reasonable brakes on, or prompts to, action. They can represent your deepest values, identity, and integrity as a person and as a professional.

Step 8. Do the right thing!

This step should go without saying, but there are many obstacles to acting ethically in practice. Doing the right thing may be difficult because of conflicting loyalties, hierarchies, cultural differences, survival needs, limited resources, and extreme circumstances like war and natural disasters. Professional ethics may seem a slim reed to grasp onto in extreme situations. But those who do follow the moral route in hard times may fare better in the long run than those who shuck their ethics, as if it were a mere moral carapace, for the "easy" thing to do. Although doing the right thing is sometimes the most difficult thing to do[15], attempting to do it allows you to develop your "moral muscles," as Mill wrote[16], and resist the seemingly irresistible.

V. Applying the Ethics Process

Now, consider the use of the ethics process in a complicated, controversial, and very sad real-life case with which one of the authors was involved many years ago.

Case 3.2 To Feed or Not to Feed?

Ms E, a 22-year-old woman ill since age 14 with severe anorexia nervosa, was brought into the emergency room in cardiovascular collapse. She was extremely emaciated, weighing less than 60 lbs., and virtually unresponsive. After receiving a bolus of intravenous glucose, she perked up just long enough to pull out her intravenous line.

Ms E had been admitted numerous times in her starved state and had spent most of her previous eight years in hospital. She had been considered one of the most "difficult" patients by specialty units of various tertiary care hospitals. All corrective therapy had failed. Drug therapy using antipsychotics and antidepressants was unsuccessful. Different psychotherapeutic approaches over many years—including cognitive-behavioural, family therapy, and even "paradoxical" therapy (admitting to the patient that she is going to die and hoping she will struggle against this pessimistic message)—had also been of no sustained benefit.

On previous admissions Ms E had received nutritional rehabilitation, including force-feeding requiring restraints and causing major disruptions on the ward. She had expressed a wish to die but not consistently so. She had recently told her family doctor she wished her suffering would soon end; at that time, she requested no forced feedings in the future. Ms E thought she was, and had always been, overweight, refusing to believe her food refusals endangered her life. Various tertiary care hospitals refused her readmission because of her previous extreme resistance and disruptiveness.

The healthcare team involved in Ms E's care considered the option of providing nutrition through a gastrostomy tube (a tube inserted directly into her stomach through a small incision in the abdominal wall). This would have entailed a minor surgical procedure and, most likely, putting her in physical restraints.

What should have been done on this admission?
How might Ms E's situation be distinguished (or not) from that of someone who is terminally ill?
How would you assess the status of her request not to be force-fed?

Discussion of Case 3.2

1. The case

The first step is to acknowledge an ethical dilemma exists. Sometimes we become so focused on what we are doing in medicine that we fail to ask, wait a minute—what are we doing here? Are we sure about this? Should we be doing something different? Once these questions were raised, the ethical moment had been recognized. The care providers for Ms E felt it was their (deontological) duty to feed her but were troubled by the consequences of doing so—for the patient primarily, and for everyone else as well.

2. The problem

This case contains a number of problems, but the central one is whether Ms E should be force-fed or not. The standard of care for patients with anorexia nervosa is nutritional rehabilitation with the aim of weight restoration and psychotherapy or other social/psychiatric support. Patients who do not respond require "higher levels of care," [17] including involuntary hospitalization and feeding by any means possible. Does the standard of care, however, require you to do so again and again with a protesting patient [18]? When might not feeding such a patient ever be appropriate?

3. The alternatives

Obviously, the central immediate problem for Ms E was her state of severe starvation and imminent vascular collapse. The alternatives were only two: emergency fluid resuscitation and then more aggressive force-feeding, or not rehydrating and not re-feeding her.

4. Applying the principles

Ms E had previously requested not to be force-fed, so this option would seem to be in agreement with her "autonomous" wishes [19]. For some people these days, anorexia nervosa is not so much an illness as a "lifestyle" choice [20]. This view is popular among some with the disorder and others resistant to the idea of psychiatric illness altogether. ("The 'psychiatric patient' is a person who fails, or refuses, to assume a legitimate social role." [21])

But what was the status of Ms E's wish not to be force-fed? Was this really an autonomous choice or was it the product of a mind unbalanced by delusions (firm, fixed beliefs unamenable to criticism or evidence) and starvation?

It can be argued that Ms E was not competent and therefore not authentically autonomous (and therefore that her case was quite distinguishable from that of a person on a hunger strike for political reasons[22]). Following her wishes would result in her death by starvation, an outcome she had not consistently or clearly requested. Perhaps her request for her suffering to be over was a wish for healing and not for death—it may have been a cry for *more* help, not less. Her failure to truly appreciate the consequences of self-starvation and prior refusal of all forms of nutritional rehabilitation, as is the case for many anorexic patients, made her prior wishes incapable ones and therefore unreliable[23].

There is no legal duty to force-feed capable starving patients who have chosen not to eat, but there is an obligation to try to offer help to incapable patients in imminent peril[24] (see Chapter 9). Healthcare professionals are generally obliged to intervene when patients under their care place themselves at risk of death by a suicide attempt or a failure of self-care in the context of a mental illness. So, the central question was: *Could Ms E have been saved by more aggressive intervention?*

5. The context

This was perhaps the most difficult and complex question to answer. It depends on one's clinical experience with such patients and whether one believes it is possible to form a therapeutic alliance with patients such as Ms E.

All of Ms E's options seemed fraught with pain and suffering. Many, including her parents, who were her substitute decision-makers in law, felt keenly that she had suffered enough. But was letting her go a mercy[25]? Or was it a negative emotional reaction to a difficult, and so, in the staff's eyes, "untreatable" patient? On the pro-treatment side was the fear of legal liability, such as negligence, if she were allowed to die. Although courts have generally ruled against forced feeding, this has usually been in the context of competent refusals of food, such as by prisoners on hunger strikes. It is an established norm for doctors that "[f]orcible feeding [of prisoners] is never ethically acceptable"[26].

6. Resolution

For most patients with anorexia in extremis, however, rescue would be undertaken without delay. This position could be generalized into a principle such as "Incapable patients in danger of dying from self-starvation should receive non-voluntary nutritional rehabilitation." This principle can be rooted in instructions made by a (previously capable) patient telling others to ignore refusals of treatment of her future (incapable) self.

This kind of advance instruction has been called a "Ulysses contract." In the ancient Homeric myth of Ulysses, the Sirens were sea nymphs whose singing so bewitched and entranced mariners passing by they would crash

continued

their vessels into the local rocks. Ulysses wanted to hear their song, so he ordered his crew to stuff their ears with wax and to bind him to the mast of his ship. They were told not release him, no matter how much he implored them, until they passed safely by the Sirens' island. Indeed, as they sailed by, the sea nymphs' song was so sweet and attractive that Ulysses struggled to loosen his ropes, begging his men to release him. They ignored him, as previously instructed, binding him even tighter until they were finally out of earshot[27].

7. Critical considerations

What are the limits to this principle? It would be inappropriate to force-feed a competent autonomous patient who expresses a clear wish not to be fed. In a "reverse Ulysses" contract, a capable patient asks *not* to be treated and so, presumably, to be allowed to die—such as the critically ill patient with advanced cancer who declines aggressive chemotherapy, preferring to risk an earlier death.

Must all prior instructions be followed?

If instructions to limit care are made when the patient is incompetent (see Chapter 7), capacity is a central issue. However, no matter what the patient's mental state, elaborate efforts to save a patient would be less than morally optimal if it is clear further feeding could no longer benefit her. Thus, if the patient were to die anyway, further feedings would be futile and should be withheld. This might be the case for an unconscious patient with a terminal illness such as advanced cancer or advanced dementia.

In other words, treatment that cannot achieve any reasonable medical goal need not be given. The duty to rescue should be a proportionate one and not an excuse to torture the dying with extravagant therapy[28]. Although anorexia nervosa is not a recognized terminal illness, Ms E was so emaciated and so entrenched in her belief she was overweight that she could not be rescued. Were they to have attempted re-feeding, the care providers in the ER might have won the day's skirmish, but the war was being lost. She was terminally ill.

8. Action required

Ms E was, in fact, not resuscitated[29]. After meeting with her family and obtaining consultations in hospital with the departments of Psychiatry and Internal Medicine and the hospital ethics committee, Ms E's physicians deemed her to be beyond rescue and decided against rehydrating or force-feeding her. Her parents were motivated by love—they felt she had suffered enough and recognized the desire to keep her alive was self-centred on their part. Ms E died shortly after admission, in the presence of her family.

On emotion and reason

Of concern is the possibility that the decision to limit care was due to an un-explored animosity of healthcare providers toward a seemingly hopeless and de-manding patient. Did they give up too soon because Ms E seemed incurable and imposed such a burden on others? Some hold that *no* patient with anorexia ner-vosa should be considered hopeless [30], but this may be overly optimistic. Would another physician in a different institution have done better? Or would she have simply suffered more? Needless to say, it is easy to be wise after the event. Cases like this are very troubling for all concerned.

One must of course try to guard against the negative reactions to patients that can lead to undertreatment. But one also cannot ignore the emotions of identifica-tion and sympathy that can lead to overtreatment.

Emotions have an important role to play in the ethics of healthcare: they cause us to *care* about what we do, as reason alone may not. Feelings, such as empathy and compassion, love and despair, can be a test as to what we should and do care about. Ethics is never simply an intellectual enterprise [31].

The Scottish philosopher of the Enlightenment, David Hume, arguing for the centrality of feeling and sentiment to moral judgment, wrote in 1738, "the rules of morality, therefore, are not conclusions of our reason." He was pessimistic about the role of rationality in disputes over ethics: "reason alone can never be a motive to any action of the will . . . and . . . it can never oppose passion in the direction of the will." [32]

Pessimistic though Hume might have been about the influence of reason on morality, he understood the importance of sympathy. It is "the chief source of moral distinctions," he wrote [33]. For example, feelings of benevolence—compassion, caring for and about others, and a concern for humanity—ground and extend our ethical judgments.

Conclusion

Ethics is a complex and sometimes confusing field. The dire situation of some pa-tients demonstrates how difficult the management of ethical dilemmas can be in the real world of everyday medicine. Facts are uncertain, wishes hard to ascertain, truth elusive, and authentic choice tenuous. Nevertheless, we should never cease seeking a sense of the emotional truth in our deliberations, that is, for better and more imaginative options—not unassailable right answers but responses that are prudent and reasonable in the peculiar and particular facts of the case.

We will now turn to the principle of autonomy that has, singlehandedly, revo-lutionized healthcare.

Cases for Discussion

Case 1: Beyond Help?

You are the primary care provider for Mr I, a 20-year-old second-year college student with a past history of depression as a teen. For several weeks, he has confined himself to his small garret-like flat, refusing visitors. His best friend was killed two months previously when a car struck his bicycle. According to others in the house, Mr I has not been carrying out his day-to-day tasks, appearing dishevelled when glimpsed. He can be heard crying and shouting day and night.

After Mr I misses several appointments, you decide to visit him at his home. Reluctantly, he lets you in. He admits having stopped taking the anti-depressant he was prescribed at the university's health service because one of his housemates told him it was a "psychiatric poison." He looks ill-kempt and admits to being very sad. Mr I acknowledges that pills and therapy are interventions that might help some people—indeed, his own episodes of depression responded to them in the past. Nonetheless, he refuses them now on the grounds that "I've seen Jesus and he can't help me. I am, as he was, as we all are," he cries, "under the control of a higher power."

Questions for Discussion
1. What is the ethical dilemma in this case?
2. What should you do?

Case 2: A Family Affair

You are a nurse practitioner on the Oncology service. Mr O, a 72-year-old male, has been admitted with nausea and ataxia. In hospital he has had several brief seizures and is now on phenytoin, an anticonvulsant. An enhanced MRI reveals a thin coating of tumour wrapped around his brainstem: he has leptome-ningeal carcinomatosis. This uncommon condition is virtually untreatable. Time to death after diagnosis is usually weeks to a few months.

He is unaware of his diagnosis but his family knows—they had an acquaintance in the MRI suite who tipped them off. The large and supportive family has formed a protective cordon around Mr O.

His wife, herself a doctor from another country, pleads with you not to tell Mr O what you know. "I know the prognosis for my husband is terrible.

We have all come to accept that. Now we only want to be able to take him home and let him die there in peace," she says with tears in her eyes. "It would be cruel and do him no good to be told his exact diagnosis. We have told him he has a seizure disorder from a brain abnormality, that it cannot be fixed, and left it at that. We think he should only be told good news; anything else would only make him feel worse. We accept that it is the family's responsibility to look after the patient. You can't do anything for him; we will do everything for him."

Questions for Discussion

1. What are the ethical conflicts here? On which dilemma would you focus if you were the healthcare practitioner in this case?
2. What of families who ask clinicians to do everything for a dying relative?
3. What should be done when deception is in the patient's best interests?

✦ 4 ✦

....

The Times are Changing
Autonomy and Patient-Based Care

Autonomy, the liberty to live after one's own law.

Henry Cockerham, 1623 [1]

Although the concept of autonomy has existed for hundreds of years, the notion that people should be free to make choices about their own lives and their own healthcare has truly revolutionized medicine over the past 60 years. In significant portions of the world, even in locales not considered democratic, the notion of patient autonomy has irreversibly changed how clinicians, patients, and the public think about acceptable medical care. We defend autonomy not as a sole principle or necessarily the overriding principle of healthcare; we do think that including it in decision-making simply improves, makes for more helpful, healthcare.

Citizens around the world are pressing for more liberty to make choices about their personal lifestyles, their family structures, and the kind of societies they want without fear or intimidation. Can they also expect healthcare, as with other hierarchical structures, to mirror these changes? Choice is an essential ingredient of modern medicine. Effective care means patients can choose, if they wish and if given the opportunity, from among different viable options. Unfortunately, the sad reality throughout the world is one of "massive inequalities in the opportunities different people have" to access proven effective medical care [2]. Autonomy cannot be considered apart from the other primary rights and conditions people must have—freedom from starvation, wars, illiteracy, crushing poverty—in order to live flourishing lives. The possibility of global ethics will recur in Chapter 13.

Case 4.1 More Surgery Wanted!

Ms X, a 60-year-old woman with early-stage breast cancer, accompanied by her 25-year-old daughter, has come to see Dr Y for a second opinion. The breast surgeon explains, as far as surgery goes, fortunately all she needs is breast-conserving surgery (BCS). Ms X does not look relieved. With her daughter translating, she replies, "That's what the other doctor said, too. But that's not what I want!" Her daughter explains she wants a modified radical mastectomy, having no confidence in BCS as one of her friends had a recurrence of breast cancer after this.

Dr Y is a little confused. She usually finds herself in the opposite position of trying to convince some women to have any surgery at all. Although Dr Y describes the morbidity associated with radical surgery, Ms X remains unconvinced. Her daughter explains this view of BCS is common in their culture.

Must Dr Y go along with the request for more radical surgery than is medically indicated?

I. The Autonomy Principle

Medicine must start by attempting to understand patient needs and wants in the context of the patient's life. Patient-based interviewing creates an atmosphere of trust whereby the patient feels respected and heard—it is an essential step in establishing rapport between the healthcare professional and the patient (see Box 4.1) [3-6].

Patient-based care

Patient-based interviewing leads to patient-based care, which is intimately bound up with the ethical notions of patient autonomy and respect for persons. If this perspective is right (and we think it is), health professionals and their institutions should incorporate their patients' views and interests into the foundation of appropriate healthcare.

Respecting patients also implies an allegiance to a patient-based notion of benefit—benefit as seen and experienced by the patient. This does not, however, entail a model of medicine as a business enterprise where the patient is a client or consumer. The business-derived notions of "buyer-beware" or "the client-is-always-right" have no place, in general, in healthcare. These are antithetical to the mutual trust and respect that serve as the foundation of patient-based care. That

> **Box 4.1**
>
> For patient-based interviewing:
>
> - First, introduce yourself to the patient.
> - To establish eye contact at the patient's level, sit on the edge of the bed or on a chair.
> - Put the patient at ease with a touch or a handshake, if culturally acceptable.
> - Avoid medical jargon and be sensitive to patient cues of fear, anxiety, and the like.
> - Allow the patient to finish their initial monologue about their concerns.
> - Facilitate communication by employing active listening by nodding, echoing, saying "umm-hmm."
> - Elicit the patient's concerns by asking, "What else?" "What other concerns do you have?"
> - If there are many issues, prioritize by saying, "You have a lot of concerns; what were you most hoping we could do today?"
> - Review with the patient: "What I hear you saying is . . ." "Is it all right if we focus on your main concern? . . ."
> - To avoid being prematurely reassuring, first listen to the whole story. Then pause and ask, "Let me see if I have this right . . ." Or, "Sounds like . . ."

said, because power and information tend to flow *away* from the patient, medicine is an uneven playing field favouring the healthcare professional. The ethical practitioner must work at levelling out that field.

> **Discussion of Case 4.1**
>
> In Ms X's community of origin, according to at least one study, it is common for women to reject BCS for the very reason she cites[7, 8]. Dr Y needs to understand Ms X's position from that of her community of origin. The resistance she faces is not due to idiosyncratic beliefs on the patient's part. It is a culturally based belief and less likely to be dislodged.
>
> At least Ms X's request for a modified radical mastectomy is aligned with the standard of care. It is much harder to convince some women who decline any surgery or chemotherapy and prefer "alternative medicine." If Dr Y cannot

persuade Ms X to change her mind, it would not be inappropriate to go along with her request for more surgery.

In this case more surgery may not be better than less surgery, but it is better than none at all[9].

The meaning of autonomy

The word "autonomy" is derived from the Greek *autonomia* or *autonomos*, meaning "having its own laws," which is in turn derived from *autos* ("self") and *nomos* ("rule" or "law")[10]. *Autonomous* patients are those capable of exercising deliberate and meaningful choices, choices consistent with their own values—making their own laws. They are persons with the cognitive and emotional "competence" or "capacity" to make decisions for themselves. (As Kant wrote, "Autonomy is therefore the ground of the dignity of human nature and of every rational nature"[11].)

Heteronomous persons, by contrast, are those who cannot, or will not, make decisions for themselves. Literally, they are subject to the laws of others. Heteronomy may occur on account of familial, cultural, or social factors that encourage an inordinate (or appropriate or acceptable) dependence on others. Persons may exhibit "decidophobia," an inability to compare alternatives and make decisions "with one's eyes open"[12]. It may also result from a deficiency of mental capacities, as in a newborn or in a comatose or a severely demented patient, or from a seeming lack of will, as in depressive or compulsive disorders. It may also relate to aptitude and interest and can fluctuate with time or conditions.

The concept of a binary choice between autonomy and heteronomy is not quite right, however. They each exist on a spectrum. The proper exercise of autonomy requires the right social conditions. Autonomy does not exist on its own or imply one must make all decisions by oneself. "[T]he obligation to make all one's own decisions . . . states an unattainable and unwise standard," warns Schneider in his book on autonomy[13]. An autonomous individual—capable, rational, well-informed—can relinquish or "waive" the right to make their own decisions in favour of a spouse, family unit, community, or the like. Alternatively, they can share the decision with, or relinquish it to, a healthcare professional, family members, or indeed, a whole community (be it secular, political, or religious)[14]. Sharing our concerns and decisions with those to whom we are the closest can help us consider alternatives in a more well-rounded way and strengthen us as integral, rooted persons. This does not have to diminish our autonomy[15].

Autonomy simply means being "authentic," being true to one's self. How one experiences and achieves this has much to do with one's family, the local culture, and mores. But there is a deep well of thought here.

> ## Box 4.2
>
> "Autonomy is essentially a matter of whether we are active rather than passive in our motives and choices—whether, however we acquire them, they are the motives and choices that we really want and are therefore in no way alien to us." [15]

The seventeenth-century French philosopher and mathematician René Descartes argued that the only statement of which one can be absolutely certain is *cogito ergo sum* ("*I think, therefore I am*"); it was a remarkably novel and radical departure from the punishing conformist attitude of the time and captures the Enlightenment sentiment in favour of self-determination. Just think how radical Descartes' dangerous idea was and still is: only the individual can (and must) decide what is right and true; everything else—family, society, religion, God—is uncertain [16].

Once the self is recognized as the fount of decision-making and the locus of certitude, other ideas naturally flow—ideas about independence of thought and action, idiosyncrasy of interpretation, the right to be "wrong" and not be sanctioned for this, and so on. This right to make choices, whether right or wrong, is a carefully guarded right and yet denied to millions throughout the world. Ensuring its availability to all is a long work in progress.

II. Autonomy as the Patient's Preference

Making the patient's own priorities and aspirations the focal point of medical care means that healthcare practitioners ought not, in general, substitute their wishes and preferences for those of patients, even if what the physician wants seems more likely to promote the patient's best interests. A successful medical encounter, however, incorporates the perspectives of patient *and* physician.

Case 4.2   A Man Who Would Live on Eggs Alone

Mr S had lived on the same street in Parkdale in Toronto for as long as anyone could remember—decades, anyway. He had survived the Nazi occupation of Poland, as had many of his neighbours on the street. But by now he had outlived them all. Mr S was a widower, had no children, and, as far as anyone on the street could tell, had no visitors either. He was fiercely independent, turning down any offers of help from his neighbours, most of whom had moved in during the past several years. That harsh winter, Mr S could be seen now and again shovelling the snow from his walk, his back bent and crooked. Then, his neighbour, Ms T, noticed snow piling up on his walk. Worried about Mr S, she knocked on his front door. Finding it unlocked, she hesitantly stepped into his house, afraid of what she might find.

What Ms T found there shocked her. Mr S was lying in a cot off his kitchen, barely able to stand. He looked terrible—pale and dishevelled, wraith-like, a ghost of his usual self. Declining her offer to help him in any way, he insisted he just needed a few days' rest. He assured Ms T he was fine: "I'm eating raw eggs every day."

This information increased her concern. She offered to take him to the emergency room at a nearby hospital, "just to get you checked out."

Mr S stood firm in his refusal of help: "No hospitals!"

Ms T sought help from a general practitioner, Dr P, who had recently moved in across the street.

Is there an ethical dilemma here?
What could Dr P do?

Discussion of Case 4.2

There is an obvious conflict in this case between Mr S's wishes and what might be called his best interests. He thinks he is fine. His neighbour is not so sure. Respecting his right to choose does not necessarily mean respecting his expressed wishes, however. Does Dr P have a duty to try to help Mr S?

Ms T has no duty of care for Mr S, but she is concerned about him as a human being who is alone and in distress. Because Dr P has not previously seen Mr S as a patient, he, too, has no duty of care for him. Nonetheless, while he may not have a *legal duty* to care for Mr S, there is a strong and simple *moral reason* to intervene once he has been informed of his plight: Mr S may die if nothing is done. In any case, Dr P would hardly have to go out of his way to offer assistance.

But what if Mr S rejects help from Dr P? Would it suffice for Dr P to do nothing, on the assumption Mr S is an independent, autonomous adult with the right to refuse medical care? From a professional perspective, such a response from Dr P would not do. Dr P could assess Mr S's mental capacity to refuse care. If Mr S's choice is not informed or freely made, Dr P would have good grounds for involving emergency services.

Not every critical situation allows a healthcare professional to refuse a patient's wishes and preferences, however. What are the circumstances that justify not intervening in a medical emergency? The courts have examined this question and the following is one such case.

III. The Case of Ms Malette and Dr Shulman

In 1979 Ms Malette, a 57-year-old woman, was brought, comatose, to the ER of a hospital in a small town in Ontario. She had been critically injured in a severe motor vehicle accident, which had killed her husband. Dr Shulman, the emergency room physician, believed a blood transfusion was required to save her life. However, Ms Malette had a card in her wallet stating she was a Jehovah's Witness and would never want to receive blood products. Although the card bore her signature, it was neither dated nor witnessed. Feeling there was sufficient uncertainty with regard to her true wishes, Dr Shulman proceeded to give her a blood transfusion.

A 1987 court found that the transfusion had been given against Ms Malette's known wishes, despite it having saved her life [17]. Found guilty of battery, Dr Shulman was ordered to pay $20,000 in monetary damages, obviously not a large sum but significant at the time to serve as a caution to doctors.

A higher Ontario Court of Appeal would later uphold this judgment placing the principle of autonomy above that of beneficence [18]; the ruling has provided direction in cases ever since. Commenting on the refusal of treatment for religious reasons, the judge wrote such an objection does not permit the scrutiny of "reasonableness" which is "a transitory standard dependent on the norms of the day." Moreover, if the patient's refusal has its basis in religion, it is "more apt to crystallize in life-threatening situations" [18].

The crucial finding of this judgment was that Dr Shulman's care was substandard because it ignored the prior expressed wishes of Ms Malette. This judicial ruling—a clear endorsement of the primacy of patient autonomy—had a significant impact not just within Ontario, but also across Canada and indeed throughout the world.

Box 4.3

"A doctor is not free to disregard a patient's advance instructions any more than he would be free to disregard instructions given at the time of the emergency."

Malette v Shulman, 1990 [18]

While medicine's central goals are to ameliorate suffering and prevent premature death (the beneficence principle), in general, these cannot be achieved at the expense of the patient's expressed wishes (the autonomy principle).

Box 4.4

"If [the doctor] knows that the patient has refused to consent to the proposed procedure, he is not empowered to overrule the patient's decision for her even though he, and most others, may think hers a foolish or unreasonable decision."

Malette v Shulman, 1990 [18]

This legal judgment makes the issue seem black and white. In hindsight, it seems unfair to assume Dr Shulman disagreed with the legal principle that competent patients have a right to refuse life-saving care. There was no evidence, for example, that he gave Ms Malette blood on the grounds of his own moral beliefs. Rather, he did so as he seemed genuinely uncertain as to her deepest beliefs.

The bottom line of *Malette v Shulman* is that clinicians in Canada who fail to respect evidence of a patient's wishes do so at their professional peril. When that evidence is unclear, however, many healthcare professionals prefer to err on the side of preserving life, and so risk sanctions for providing non-consented treatment, rather than to allow an incapable patient to die.

Malette v Shulman affirmed

In another Ontario case, concerned with refusal of antipsychotic treatment, the court wrote that the best interests standard (the patient's "well-being" from the medical perspective) cannot be used to overrule a psychiatric patient's wish to refuse treatment [19]. Were that allowed, it would violate "the basic tenets of our legal system" and fail to be in accordance with the "principles of fundamental justice." The law across Canada, and in many other jurisdictions as well, is clear: it assumes patient competence unless proven otherwise. Although the patient may now be "mad," bad, or just plain ill, it is the patient's prior expressed capable preferences that ought to guide care.

Box 4.5

"The patient's right to forego treatment, in the absence of some overriding societal interest, is paramount to the doctor's obligation to provide medical care. This right must be honoured, even though the treatment may be beneficial or necessary to preserve the patient's life or health, and regardless of how ill-advised the patient's decision may appear to others."

Fleming v Reid, 1991 [19]

If you believe this to be an outdated issue, a case reported in the *New England Journal of Medicine* in November 2017 indicates this is still very *au courant* [20]. An unaccompanied 70-year-old man with no identification arrived at an emergency room in Florida, unconscious. On his chest was a tattoo declining cardiac resuscitation. Efforts to treat possible causes of his decreased level of consciousness were unsuccessful. Unable to discuss goals of care with him and unsure whether the tattoo represented a genuine advance directive, staff decided to ignore its instruction but then asked for an ethics consultation. The consultant recommended that further resuscitation be discontinued despite the uncertainty. The tattoo, it seemed, was a pretty clear (and indelible) way of making one's wishes known. (See Case 1 at the end of this chapter for a similar case.)

The ready acceptance of advance directives in Canada is not mirrored in all jurisdictions, however. In some US states, for example, advance directives refusing life-saving care, such as a blood transfusion, must meet a high level of scrutiny—"clear and convincing evidence" of an "informed refusal"—before they will be followed by physicians [21]. And in some places in the world advance directives are not allowed or only allowed in restricted situations [22]. It cannot be said there is any unanimity on this issue. What follows, therefore, reflects largely North American attitudes towards advance directives.

IV. Choices: The Good, the Bad, and the Ugly

The "good": The right to choose

Patients, by the principle of autonomy, have a right to make choices about the kind of healthcare they receive. Patients can choose to have or forego any medical intervention "within reason." They can choose, for example, what kind of dialysis to go on or opt not to go on it at all. The right to a second opinion is an important corollary, as is the right to information. Patients can ask for almost anything. Whether they will obtain it depends on the urgency of their problem, where they live, the alternatives, and whether they can afford to wait—in short, it depends on availability and the standard of care.

Yet paternalism persists in some areas of medicine—almost unchallenged.

Case 4.3 Ligation Litigation

A 22-year-old unmarried woman, Ms Q, is pregnant for the second time with a Caesarean section already scheduled. Well on in her second trimester, she requests to have her "tubes tied" at the time of the delivery. The obstetrician, Dr R, refuses to do this procedure, citing her young age and unmarried status.

"How do I know you won't change your mind in a few years?" the obstetrician says to her.

What is the ethical dilemma here?

Discussion of Case 4.3

This is an all too common doctor-knows-best scenario [23]—although perhaps less common now than in the past [24]. The conflict is between the nonmaleficence principle and the autonomy principle. Although the obstetrician has his reasons, from the autonomy perspective these may be insufficient to support his refusal to perform a tubal ligation on Ms Q. If she understands and appreciates the proposed procedure, this should suffice. Dr R can provide information and send her away to think about it, but ultimately the choice is hers to make. (Informed choice should be a *process* of communication anyway, not a one-time event.) Patients may regret a procedure they undergo; the best a clinician can do is make a reasonable attempt at explanation and hope the patient comprehends the procedure and its likely outcomes (especially, in this case, the irreversibility of the ligation).

The professional reluctance to grant a competent adult patient's request for surgical sterilization may be a holdover from certain cultural and religious objections to non-therapeutic sterilization and may be hard to eradicate. Another explanation is surgery is different from other types of healthcare [25]. Surgeons need to harm patients in the act of doing surgery to help them achieve their desired outcome. This may be one reason why surgeons tend to still take a paternalistic approach to the patient–physician relationship.

Thus, this is an area where the doctor's peers would probably act similarly. "Any experienced, wise gynecologist," it has been argued, will routinely refuse a tubal ligation for a woman younger than 25 years old [26]. In their view, women have other, very effective, safe, and non-permanent methods of birth control. Requests to have their "irreversible" sterilization reversed are not unusual when some enter a new relationship years later. Physicians following a young person's wishes fear litigation from a "regretted" tubal ligation. While tubal ligation is a litigation-prone procedure, this is usually on account of an unwanted pregnancy from a negligent (such as ineffective) ligation, not because the gynecologist has acquiesced to the request for sterilization from a young woman. Young men would have similar difficulty getting a vasectomy, so the problem is not simply one of sexism and is not discipline specific.

continued

> It is certainly within the standard of practice of doctors to provide only those procedures that are considered appropriate. Surgeons cannot and should not be required to perform a surgical procedure they consider inappropriate or unsafe. Their reasoning should, however, reflect a reasonable professional standard of care rather than their own personal distaste.

Clinicians may find it challenging to decide which requests are legitimate and which are not. Cosmetic surgery for a child with a cleft palate? Yes, obviously, as it is in the child's benefit. Gender confirmation surgery? Yes, as research supports its use in transgender persons as a necessary medical procedure, and it is starting to be covered under provincial medicare plans. Limb removal in a patient with body identity integrity disorder? No, as it seems to be a psychiatric disorder requiring a different sort of intervention.

What is an acceptable medical intervention is not something fixed in cement but depends, in part, on wider social trends. Physicians may feel they are skating on thin ice at times. Sometimes, unavoidably, they are. Times change. The best one can say in such circumstances is to keep up with the times (what is a reasonable change in practice and what is not?) and seek advice from peers.

The "bad": The right to foolish choices

Autonomy and the freedom to exercise choice mean, among other things, the freedom to make "bad choices." By and large, it is up to individuals what harms (and benefits) they are prepared to take on. Citizens in our society have the liberty to engage in risk-prone activities (such as driving fast cars, eating junk food, and smoking)—so long as such activities do not harm others. There is an old adage that your right to swing your fist ends where my nose begins. The moral difficulty for clinicians is in determining how to handle patients' more controversial wishes.

Case 4.4 "Don't Touch My Arm!"

"Whatever you do," the 64-year-old patient, Ms N, warned her anaesthetist, Dr Y, "don't touch my left arm. You'll have nothing but trouble there!" Dr Y accepted this cryptic prohibition without seeking further clarification. Soon after Ms N's elective surgery for a prolapsed bladder began, he lost intravenous access in her right arm. Ignoring the patient's prior stated request, he started a new IV in her left arm. The operation was completed without incident[27].

Unfortunately, the IV in Ms N's left arm went interstitial post-operatively. A toxic fluid leaked into the surrounding arm tissue, resulting in a significant injury to her arm. At trial, no evidence was presented of any medical reason for her left arm not to have been touched. On the other hand, no evidence was offered supporting the necessity of starting an IV in that arm. Ms N successfully sued Dr Y for battery (non-consensual touching) [28].

What is the rationale for this judicial ruling?

Discussion of Case 4.4

This case again highlights the issue of autonomy versus beneficence. Although Dr Y was acting beneficently from his perspective, he did so at the cost of ignoring his patient's stated wishes. That Ms N was alert and there was no question regarding her mental capacity constitutes the distinctive difference of this case from that of Mr S in Case 4.2. Patients have a right to idiosyncratic beliefs. In this case, the arm injury was entirely fortuitous: the patient had no foreknowledge that harm would ensue if the doctor touched her left arm. Nevertheless, her instructions were explicit and were accepted by the anaesthetist. Intraoperatively, he should have sought IV access anywhere else but Ms N's left arm.

The surgeon was found guilty of battery—a charge that protects patients from unwanted physical touching. "Lacking consent, all surgery is battery" [29]. A judge has commented, "This [consent] is not a mere formality; it is an important individual right to have control over one's own body, even when medical treatment is involved. It is the patient, not the doctor, who decides whether surgery will be performed, where it will be done, and by whom it will be done" [30].

As the old saying goes, "The doctor proposes, the patient disposes."

Of course, it would have been quite appropriate to question this patient *before* surgery about her unusual request. Why did she not want her left arm touched? If she persisted in her prohibition and her doctor felt this to be unsafe, he could have declined to act as her anaesthetist (much as a surgeon should refuse to operate if asked to do so with one hand tied behind their back). *If a patient's request is inherently unsafe and abiding by it exposes the physician to negligence or unprofessional conduct, the healthcare professional has no duty to acquiesce.* In fact, they ought not to comply with it. However, waiting until the patient is asleep under anaesthetic is not the best time to question or override a patient's prior stated wish.

The principle of autonomy allows patients to set their own goals and define their own ways of living (and dying). While some will be straightforward, others will seem unusual and perhaps eccentric. Unless seriously deranged, these choices should be explored, not simply dismissed. Seemingly competent and autonomous patients can choose irrationally by

- thinking about the immediate future and ignoring long-term risks,
- believing that nothing bad will happen to them,
- acting on unreasonable fears that make them avoid necessary treatment,
- exhibiting extremely eccentric beliefs, or
- adhering to unusual ways of interpreting information [31].

None of these reasons is sufficient on its own to not honour a patient's wishes. They do suggest something may be amiss with the patient's cognitive state and act as red flags for the prudent clinician to probe those patient beliefs more thoroughly. Seemingly irrational choices made by patients can authentically spring from deeply held convictions, while others are products of their defence mechanisms, such as denial, in the face of difficult life events.

Yet others may spring from a different understanding of science and the world. The idea that we live in a world of "post-truth," that there are "alternative facts," is a popular but mistaken idea [32]. But there are alternative ways of coping with and adapting to the world—and one culture cannot claim to have the only or a privileged access to the "Truth" [33]. Allowance must be made for these alternative perspectives rather than rejecting them out of hand (see Chapter 17). The challenge for healthcare professionals is to recognize when rejections of life-sustaining treatment must be respected and when they ought to be challenged.

The "ugly": self-destructive wishes

Abiding by the autonomy principle can cause some healthcare professionals to feel like handmaidens to less-than-optimal goals of their patients, ones that can border on the self-destructive. This may be something quite different from what they expected when they entered their training program. Is it not their job to save lives rather than imperil or end them?

Case 4.5 Tranquillizer Trap

An 84-year-old woman, Ms K, has a history of coronary disease. She requests her usual prescription of triazolam, a short-acting benzodiazepine she has taken for years for insomnia. Despite repeated efforts on your part to wean her from this drug, Ms K insists on taking it. Her fervent wish is for a good night's sleep. And, oh yes, she has tried "everything" already to help her sleep. "Only *this* little pill works."

Should you prescribe "this little pill" yet again?

Discussion of Case 4.5

Elderly people, in Canada and elsewhere, are notoriously overmedicated[34]. This patient risks falling and confusion secondary to her use of a benzodiazepine, problems not infrequent in her age group[35]. Many long-time users of hypnotics and anxiolytics are not readily weaned from them ("But, doctor, I can't sleep a wink without them."). They can hang on to their drugs as tenaciously as if their lives depended on them ("You'll pry them from my dead hands.")[36].

In this case there is a clash between autonomy, nonmaleficence, and beneficence. You should try to balance the task of getting Ms K to agree to reduce the risks to her well-being (which such patients typically downplay) by coming off such medication against the risk of becoming embroiled in a power struggle and losing her as a patient. If you refuse her request, Ms K could go to another physician. By being the prescribing physician, you can at least continue to monitor her use.

You should try, once more, to remind Ms K of the risks of hypnotics and discuss alternatives with her. In doing so you will satisfy the nonmaleficence and beneficence principles. You will also satisfy the autonomy principle if you take the patient's preferred goals into account.

This could be one more battle you are unlikely to win. If you decide to continue prescribing the medication, you should do so *safely*: prescribe limited quantities each time, have a discussion about associated risks on a regular basis, document these discussions, making it clear that the patient is making an informed choice, and continue efforts to wean her off. Of course, it goes without saying that patients such as Ms K should be carefully and regularly monitored for the development of such adverse effects and a more urgent discussion undertaken if such symptoms do emerge.

Box 4.6

"Ultimately, good medicine is about doing right for the patient. For patients with multiple chronic diseases, severe disability, or limited life expectancy, any accounting of how well we're succeeding in providing care must above all consider patients' preferred outcomes."[37]

Although healthcare practitioners may have ideal guidelines in mind when treating a patient (for example, "a patient should not be on benzodiazepines indefinitely"), such guidelines must take into consideration the patient's goals (for example, the older patient using a sleeping pill may prefer to accept the risks of impaired memory for the benefits of restored sleep).

Reversible factors

The modern allegiance to patient autonomy should not be an excuse for abandoning a patient. It is the clinician's job—their fiduciary responsibility—to explore the choices a patient makes, to invade that person's privacy (with their consent, of course) to make sure the patient is not cast off in their autonomous shell. We've said this before but it bears repeating: you should always consider, but not always abide by, the patient's wishes.

Some patients' wishes seem to defy comprehension. (For example, why would the patient in Case 4.4 not want an IV in her left arm? Well, maybe she'd had a previous bad experience with an intravenous in that arm and some doctor had said, "Don't ever let them start a line in there.") The careful clinician will make sure a patient's decision to forego care, or to embark on a course that will lead to harm or death, is not influenced by modifiable, reversible factors, such as social deprivation, psychiatric illness, isolation, or substance abuse[38].

The tale of Diogenes, an ancient antisocial Greek philosopher, living in less than pristine conditions in a barrel, is instructive here. "Diogenes syndrome" has come to refer to those usually solitary, typically elderly, individuals who fail at self-care and live in squalor and neglect[39]. Many suffer from a mental disorder. There is sometimes a reluctance to intervene because of a misguided respect for autonomy. On the other hand, some people can simply have different preferences. It has been said that when Alexander the Great asked if he could help, Diogenes replied, "Yes. You could move aside; you're blocking the sunlight"[40].

It should be noted that many patients (and not just the elderly) with mental disorders are sometimes undertreated for their physical maladies[41]. This may reflect the stigma attached to mental illness. Allowing mentally disordered patients the "right" to their self-neglecting actions may say more about our negative attitudes towards them and the limits of caring in our society than it does about any support for patient autonomy.

Why would a patient refuse appropriate, basic nursing care? The following is one such case.

Case 4.6   This Lady's Not for Turning

Ms W is a 56-year-old woman with a long history of disabling and destructive rheumatoid arthritis, causing her hands and feet to be cruelly contracted.

Despite numerous surgeries she is unable to bear weight; even sitting is painful. She is admitted to hospital for yet another attempt at corrective surgery. Unfortunately, she develops C. difficile colitis and, later on, large sacral pressure sores. Now Ms W is refusing to be turned in her bed. The patient has no significant family members to be called upon. After several weeks of intense but fruitless negotiation, the hospital ethicist is asked by the treating team to see her.

The team asks the ethicist, "Could Ms W be turned despite her wishes not to be?"

Discussion of Case 4.6

Ms W is alert but sad. Confined to bed for almost a year, she had managed with live-in help at home. She hates her life: restricted, inactive, and isolated. Asked why she is refusing treatment for her pressure ulcers, she complains about the care on the ward. At first the staff hardly turned her at all.

"Now that my condition is so bad," she whispers, "they blame me for the problem!" Some turn her more roughly, without attending to her pain. She acknowledges her situation is far from ideal.

With this the ethicist has to agree: Ms W has large necrotic pressure ulcers on her sacrum and buttocks. Moreover, the odour from them is noticeable as soon as one arrives on the ward and is almost unbearable. *Horribile dictu*, the ethicist also notices small black flies flitting about the patient.

The ethical dilemma in this case seems to pit nonmaleficence and autonomy against beneficence and justice. Could it ever be acceptable for a patient to refuse basic nursing care, such as sacral ulcer care? Providing care would cause her agony and would run contrary to the patient's autonomy, but not doing so would certainly cause her harm as well.

There is also the issue as to whether her refusal of care has an unfair impact on staff and other patients (and so is unjust to them). Her refusal of care is draining for the whole ward. She is literally rotting in her bed "with her rights on."

As far as context goes, there is no precedent in the hospital for such a refusal. No policies seem applicable, but failing to accept basic nursing care seems a grave offence to the nursing staff especially.

This case, the ethicist writes in the patient's chart, has gone on far too long: other patients are disgusted by the odour, staff are alienated from the patient, nurses and trainees fail to turn up when expected, and even the attending surgeon has not been around for days. A difficult situation has

continued

literally festered. Discussion with staff allowed them to examine their own attitudes to a "hateful patient" [42]. The team was encouraged to explore how Ms W might be treated more humanely, for example, by treatment under anaesthesia. Psychiatry, Advanced Nursing Care, [43] and Palliative Care were also consulted for other appropriate options.

Ms W's right to refuse was limited, as it threatened to undermine the welfare of other patients. However, exploration with the patient revealed her main goal for treatment was to be pain free. Ms W experienced her care as torture. She was not really refusing care, only excessively painful care. As even the lightest touch provoked a pain response from her, the resolution of the issue required some concerted efforts and imagination in order to treat her humanely. At the end of the day, this case wasn't really about the right to say no but rather about the limits of beneficence and how distant the team was from understanding the patient's experience of her illness. But the flies definitely had to go. It was simply undignified [44].

Autonomy has its limits [45]. There is only so far a patient in an institution, where the welfare of other patients is at stake, can refuse care.

Box 4.7

Limits to autonomy include

- requests for illegal or unprofessional care (see Chapter 10),
- patient incapacity (see Chapter 8),
- limited resources (see Chapter 13),
- limited knowledge and expertise (see Chapter 9), and
- social welfare/public health interests: control of contagious disease, violent persons, terrorism, and the protection of the public generally (see Chapter 7).

Conclusion

When a patient and a doctor clash, whose view should prevail? The answer is often neither view on its own. Instead, the participants ought to try principled negotiation; common ground should be sought through mutual understanding and respect.

> ### Box 4.8
>
> "I don't know is not a shameful admission; add but I'll work on it, and it can signal the beginning of a meaningful engagement. Our patients say this is what they hanker for." [46]

By examining one's own feelings and the patient's feelings, expectations, worries, and altered functioning in the world as a result of illness, the self-reflective clinician will be better able to devise a treatment plan that combines the patient's goals with the physician's obligations. This finding of a common ground by dialogue avoids unnecessary power struggles and simplistic kowtowing to the patient's expectations [47]. In the face of uncertainty, shared decision-making is the right way to go [46].

Cases for Discussion

Case 1: The Significance of an Order [48]

Ms C is a 42-year-old woman diagnosed with breast cancer in 2008. Found to have bony metastases four years later, she undergoes hormonal treatment in conjunction with chemotherapy and radiotherapy. Two years after this she is admitted to hospital with esophageal stricture, dehydration, dysphagia, and poorly controlled pain.

A do-not-resuscitate order had previously been entered on her medical record.

In the emergency department, Ms C receives small doses of morphine intravenously. Upon transfer to the ward, the patient is inadvertently given hydromorphone instead of morphine. (Hydromorphone is six to seven times as potent as morphine.) Shortly thereafter she is found not breathing.

Questions for Discussion

1. Should Ms C's previous wish not to be resuscitated be followed? Why? Why not?
2. Does such an order preclude the use of naloxone that may reverse narcotic overdose?
3. Does the fact that an error may have been the cause of her decline make a difference?

Case 2: A Hypnotic Request

Ms K, the 84-year-old patient encountered in Case 4.5, refuses alternative means of sedation. The following year she suffers a myocardial infarction for which she is hospitalized for three weeks. Her illness is complicated by congestive heart failure and arrhythmias. Upon discharge she once again requests triazolam.

Examination reveals an elderly woman in no acute distress but with subtle changes in her mental processes; Ms K seems more confused than before her myocardial infarction. You discover she has been using higher daily doses of triazolam to cope with feelings of anxiety and panic over her diminished stamina. Worried that her overuse of this drug might be contributing to her mental state, you decide to involve a community Geriatric Psychiatry team to help her cope better with her losses and end her dependence on the drug. Ms K refuses to see them. She's seen psychiatrists before and knows they will want to stop her triazolam.

Questions for Discussion

1. What are the ethical issues here?
2. How would this situation be best managed?

Reasonable Persons

The Legal Roots of Informed Consent

Every human being of adult years and sound mind has a right to determine what shall be done with his own body; and a surgeon who performs an operation without his patient's consent commits an assault for which he is liable in damages. This is true except in cases of emergency where the patient is unconscious and where it is necessary to operate before consent can be obtained.

Benjamin Cardozo, 1914[1]

While the basic rationale for medical consent is ethical at its core, born of a respect for individual autonomy, in modern medical practice consent is inextricably bound up with legal precedents and justifications[2]. In this and the next chapter, we will examine the notion of informed consent both from legal and ethical points of view. In this chapter, we will review the types of consent in medical practice and the legal history which has shaped this concept over the past 100 years. In the next chapter, practical aspects and challenges of "informed consent" in medical practice will be discussed.

I. Medical Consent

Most discussion involving consent in medicine revolves around the concept of "informed consent." This is quite appropriate, since "informed consent" represents one of the main pillars of modern medical practice. Many working in healthcare, however, may be surprised to learn that much of the consent obtained in medicine is invisible and not of the "informed" variety. This common form of consent reflects the natural requirement to obtain permission from patients when interacting with them in a medical context and occurs every time a healthcare provider takes a history, performs an examination, or orders a test. It is best referred to as simple consent.

Case 5.1 A Simple Question

A clinical clerk who has been reading about informed consent in preparation for her Surgery rotation asks a disarmingly simple question: "I know we need to get informed consent from patients if we operate on them, but how come we don't get consent when we examine them in the ER or take their blood or take an X-ray?"

Is the student correct?
Should consent be obtained from patients for routine matters of healthcare?

Simple consent: implied and express

Two types of simple consent typically take place in medicine: implied and express consent. The latter can be either oral or written.

Implied consent takes place when a patient's action or behaviour *implies* they voluntarily agree to what a healthcare provider is doing. When patients make appointments with physicians or come to the emergency room, they are tacitly consenting to providing medical information and undergoing an appropriate physical exam. When the venipuncture technician approaches and a patient rolls up their sleeve, they are implicitly consenting to having blood taken. In many medical interactions, implied consent is ethically and legally sufficient. It is appropriate in circumstances when there is no significant risk or likelihood of discomfort to a patient.

If there is uncertainty around whether implied consent is sufficient, or if the intrusion on a patient is somewhat more significant (for example, examination of intimate areas, such as genitalia, breasts, or anus) or carries some risks (even minor procedures, such as suturing a wound or treating skin lesions with liquid nitrogen), then express consent should be sought. Express consent may also be requested when the information being sought is a bit more sensitive or personal or may not appear immediately relevant to a patient (such as, "Sometimes problems like this have to deal with sexual activity. Do you mind if I ask you a few questions around that?").

Most physicians detect instinctively when express consent is required and seek clear verbal permission to proceed. Like implied consent, express consent is frequently not recognized as such and may be sought several times in the course of a physician–patient interaction ("I really should have a look at that area in your groin that you mentioned, all right?"). Express consent occurs when the patient nods their head in agreement or says, "Sure, go ahead."

In everyday medical practice, the line between implied and express consent may sometimes be blurry. A healthcare practitioner may believe that a patient tacitly consented, when they did not (such as, "It was OK that Dr X did such and such, but it would have been nice if they had asked permission first.").

Up to this point we have been discussing primarily express *oral* consent. Express *written* consent is useful when there is a perceived need for written confirmation or documentation. It makes it easier to prove consent was provided. It is useful when there is concern a patient may not recall or may dispute that permission was given or if there are appreciable risks associated with a procedure[3]. Sometimes a note in the chart at the time indicating the patient consented is sufficient, while at other times it may be best to have the patient sign a formal consent form, such as when obtaining consent for medical treatments or surgical procedures. Although we have primarily been discussing consent for treatment up to this point, it should be noted that there are numerous other circumstances when express written consent should be obtained, such as when medical records are to be transferred to another physician or when photographs are taken for the purposes of research or teaching (see Chapter 11). On its own, however, a signed form is only as good as the conversation that preceded it.

Discussion of Case 5.1

The student's question, while understandable, actually contains a mistake. Consent does exist in all these circumstances. It is simply frequently not appreciated or perceived as such, because it is implied or casually obtained in a conversational fashion.

Box 5.1

Types of consent in everyday practice:

- Implied consent
- Express consent (oral or written)

II. Informed Consent: A Brief Legal History

Consent is front and centre in most patient–physician interactions and is embedded in an ethical framework recognizing the centrality of patient autonomy in healthcare. While it is important not to confuse our ethical obligations with our legal ones, the jurisprudential history of informed consent is both edifying and important for practising physicians to understand. Physicians should be aware of their legal obligations.

The concept of medical consent for procedures has evolved gradually over the past 100 years in both Canada and the United States. While decisions in Canadian and American jurisprudence do not establish precedence for one another, they do influence each other. It is not uncommon for decisions in one country to refer to decisions in the other. A ruling by a senior court "casts a shadow" on rulings elsewhere. The term "informed consent," for example, was originally coined in an American context in 1957[4, 5]. We will therefore discuss the evolution of consent as it has evolved in the context of both countries.

Schloendorff

One of the first and most influential legal cases involving consent was the American case of *Schloendorff v Society of New York Hospital* in 1914[1]. While being investigated for abdominal pain, Mary Schloendorff was diagnosed with a mass on her uterus. Although she refused the recommended surgery to remove this, she did consent to undergoing an examination under anaesthesia to allow for better characterization of the mass. Despite her clear instructions prior to the procedure, the mass was removed. Post-operatively she developed gangrene of her left arm and required amputation of some fingers. She subsequently filed suit against the surgeons and hospital for having performed surgery against her wishes. The case was decided in her favour and included one of the most well-known articulations of patient autonomy in North American jurisprudence:

> Every human being of adult years and sound mind has a right to determine what shall be done with his own body; and a surgeon who performs an operation without his patient's consent, commits an assault, for which he is liable in damages.
> *Schloendorff v Society of New York Hospital*[1]

The decision in favour of Mary Schloendorff was based not on a finding of medical negligence that resulted in the loss of her fingers, but rather on the lack of consent for the surgeon to remove the tumour in her uterus. It was not negligence, but rather battery. Had she consented to the procedure in the first place, but still lost her fingers, she likely would not have won the case. The case underlined the importance of "consent" in general for medical procedures, but did not say anything about "informing" a patient about hazards of a procedure.

Salgo v Leland Stanford Jr: consent vs informed consent

Informing patients about the risks of a procedure was at the heart of the 1957 American case of *Salgo v Leland Stanford Jr,* when the term "informed consent" was first introduced[5]. Mr Salgo was suffering from weakness and pain in his lower extremities. Believing this to be a result of poor blood supply to his legs, his physicians advised translumbar aortography to demonstrate vascular blockage. Mr Salgo consented to this test, which involved introducing a needle through the lumbar region of the back into the aorta and injecting intravascular dye. A vascular obstruction was indeed confirmed.

However, when Mr Salgo awoke the next day, he found himself paralyzed from the waist down—permanently so—as a result of the procedure. He sued, arguing he had not been adequately informed of the perils of the procedure, specifically that there was a risk of paralysis. His physician (one of the defendants) argued Mr Salgo would probably have declined the procedure, had he been informed of the small risk of permanent neurologic damage. In contrast to *Schloendorff,* the court did not question whether "consent" had been obtained, but rather whether the consent was adequately informed. The court found in favour of Mr Salgo— again not because of any negligence in the execution of the procedure, but rather because the patient had not been adequately informed of the associated risks.

Box 5.2

"A physician violates his duty to his patient and subjects himself to liability if he withholds any facts which are necessary to form the basis of an intelligent consent by the patient to the proposed treatment."

Salgo v Leland Stanford Jr, 1957 [5]

The *Salgo* case was not so much concerned with whether Mr Salgo had consented to the procedure, but rather whether he had been adequately informed in order to "intelligently" consent [6]. While this case established a duty on the part of a physician to inform a patient about relevant facts of a procedure, it did not clarify specifically *what* needed to be disclosed. In *Salgo,* the standard for disclosure took the perspective of the physician, emphasizing what a *reasonable physician* would deem appropriate to impart (the so-called "objective" standard for disclosure).

This view was gradually challenged by a number of cases over the subsequent 15 years. Especially noteworthy was the US case of *Canterbury v Spence* in 1972 [7,8]. *Canterbury* involved a complicated and protracted 12-year litigation dealing with partial paralysis following surgery on a ruptured disc. Dr Spence contended that Mr Canterbury would have declined the much-needed surgery had he been informed of the small risk of paralysis. Therefore, he had not disclosed the risk. The court rejected this paternalistic approach, arguing that a physician has an obligation to disclose the material risks of a procedure to a patient—that is, risks *a reasonable person* would want to know in order to decide on surgery.

Box 5.3

"[A] risk is thus material when a reasonable person in what the physician knows or should know to be the patient's position, would be likely to attach significance to the risk or cluster of risks in deciding whether or not to forego the proposed therapy."

Canterbury v Spence, 1972[8]

The net result of *Canterbury* was a change in the standard for disclosure from a *physician-based* to a *patient-based* standard. Disclosure was no longer dependent on what a competent physician would normally disclose, but rather what a competent patient needed to know to make a rational decision[8].

Box 5.4

Three key US legal cases on consent:
1. *Schloendorff v New York Society* (1914)
   • Consent to perform procedures is necessary
2. *Salgo v Stanford Leland* (1957)
   • Informed consent is physician based
3. *Canterbury v Spence* (1972)
   • Informed consent is patient based

III. Informed Consent: The Canadian Context

The notion of informed consent underwent further refinement in two closely watched and now widely cited Canadian cases, *Hopp v Lepp* (1980)[4] and *Reibl v Hughes* (1980)[9].

Case 5.2 New Grads and Small Centres

Dr N is a newly graduated general surgeon doing a locum at a regional hospital. On his first day on call, he assesses Mrs S, a 57-year-old married woman with two adult children, who has a high-grade bowel obstruction. She has received several doses of IV morphine for pain. After thorough assessment and investigations, Dr N advises emergency surgery to prevent a bowel perforation. He explains to Mrs S and her family in detail the nature of the surgery, risks and benefits, alternatives and possible consequences of not doing surgery.

Clearly in distress, Mrs S signs the consent form, pleading, "Please, just fix this problem!" Her family are struck by how awfully young Dr N looks. "How many of these procedures has he done?" they wonder aloud. Maybe they should take Mrs S to somebody more experienced at a larger centre for surgery?

What should Dr N tell the family with respect to his experience?
Is Dr N legally at risk if something goes wrong with Mrs S at the smaller centre?
Given that Mrs S has had several doses of morphine, is her consent legitimate?

Hopp v Lepp

Dr Lepp, a newly minted orthopaedic surgeon in Lethbridge, Alberta, carried out a hemilaminectomy on the 66-year-old Mr Hopp for persistent back pain in the lumbar region[4]. Prior to the surgery, the patient had inquired whether he would be better off going to a larger centre with more resources. Dr Lepp indicated that the surgery could be done just as well in his centre, that it was a "simple" operation, and that Mr Hopp "would be up and about in six to ten days." He did not inform the patient this was his first such procedure since obtaining a specialist licence.

Appropriate investigations carried out beforehand had demonstrated a lesion between the third and fourth lumbar vertebrae. Although surgery was uneventful, post-operatively, Mr Hopp's pain did not improve and so he was subsequently referred to Calgary. After more investigations, further nerve blockage at his third and fourth vertebrae was identified. Mr Hopp subsequently underwent a more extensive decompressive laminectomy in Calgary. This unfortunately resulted in damage to some nerve roots, leaving him with a permanent disability. The court did not find any negligence on the part of Dr Lepp either in the way he carried out the procedure or in his referral of the patient to another physician in a larger centre. It did find that he misled Mr Hopp as to the gravity of the initial procedure and had not adequately informed him of the risks of the initial operation. This case addressed, in large part, the scope of disclosure a physician must make.

Box 5.5

When obtaining informed consent, "a surgeon, generally, should answer any specific questions posed by the patient as to the risks involved and should, without being questioned, disclose to them the nature of the proposed operation, its gravity, any material risks and any special or unusual risks attendant upon the performance of the operation. However, . . . the scope of the duty of disclosure and whether or not it has been breached are matters which must be decided in relation to the circumstances of each particular case."[4]

There were two important outcomes from *Hopp v Lepp*. First, both the original decision and the subsequent Supreme Court of Canada ruling agreed Dr Lepp was under no obligation to notify his patient that this was his first operation since obtaining his specialist licence. It was felt he was duly qualified to perform the surgery, having performed many such operations with minimal supervision during his residency. Second, both judgments also concurred there was no duty on the part of Dr Lepp to inform Mr Hopp there might be complications which would necessitate transfer to a larger centre. The court agreed that such a procedure could be performed just as well in Lethbridge as in Calgary. While there was a possibility of an outcome which could require transfer to a larger centre, it was considered merely a possibility, not a probability.

Box 5.6

"It would be ridiculous to require a licensed specialist to tell a patient (at least without being asked) how many operations of the kind in question he had performed when it was clear that he was not inexperienced."

Hopp v Lepp, 1980[4]

Discussion of Case 5.2

As in *Hopp v Lepp*, Dr N is under no legal obligation to spontaneously disclose how many laparotomies for bowel obstruction he has performed. However, he is under an ethical obligation to respond to their query about his experience. This not uncommon occurrence for young MDs is something they should learn to address openly and respectfully.

Dr N should explain clearly that he is a newly graduated general surgeon who has performed many such operations during his training. Assuming he feels confident and capable of performing this surgery in the regional hospital, he should reassure the family that he believes there is no compelling reason to send Mrs S to a larger centre. He can explain that transferring the patient will necessitate a significant delay in surgery along with all the inconvenience of having to commute to or find accommodations in the larger city. Finally, to further reassure the patient and family, he can suggest he'll ask one of his senior colleagues to either be available or in attendance to assist with the surgery. In most such cases, a respectful and honest discussion with the family will earn their trust and reassure them.

The question regarding whether the patient, having received morphine, has given valid consent will be discussed in greater detail in the next chapter. The short answer is that opiate analgesics generally do not vitiate informed consent, certainly no more than many other factors affecting patient judgment.

Case 5.3 How Not to Get Informed Consent

....

You are a first-year resident in your first week of a General Surgery rotation in July, assessing Mr M, a 50-year-old refugee from Sudan with acute cholecystitis. He is a manual labourer, speaks little English, and clearly has a limited understanding of what is going on. After discussing the case with the attending surgeon, you are instructed to admit Mr M and obtain consent from him for laparoscopic cholecystectomy to be done first thing next morning.

    Despite explaining to the attending surgeon that you are new to Surgery and have not had any experience with obtaining consent for surgery, you are told to nonetheless get consent. "Just tell him he needs his gallbladder out and that the risks of the laparoscopic surgery are 1% risk of bleeding and infection and a 0.1% risk of a common bile duct injury. You can do that, can't you? I'm caught up in the OR. Reassure him it's a safe operation and he should be back to work in two to four weeks." She sounds a little exasperated.

What should you do in this situation?

Reibl v Hughes (1980)

The 1980 case of John Reibl is the most influential and well-known case involving informed consent in Canada. At the time, Mr Reibl was a 44-year-old employee at the Ford Motor Company. Having worked there for over eight years, he was within 18 months of earning a full pension. During the course of investigation for headaches, he was referred to a neurosurgeon, Dr Hughes, who diagnosed an 85% stenosis in the left carotid artery. Although the carotid stenosis was not the source of his headaches, Mr Reibl was advised by Dr Hughes to have surgery to "remove" the narrowing, as this posed a risk for stroke. The patient was led to believe the risk was significant if he did not have the surgery. The procedure, a "carotid endarterectomy," carried a well-documented incidence of perioperative stroke (4–14 per cent) and death (2–4 per cent)[9]. He appeared to have been told only in vague terms about the procedure and the associated risks. Dr Hughes did not inform Mr Reibl about the risk of a perioperative stroke and what that could mean.

    After signing the consent, Mr Reibl underwent surgery a few days later. Either during or shortly after the surgery, he suffered a debilitating stroke, which left him paralyzed on his right side. He subsequently sued Dr Hughes, averring that had he understood the risks of the procedure, he would not have agreed to the surgery—especially as he was eligible for a full pension in 18 months. A lower court found in his favour, concluding that a reasonable person—informed of those risks for a procedure not urgently needed, and within 18 months of a full pension—would have waited. The court awarded Mr Reibl $225,000 (about $750,000 in 2018 dollars).

This judgment was upheld in a subsequent appeal to the Supreme Court of Canada. The decision involved an extended examination of the concept of disclosure in the context of consent for medical treatment. Specific issues addressed were the duty to disclose and the scope of disclosure required for an individual patient to make an adequately informed decision about their care.

Drawing on reasoning from its recent decision in *Hopp*, the SCC sided with Mr Reibl in agreeing with the lower court that a reasonable person in his circumstances, had he been adequately informed, would most likely have declined the surgery proposed by Dr Hughes at that time. This was the first time the "reasonable person" standard was applied to consent in a Canadian context.

Box 5.7

"In my opinion, a reasonable person in the plaintiff's position would, on a balance of probabilities, have opted against the surgery rather than undergoing it at the particular time."

Reibl v Hughes, 1980[9]

Discussion of Case 5.3

Quoting numbers at a patient is not, of course, sufficient or appropriate when obtaining informed consent. Informed consent is a process, a discussion, and an exchange of information between the patient and physician. It is also not purely about "consent." It is about "choice." Many who write on the topic prefer to call it "informed choice." Regardless of terminology, the process requires both the physician and the patient to be "informed."

A first-year resident, new to a service, who has never obtained consent for surgery, is clearly not "informed" and so should not obtain consent from this patient. While it may be common practice for very junior residents in teaching institutions to obtain consent for procedures of which they have little or no knowledge, when seen from the perspective of the patient, this is simply not ethical. Regardless of whether it would hold up in a court of law, the patient deserves an *informed* physician to explain the nature of the procedure, the alternatives, prognosis, and risks—as well as to respond to questions and concerns.

The delegation of part or all of the informed consent process to resident trainees, physician assistants, and other healthcare workers has recently come under closer scrutiny. In a 2017 case, the Pennsylvania Supreme Court narrowly ruled that the physician who performs an operation has the primary duty to obtain consent for the operation [10]. Based on a narrow interpretation of state law, the ruling undermines the common practice of delegating the responsibility to obtain informed consent to other members of the healthcare team [11]. If such an interpretation of physician responsibility becomes widespread, it may have a significant impact on how future physicians practise and the way in which residents learn the skills of informed consent. While unlikely to have much influence in Canada, this ruling does raise important ethical questions as to the delegation of responsibility in medical care, in particular when it comes to obtaining informed consent.

There are a few ways you can negotiate this situation. First, there may be a senior resident around who can help with the consent. Or you can simply be honest and upfront with the surgeon and explain you feel you cannot do justice to the consent process, but would be very keen to observe and learn how she would obtain it.

Most surgeons will understand your hesitation and ultimately welcome the opportunity to teach house staff about the consent process. Such an approach demonstrates not only your commitment to patient care, but also an awareness of your limitations and abilities as a learner, which will serve you well in the long term.

Box 5.8

"Achieving high-quality informed consent is complex." [11]

IV. Significance of *Reibl v Hughes*: The Modified Objective Standard

The phrase "a reasonable person in the plaintiff's position" is referred to as the "modified objective test" in Canadian jurisprudence. It is a nuanced phrase containing a great deal of meaning. The "reasonable person" represents the "objective" component of the test and helps shield physicians from purely subjective claims of negligence or battery on the part of patients. It prevents patients with unwanted or poor outcomes from saying in hindsight they would not have proceeded with the treatment. It also protects physicians from patients who may have "idiosyncratic and unreasonable or irrational" expectations no physician could fulfill [12].

The expression "in the plaintiff's position" is the "modified" side of the test. It provides a degree of protection for patients by ensuring there is consideration of their individual situation. It recognizes that not all patient circumstances are identical and that consent depends, in part, on the unique context of a given patient. Mr Reibl's unique circumstance was that he was within 18 months of obtaining a full pension. The court agreed with him that a reasonable person in his position (that is, soon to obtain a full pension) would have, on the balance of probabilities, declined the surgery, at least up until he had received the pension.

This recognition of a plaintiff's unique circumstances can have a dramatic impact on the outcome of a case. A patient making her living playing piano, for example, would have good reason to be particularly averse to any procedure potentially compromising the dexterity of her fifth finger. Together the phrases "a reasonable person" and "in the plaintiff's position" balance the interests of both patients and physicians by acknowledging the unique circumstances of patients, while safeguarding physicians from excessively subjective claims.

Finally, there is one important distinction at play here. The law differentiates the scope of disclosure from the causation associated with that disclosure. For a physician, the scope of disclosure is what a reasonable person in the patient's situation would want to know in order to make a decision about treatment. The modified objective test is a test of causation—that is, whether the patient would have made the same decision had they been adequately informed about the treatment. This is illustrated in the following example.

Case 5.4 "You'll Be Back to Work in No Time!"

Dr X, a surgeon, diagnoses Mr Y with acute appendicitis and advises an appendectomy. Although he explains the nature of the surgery, he glosses over the risks by saying that it is a very common procedure that should allow him to be home in a day or so and back to work in a week.

At the time of surgery, Dr X finds a badly perforated appendix. He removes it and treats the patient appropriately with antibiotics post-operatively. Unfortunately, Mr Y develops an extensive subcutaneous necrotizing infection of his abdominal wall that subsequently requires multiple procedures, debridement, and skin grafts. After six weeks in hospital, he finally goes home, unable to resume work for another six months until he has fully recovered.

Mr Y subsequently sues Dr X for failing to adequately inform him of the risks associated with the surgery.

Did Dr X adequately obtain informed consent?
Should Dr X have explained to Mr Y the remote risk of a developing a necrotizing abdominal wall infection?

Discussion of Case 5.4

Dr X did not provide adequate information to Mr Y to obtain informed consent. An appropriate discussion would have included more detail as to the nature and gravity of the surgery, including common or material risks. Dr X should also have mentioned any accepted alternative treatments, as well as the risks of not having surgery. Finally, Mr Y should have had the opportunity to ask questions about the treatment.

The inadequacy of Dr X's disclosure of risks notwithstanding, it is possible the courts would not find in favour of Mr Y. Although Dr X may not have provided sufficient information to obtain informed consent, this fact would not likely be causative for the patient to decline the operation. In other words, the courts would very possibly conclude that a reasonable person in Mr Y's circumstance, even if he had been adequately informed of the risks, would still most likely have opted to proceed with the surgery.

Since necrotizing subcutaneous infections are not typically associated specifically with the type of procedure performed, it is unlikely that courts would expect Dr X to explicitly mention it as a risk associated with appendectomies.

Case 5.4 illustrates how the "reasonable person" standard serves to protect physicians from excessive subjective bias which might accompany patients who have bad outcomes. That said, even if a reasonable person in the circumstance would still have proceeded with a procedure, physicians nonetheless have an ethical obligation to provide a thorough explanation of the procedure, its risks and alternatives. It is a sign of respect for the autonomy of another individual, part of doing right.

Box 5.9

"As a rule of thumb a physician would be well advised to pose and answer the following question: If I were this patient* what would I want to know before deciding whether to agree to the proposed surgery or treatment? If there is any doubt about the answer, disclosure should be made." [13]

* A variant on this is to ask, "If the patient were my best friend . . ."

Case 5.5   What You Don't Know Won't Hurt You

A 55-year-old female patient, Ms G, has a five-month history of a sore shoulder. Her physician, Dr H, has prescribed duloxetine, an antidepressant commonly

continued

used to treat chronic pain as well. Dr H did not inform Ms G this is a psychotropic medication, nor did he warn her about its possible side effects.

Only on discussion with a relative who is a nurse does Ms G realize the
dizziness, upset stomach, and racing heartbeat she has experienced for the
past week could be due to the drug. The physician later explains it is not his
practice to warn people about medications he has frequently used successfully before.

Is Dr H's response acceptable?

Discussion of Case 5.5

Dr H's actions are clearly not acceptable. It can sometimes be difficult to decide
what side effects of medications to discuss with patients, especially if they are
vague and non-specific. Some patients want to be informed about "all possible
side effects"—an impossible task [14]. In such discussions a patient should be informed of common adverse effects, as well as any serious, but less common,
risks. In general, the more serious the possible side effect, the more important
it is for a clinician to disclose such information to a patient.

If in doubt, it is better to err on the side of caution and inform the patient.
Clinicians should also be aware of different ways of communicating the benefits
and harms of drugs. For example, studies have shown using a succinct percentage
format or a simplified "drug facts box" often improved patient understanding and
resulted in better choices [15, 16].

On the subject of psychotropic prescribing, a source of concern is the
widespread use of antipsychotics for behavioural and psychological symptoms of dementia (BSPD). Off-label use of the newer "atypical antipsychotics" is particularly prevalent. While the evidence for the efficacy of these
drugs over others is scant, physicians may turn to them as a last resort
when other ways of ameliorating the patient's symptoms have failed [17].
However, physicians are not always assiduous in obtaining informed consent for their use, despite potential serious adverse effects, such as stroke
or worse. Given the risks associated with these drugs, some have argued
for written consent to be obtained from a substitute decision-maker prior
to their use [18].

Failing to adequately inform patients or their substitute decision-makers
of possible adverse effects of medications might not pose a significant legal
risk to physicians, but can lead to formal complaints and unhappy patients.

Arndt v Smith (1997)

While deference to a patient's unique circumstances provides a degree of protection for patients, it can cut both ways, as was the case in *Arndt v Smith*[12]. In British Columbia in 1986, Ms Arndt was 12 weeks along in a much-wanted pregnancy when she contracted chicken pox. Wary of conventional medicine, she wanted to keep interventions to a minimum. For example, she declined a prenatal ultrasound and planned to have only a midwife help with the delivery. Perinatal infection with chickenpox can be associated with profound cognitive and physical disabilities, known as congenital varicella syndrome. Her family physician, Dr Smith, not wanting to cause excessive worry and alarm, downplayed the risks. She explained the fetus could suffer some abnormalities of the limbs and skin as a result of the infection, but that the risks were relatively remote. Dr Smith reassured Ms Arndt this was not an indication for abortion.

The child was born, however, severely disabled from congenital varicella syndrome. She has spent much of her life in hospital. The parents filed a wrongful life suit against Dr Smith, alleging that had they known about the risks to the fetus from the infection, they would have opted for abortion.

The case eventually went to the Supreme Court of Canada where the decision made rested largely on the reasoning set out in *Reibl*. Here the court decided that a reasonable person in Ms Arndt's circumstances, even if she had been more fully informed by her physician of the risk and significance of congenital varicella syndrome, would most likely not have aborted her fetus.

Conclusion

The evolution of the legal concept of informed consent over the past 100 years mirrors the recognition over the same time period of the increasing importance of patient autonomy in healthcare. It provides an instructive and valuable background when addressing issues of choice and consent with patients.

In the next chapter we shall explore in more depth the concept of informed consent and examine how truthtelling and trust are manifest in the respect for patients.

Cases for Discussion

Case 1: Lost in Translation

Ms W, an elderly Asian woman, has been diagnosed with an early rectal cancer. In the course of preparing her for surgery, Dr R explains the nature of the surgery, the risks, and the possible need for a colostomy. With her oldest

continued

son translating, Ms W happily agrees to the surgery. Afterwards, the medical student Dr R is supervising, who also speaks Cantonese, mentions that the son did not inform Ms W of the possible need for a colostomy. When asked about this, the son explains his mother would likely not agree to the surgery if she knew about the risk of colostomy. He adds that it is customary for him to make these sorts of decisions on his mother's behalf.

"Besides," he says, "it's not certain she'll need a colostomy. No need to worry her unnecessarily, if it's only a possibility."

Questions for Discussion

1. Is it acceptable for family to make decisions on behalf of elderly non-English-speaking family members?
2. What should Dr R do?

Case 2: Taking One for the Family

Mr L is an elderly man treated for acute leukemia. He is quite debilitated from his most recent round of chemotherapy which, unfortunately, appears to have failed. Dr B suggests the next best option is a bone marrow transplant. After Dr B explains in great detail what is involved and the risks associated with this procedure, Mr L sighs loudly and asks where he should sign.

Concerned about his attitude, Dr B inquires more deeply about Mr L's real wishes. "In all honesty, Doc," says Mr L, "I've had a long and happy life. If it was up to me, I'd just opt for some pain medication and let nature run its course. I'm not afraid to die. But my family will never let me do that. They want to keep me alive at all costs."

Questions for Discussion

1. Is Mr L's consent valid under these circumstances?
2. If not, what should Dr B do to ensure genuine consent on Mr L's behalf?

✦ 6 ✦
....

Informed Choice and Truthtelling

The Centrality of Truth and Trust

Words which burnt like surgical spirit on an open wound, but which cleansed, as all truth does.

Lawrence Durrell, 1960 [1]

While the legal and historical aspects of informed consent are both important and instructive, it is imperative not to lose sight of its ethical underpinnings: namely, a deep and abiding respect for the autonomy of individuals. The word "consent" is often interpreted as primarily to do with providing permission to carry out a treatment or procedure. But that is not the full story. Patients may, for very good reasons, decline a recommended treatment: so-called "informed dissent" [2,3]. Thus, there is an increasing trend to use the term "informed choice" [4], a term which also encompasses shared decision-making.

While the legal requirements of informed choice afford important safeguards, both for patients and physicians, they do not satisfy all the ethical requirements. The process of informed choice is a complex phenomenon influenced not just by the type and circumstances of the proposed treatment, but also by patient and physician factors. It demands of physicians that they be honest and truthful with patients, while also respecting their ability to understand and assimilate information. The imbalance of knowledge and power in the physician–patient relationship, as well as the gravity of the matters involved, render patients uniquely vulnerable during this process. Having long recognized these challenges, the courts have imposed a fiduciary duty on physicians [5]. This is reflected in the recognition by physicians and patients of the crucial role of truthtelling and trust in the consent process.

I. Disclosure and Truthtelling

Although doctors and other healthcare professionals acknowledge the importance of telling the truth, medicine has long been known for its parsimonious approach to doing so. After all, to "doctor" something has long meant to disguise, tamper with, or falsify it[6].

Law and social custom used to be quite deferential when it came to the common practice of "doctoring the truth." Until 40 or 50 years ago, even in Western democratic societies with some sort of commitment to "informed consent," deceptive actions by physicians were commonly sanctioned as acceptable practice.

In a 1954 case from Ireland, for example, a gynecologist opted not to inform a patient of a large needle left accidentally in her perineum following an episiotomy because he thought it might cause her "excessive worry." In a show of paternalism and class discrimination typical of that era, the judge justified the deception by noting that the "husband and wife were of a class and standard of education which would incline them to exaggerate the seriousness of the occurrence and to suffer needless harm"[7].

The changing practice of honesty with patients

A landmark study from 1961 revealed the prevailing attitudes at the time. In his survey of 219 physicians in the United States, Oken found that 90 per cent would *not* disclose the diagnosis of cancer to a patient[8]. This study, carried out around the advent of informed consent, reflects an era of medical paternalism, when doctors made decisions for competent patients.

A shift away from this "doctor knows best" attitude was evident less than 20 years later in 1979, when a study of 264 American physicians found that 97 per cent *would* disclose a cancer diagnosis to their patients[9]. There were many reasons for this, including consumerism, the rise of popular movements, and a more optimistic view of cancer treatments, which was encouraged by medical success stories. Other studies, however, suggested a less than complete conversion to medical candour. In another US study, for example, physicians who reported commonly telling cancer patients the truth said they did so in a way intended to preserve hope and "the will to live"[10].

What patients want

The majority of empirical studies have indicated patients do want to know the truth. Studies as far back as 1950, reviewed in Oken's 1961 paper, revealed that 80 to 90 per cent of patients wanted to be told if the examination revealed a diagnosis of cancer. Typical of the studies examined was one conducted in 1957 in which 87 per cent of a group of 560 cancer patients and their families felt a patient should be told the truth[11].

An American survey in 1982 by the President's Commission on Ethical Problems in Medicine revealed that 94 per cent of patients wanted to know "everything" about their condition, 96 per cent wanted to be informed of a diagnosis of cancer, and 85 per cent wanted to be told a realistic estimate of their time to live, even if this was less than one year[12]. In a 2006 study, 89 per cent of patients with cognitive complaints wanted to be told if they suffered from Alzheimer's disease[13], and over 80 per cent of patients with amyotrophic lateral sclerosis wanted as much information as possible[14]. Studies of older patients, sometimes thought to be less interested in the truth, have shown that almost 90 per cent would want to be told a diagnosis of cancer[15].

Case 6.1 A Dark Secret

A 20-year-old female student has recently become a patient in your primary care practice. She has been well, other than undergoing surgery as a young teen for what she was told were "diseased reproductive organs." She knows little else about that surgery.

When her medical records are received, there is a letter from her pediatricians stating that "she" is, in fact, genetically a male with Androgen Insensitivity Syndrome. (In this disorder of gonadal dysgenesis, patients usually have an XY karyotype with inguinal testes and a female phenotype. Due to lack of responsiveness to testosterone in utero, male genitalia do not form. Children are often not diagnosed until puberty, when they fail to menstruate. The testes are removed during adolescence because of an increased risk of testicular cancer.) The patient's family and her physicians had decided not to tell the patient of her "true sex," feeling it would possibly cause great psychological trauma. The letter urges future healthcare providers not to tell her.

What, if anything, should you say to this patient?

"Done for her own good": this was a common paternalistic refrain heard from those who would act in deceptive ways. Patients, especially when ill, were presumed to have difficulty handling the unvarnished truth. It was often the doctor's duty to keep the "whole truth," or even a "partial truth," from them[16]. Some cultures and families believe truthtelling is cruel because it may cause worry in the ailing or frail patient (see Chapter 17). This "protective deception" has strong cultural roots and may have had some credence in times and places where medicine could offer little tangible help to patients. However, even when patients cannot be helped, the truth can be important for them all the same.

The principle of respect for persons—encouraging valid choice, promoting patient empowerment, supporting authentic hope—calls for honest disclosure. Doctors who withhold critical information from patients are denying them the opportunity to live and die as they see fit—a practice that disallows patients an opportunity to cope and hope on their own terms. Hope does not require dishonesty [17]. In a study done before any treatment for multiple sclerosis existed, patients with the disease felt they had a right to know what was wrong with them. Some were angry about being asked why they wished to know. One said, "Do I have to explain why? Just so that I know" [18]. Patients have a right to know the truth about their own health.

Whether patients *do* anything with medical or "personal health information" is a separate issue. A patient's desire to take an active role in making decisions about treatment "may be less strong than [simply] the need for clear and accurate information" [19]. Very ill patients may want someone to look after and guide them, but this does not necessarily mean a preference for ignorance or deception.

Discussion of Case 6.1

Androgen Insensitivity Syndrome is a dark secret for some [20, 21]. In the past, the diagnosis was commonly not disclosed to those with this condition. Those who participated in the original diagnosis of this patient may regret failing to consider when and how her condition should be revealed to her later in life.

Interestingly enough, when this patient was told the truth, her longstanding feelings that she was "different" from other women were confirmed. She was relieved to find a physical basis for her feelings. Indeed, she laughed when told about her condition! So much for the expected devastating effects of telling the truth. She did, however, express anger towards her previous doctors and her parents, who had deceived her for so long.

The importance of truthtelling

It is easy to tell one lie, but hard to tell only one, as Sissela Bok wisely observed in her seminal book, *Lying*. Deceit in medicine is particularly insidious, as it tends to proliferate and undermines trust between the healthcare provider and patient [22]. Lies from a health professional, even if done with the best of intentions, can seem particularly shocking when revealed to the public eye; they undermine public faith in medicine.

There are a great many additional reasons for being truthful with patients: it improves health outcomes, lessens risks to patients, and reduces litigation [22-29]. More importantly, being honest and truthful with patients demonstrates a basic respect for them and fosters the covenant of trust so crucial to the therapeutic relationship [30]. Nowhere is this more important than in the process of helping patients make informed choices about their care. As we will discuss in the next section, truthtelling is critical to the duty of disclosure required for truly informed choice. One cannot imagine modern medicine without the essential components of veracity and honesty.

Box 6.1

....

Some benefits of telling the truth to patients:

- It promotes good outcomes.
- It reduces risks of harm to patients.
- It shows respect for and promotes trust.
- It encourages shared decision-making.
- It reduces litigation.

II. The Elements of Informed Choice

Modern ethics and the courts have repeatedly acknowledged three key requirements of informed choice: adequate and truthful disclosure of information, capacity to understand and make decisions, and voluntariness of choices made [31]. Some authors add fourth and fifth elements, namely, patient comprehension and formal signed authentication [32]. It can be argued that comprehension is subsumed within the disclosure, insofar as provision of information to a patient without regard as to whether it is understood is not truly disclosure. This will be touched on further below. Signing a consent form is primarily a legal consideration and, while important, merely documents the consent process. The actual consent is based on the discussion leading up to formal documentation.

Box 6.2

....

The three elements of informed choice:

1. Disclosure of adequate information
2. Capacity to understand and make decisions
3. Voluntariness of the decision-making process

Case 6.2 "If I Had Only Understood"

....

Mr K is an 80-year-old widower, originally from Peru, now living in a supportive housing facility. After an incidental finding of a left-sided kidney mass, he is referred to a urologic surgeon for removal of the kidney. Dr U explains the

continued

rationale for the procedure and outlines the main risks including pain, bleeding, infection, and the risk of renal insufficiency post-op that might necessitate dialysis. Mr K consents and surgery is booked. The procedure is uncomplicated and the pathology confirms an early kidney cancer, which appears to have been adequately resected.

Unfortunately, in the weeks after the procedure, Mr K's remaining kidney function deteriorates, forcing him to go on dialysis. This necessitates placement of a dialysis catheter, with trips to and from the dialysis unit three times a week for 4 to 6 hours at a time. His diet and fluid intake is restricted and his entire life now seems organized around dialysis.

Mr K complains bitterly that if he'd understood what dialysis involved, he would never have proceeded with the surgery.

Was Dr U's disclosure of risks adequate?
Did Dr U have an obligation to ensure that Mr K understood what dialysis entailed?

Disclosure

The principle guiding disclosure in consent is what "a reasonable person in the patient's position" would want to know. In practice, this means patients should be informed about the nature of the treatment, its gravity, and any reasonable alternatives (including the "zero option"—the option of doing nothing). They should also be given an explanation about the prognosis with and without treatment, as well as any common, unusual or material risks associated with the procedure. Finally, any questions patients may have about the treatment or its alternatives should be addressed.

What constitute material risks? A frequently cited definition is "significant risks that pose a real threat to the patient's life, health or comfort"[4].

In general, material risks are those known to be associated with a given treatment and which may have a serious impact on a patient. For example, if paralysis or loss of a limb is an uncommon but associated risk of a given procedure, then this should be disclosed. In the case of *Reibl v Hughes* (discussed in Chapter 5), the risk of stroke after carotid endarterectomy was clearly material, as it is a serious and well-documented complication associated with the procedure[33]. If a complication is one not typically associated with a procedure, say, a stroke after gallbladder removal, then it would not constitute a material risk.

The comments above notwithstanding, there is no algorithmic approach to satisfy all situations when it comes to disclosure of information. Even from a legal perspective, exactly what should be disclosed is in part dependent on the specifics of the patient.

Box 6.3

....

"It should be added that the scope of the duty of disclosure and whether or not it has been breached are matters which must be decided in relation to the circumstances of each particular patient."

....

Hopp v Lepp, 1980 [34]

From a practical and ethical point of view it makes sense that the amount or intensity of disclosure is also influenced by the urgency of the situation. Consent in the emergency room for an acute surgical problem is very different from consent in the office for a more routine elective problem (for example, biliary colic) [35]. In the case of a purely cosmetic plastic surgical procedure, the scope of disclosure is likely to be even more broad and exhaustive, since the surgery is not, strictly speaking, medically necessary [4]. In each case, the scope of disclosure is likely to be greater as the urgency of the situation decreases. While one should not unduly alarm patients with every possibility, doctors should also not provide false reassurances. This is especially so for those elective, cosmetic, or experimental interventions not typically required for the patient's well-being.

Box 6.4

....

"In the case of elective surgery, there can be no justification for withholding information." [36]

Discussion of Case 6.2

....

Dr U appears to have done a satisfactory job disclosing the relevant and material risks of the procedure. But it is clear there was a failure of some sort in ensuring that Mr K really understood what "dialysis" entailed. When it comes to ensuring a patient comprehends the risks of a procedure, the courts have given mixed messages. On one hand, they recognize that obligating physicians to ensure that patients understand all the information given to them "would place an unfair and unreasonable burden on the physician" [37, 38]. On the other hand, they argue that a physician needs to ensure that a patient comprehends the repercussions of an outcome [4, 39].

continued

Regardless of the legal views, it is clear that a physician has a moral duty to make sure a patient has a reasonable understanding of what is proposed and what certain outcomes might mean on a practical basis. Just telling Mr K that he might need dialysis, without explaining what dialysis involves, is hardly fair and respectful to him. Disclosure without explanation, even if truthful, is not really disclosure at all.

Box 6.5

Informed Consent (choice) requires discussing

- the exact nature of the proposed treatment,
- alternative treatments,
- the prognosis with and without treatment,
- the risks and benefits of the treatments and alternatives,
- any serious risks, even if unlikely, and
- any questions or concerns the patient may have.

Capacity (and competency)

Case 6.3   "Thanks but No Thanks!"

Mr P is a 55-year-old divorced bank employee living on his own, who comes to the emergency room late one evening on the advice of his chiropractor because of abdominal pain. Workup demonstrates a large amount of free air on X-ray. After confirming peritonitis on exam, Dr D, the general surgeon on call, advises immediate surgery. She explains all the relevant aspects of the surgery, including the risks, benefits, and prognosis with and without surgery.

Mr P thanks Dr D for her time and consideration, but declines the surgery. He explains he has had similar pain on many occasions; the pain generally resolves with a glass of warm soy milk. Besides, he has lots of yard work to do the next day. Dr D then restates the seriousness of the condition and the risks of not having surgery—including the very real chance of dying. Although their discussion is very cordial, Mr P still declines the surgery. Besides, he emphasizes, he does not want to miss the finale of his favourite TV show.

What should Dr D do?
Would it be a sign of Dr D's abiding respect for autonomy to accept Mr P's refusal?

Mental capacity will be discussed in depth in Chapter 8, so only a few comments will be made here. For a person to make an informed choice about a treatment, they must possess the mental capacity to understand and process the information provided. Capacity is rarely an all or none phenomenon, but frequently a matter of degree. A patient may be capable of consenting to a minor procedure or test, but not to open-heart surgery. In general, "the more serious the condition, the greater the capacity required" [40, 41].

Adults are presumed to be mentally competent. The capacity of patients who consent to reasonable treatment (for example, repairing a perforated viscus) is rarely questioned. By contrast, if a patient declines what appears to be reasonable treatment, most healthcare providers will entertain doubts about their decisional capacity. The bar for assessing mental capacity should rise or fall depending on the potential consequences of decisions regarding a serious condition.

Discussion of Case 6.3

Dr D has made a very reasonable attempt to explore Mr P's views and persuade him he needs an operation. One could argue the principle of autonomy implies Mr P's wishes should be respected, even if this may lead to considerable morbidity or his death.

However, Mr P is quite sick, and there is something not quite right about his cavalier attitude towards a life-threatening illness. A psychiatrist is consulted and concludes, under the circumstances, that Mr P lacks capacity, insofar as he does not appreciate the foreseeable consequences of his decision. No substitute decision-maker can be found. After further discussion, Mr P is admitted involuntarily and taken to the operating room where he undergoes an uncomplicated repair of a perforated duodenal ulcer. Interestingly, he does not protest or resist the decisions made that night and ends up making an excellent recovery. When later asked about his pre-surgical reasoning, he cannot recall refusing surgery. (Such amnesia is not at all unusual in very sick patients.)

This case demonstrates that a patient may have all the trappings of capacity (such as living alone, managing his own finances), but on a given night, for whatever reasons, may lack insight into his situation. Making a decision like this on a patient's behalf should never be taken lightly. However, neither should a physician just wash their hands of responsibility out of reverence for patient autonomy.

Voluntariness

For patients to make truly informed choices, they must obviously do so voluntarily. But the concept of voluntariness is more complex than it may initially appear.

Case 6.4 Ratcheting up the Rhetoric

After investigations for recurrent episodes of dizziness and vision changes, Mr Z, a 65-year-old widower, is found to have suffered multiple small strokes due to atrial fibrillation. A cardiologist, Dr M, advises that he start a blood thinner, warfarin. Mr Z is reluctant, explaining that because he has a very active lifestyle (skiing, squash, and karate), he is concerned about the risks of bleeding. He prefers to use ASA to prevent further strokes.

In order to impress upon Mr Z the seriousness of the situation, Dr M ratchets up his rhetoric. ASA won't do, he says. He warns him there is a real chance he'll suffer a massive stroke and end up in a long-term care facility, unable to control his bodily functions, drooling and being spoon-fed Pablum by his children.

Is scaring a patient reasonable in some circumstances?
How do we draw the line between persuasion and coercion?

Voluntariness means an absence of "undue influence"[42]. Is a physician, family member, or other person involved in a patient's care exerting so much influence as to potentially compromise the freedom of the patient to choose a treatment? This may be an explicit coercive threat, such as, "If you don't agree, we will have to put down a feeding tube." More likely, it could be a subtle and implicit one, such as, "We can't keep you in an acute care bed indefinitely." Although there is certainly a role for persuasion, it is not always easy to draw a clear line between reasonable persuasion and undue influence. There may be situations, such as Case 6.3, where a more aggressive approach to persuade someone is not just reasonable, but morally necessary.

Box 6.6

"In some cases, professionals are morally blameworthy if they do not attempt to persuade resistant parties to pursue treatments that are medically essential, and such persuasion need not violate respect for autonomy."[32]

Manipulation can also influence a patient's voluntariness of choice. Manipulation differs from persuasion in that it may involve a degree of dishonesty or disingenuousness on the part of a physician or family. This may occur in the way information is presented (such as overemphasizing the benefits or downplaying the risks) regarding a given treatment.

The psychologists Kahneman and Tversky, among others, have described a phenomenon known as the "framing effect"—namely, the impact that presenting the same information in different ways has on the decisions people make. For example, when physicians were told there was a 90 per cent one-month survival with surgery, 84 per cent advised surgery for their patients. However, when the same information was framed as a 10 per cent one-month mortality with surgery, only 50 per cent of physicians recommended surgery. If physicians can be so dramatically swayed by the way information is framed, one can only imagine how this can influence patients [43, 44].

It could be argued that, on some level, no patient can make truly voluntary decisions, as all patients are inherently vulnerable and under duress by virtue of both their medical illness and their lack of knowledge. And it is undoubtedly true that physicians have enormous power to influence how a patient decides. This is not necessarily a bad thing. Patients benefit from the guidance and experience of physicians. Even physicians who become patients want and need to be guided in their care [45]. This is why the concept of "trust" is so central to the process of informed consent, as we will discuss in the next section.

Discussion of Case 6.4

Undoubtedly Dr M is justified in ensuring Mr Z truly understands the possible consequences of his decision to refuse anticoagulation. However, in his zeal to impress upon Mr Z the gravity of the decision, he has pushed things a little too far and is verging on coercion.

Ultimately, it is the patient's decision whether to start anticoagulation. His concerns over its use in the context of his active life are quite reasonable. An honest, but non-coercive, discussion is much more likely to be effective in impressing upon Mr Z the benefits and risks of anticoagulation. But in the final analysis, if the patient prefers not to take warfarin, that is his choice. It may actually be the right one for him. It would not be the first or last time that the wisdom of a patient prevails.

III. Consent as Trust

The reality of informed choice is that when patients come to see physicians they are frequently sick, weak, and exceedingly vulnerable as a result of their condition [46]. Patients dealing with cancer or other life-threatening conditions may be anxious and distraught [47]. The elderly may be hopelessly confused and disoriented—both by the healthcare system and by the complex terminology and descriptions of their illness. The phenomenon of miscommunication is familiar to every physician (that is, what is said is frequently very different from what is heard), and illustrates clearly just how vulnerable and dependent many patients are[48].

There is, in addition, a vast gulf in knowledge and experience between patients and physicians. It takes physicians many years to learn the intricacies of treatments and their consequences. Can we expect patients to absorb and process much of this in a few days or weeks[47], especially taking into consideration the effects of serious illness on a patient?

As well, physicians are frequently time-constrained or distracted by other competing issues. Some may not be skilled communicators. Others, lacking empathy and emotional intelligence, may not pick up on subtle patient signals. Physicians, being human after all, may simply forget pertinent information or be impatient or inappropriately delegate the process to unsupervised trainees. In truth, there are so many factors able to corrupt or vitiate the process of informed choice that it is truly remarkable that "surgeons and patients . . . negotiate their way through these complexities with reasonable success"[49].

In a series of studies over 10 years, Martin McKneally, a thoracic surgeon, assessed qualitatively the perspectives of patients and surgeons on the experience of informed consent[49-51]. One important insight was the observation, from both patients and surgeons, that the complexity of surgical decisions renders the process of informed choice dependent primarily on trust: patients have trust in the hospital, in their healthcare team, in their surgeons, and in the entire system. McKneally and colleagues discuss an "entrustment model" of informed consent and ultimately the need for a "leap of trust" on the part of patients in order to proceed with surgical treatment[50]. Many patients acknowledge they do not see themselves making informed choices about treatment, as much as they make informed choices about putting their trust in the surgeon, the team, and the system.

Box 6.7

"Trust in the competence and commitment of their caregivers and in the expertise they came to associate with the institution where they were treated carried them across the chasm of doubt that lies beyond rational analysis and decision-making."[49]

McKneally's work illustrates that "traditional relations of trust" that used to exist between patients and physicians are still very much at the front and centre of the patient–physician relationship[52]. This trust also plays an important role in strengthening the physicians' commitments to their patients[49]. The codification of the doctrine of informed consent in statutes and laws is not a substitute for this trust. It simply provides some guidelines and safeguards for both parties when embarking on a treatment journey together.

Informed choice varies according to circumstances.

McKneally's work also illustrates how informed consent varies according to the specific medical circumstances. Consent for treatment with anti-hypertensives is very different from consent for cancer surgery. This is not only because the risks and benefits of the interventions differ, but also because the circumstances of the patient, the treatment, the role of the physician, and the degree of trust all differ as well. To apply a common legal and ethical approach to all situations of informed choice is not just unrealistic, but also potentially harmful. A patient with esophageal cancer deciding on surgery needs much more guidance (and so, more trust), than a patient weighing whether or not to get a flu shot.

Box 6.8

....

"One version of informed decision-making and consent does not fit all candidates for operative treatment." [51]

IV. Other Special Circumstances

Although we have touched on many of the key aspects of informed consent in the preceding discussion, there are a number of special situations warranting some discussion.

Emergency situations: An exception to consent?

The only real exception to obtaining consent for treatment is in emergency situations, where a patient is incapable of consenting (as delirious, obtunded, or unconscious) and a delay in obtaining consent for treatment might lead to significant harm. Under these circumstances, it is presumed a person would want everything done to prevent death or loss of limb or vital organ. This is not a discretionary action or merely a matter of convenience on the part of a physician, but an actual duty to provide care. In a way, even emergencies are not true exceptions to consent—since consent is presumed.

The duty to treat notwithstanding, there are some restrictions on the emergency exception to consent. First, unless there is a compelling need to proceed immediately, the healthcare provider should seek out a substitute decision-maker.

Second, healthcare professionals should obviously respect a patient's previously expressed wishes, as communicated in an advance directive or by a substitute decision-maker. For example, healthcare professionals should abide by the request of patients with an advanced disease, such as end-stage cancer, who have previously made it clear they do not want to be resuscitated. In such situations, especially if the refusing patient is a stranger to the clinician, it may be prudent for physicians to obtain a second opinion from colleagues or allied healthcare professionals.

Waiver of Consent

> ### Case 6.5 "I Trust Ya, Doc"
>
> Mr N is a 38-year-old male with a history of a few episodes of biliary colic. He is seeing Dr J and in the process of arranging an elective laparoscopic cholecystectomy. As Dr J begins explaining the nature and risks of the procedure, the patient says, "No need to go into details, Doc. I trust you completely. If you told me everything that could go wrong, I'd probably run like heck." Although the surgeon makes a few more attempts to explain the procedure, Mr N interrupts each time and asks, "Where do I sign?"
>
> *Is it acceptable to proceed with consent in this way?*
> *Is there anything else Dr J should do?*

It is not uncommon for patients to express a desire to waive the details of consent. For example, a patient may be fearful of hearing about complications or may feel self-conscious about their ability to understand the explanations. While one may want to support, *prima facie*, a patient's wish to not know the details, it is important to explore the reasons for this, as the concerns may be misguided or mistaken.

Patients need to have some understanding about the proposed treatments or procedures. In the case of cardiac surgery, for example, a patient should know that they may wake up on a ventilator in the ICU and may need regular bloodwork or physiotherapy. Information about the surgery and possible complications is also important to ensuring a good recovery.

Healthcare professionals should acknowledge and adjust their explanations to address the concerns of the patient. Reassuring patients about their ability to understand or assuaging their fears, by emphasizing the experiences of other patients and of the team's expertise and the precautions taken, can go a long way to helping them overcome their anxieties about being informed. Physicians have an obligation to make their best efforts to ensure patients understand what they are getting into.

Discussion of Case 6.5

Most physicians will be familiar with patients like Mr N. While their trust and respect for physicians can be quite flattering, this does not abrogate the need to ensure they understand that to which they are consenting. Dr J should let Mr N know it is important from both an ethical and recuperation point of view to be provided with some basic information about the procedure. In deference to the patient, Dr J might choose to gloss over some of the details about laparoscopic technique, but she should let Mr N know that the procedure is done under a general anaesthetic, that there can sometimes be problems post-operatively, such as bleeding, bile leaking, or even injury to the biliary system—and that sometimes further procedures (such as ERCP or surgery) may be needed.

Although there is a danger these explanations violate in part Mr N's wish to remain ignorant of the procedure and its risks, few would argue that it is unjustified or inappropriate. Given this is an elective procedure, it could be argued Mr N's disinclination to receive information about the outcomes of surgery may indicate he is not yet ready to have it.

Opiate analgesics and consent

Do opiate analgesics compromise informed consent? At many institutions, for example, patients who receive sedation while undergoing colonoscopy are instructed not to drive or make "important decisions" until the next day. This is presumably based on concerns their cognition and decision-making ability could be impaired. It is noteworthy that at the same institutions, patients in the emergency room may receive significantly more sedating medications, yet then be asked to consent to major surgery (see Case 5.2).

There is no doubt opiates affect cognition to some degree. However, whether they impair an individual's ability to make an informed choice is unclear. A recent review of the subject revealed, not surprisingly, conflicting results[53]. Attempts to empirically prove or disprove whether administration of opiates for pain vitiates informed choice are limited by the fact that capacity for consent varies according to circumstances, and that it does not lend itself to being easily measured. Moreover, the presence of pain itself may impair decision-making capability[53]. What impairs judgment more: pain or opiates? Should all patients in pain who receive opiate analgesics require substitute decision-makers? If so, this would significantly impact much of acute care medicine. Consider for example the situation of women in labour consenting to Caesarean sections! One can even argue that withholding analgesics in order to obtain consent is unethical or even coercive[54].

Given all the other factors potentially compromising informed choice, it is hard to see how the administration of opiates (given in reasonable doses, of course) for control of pain would in and of itself significantly alter the capacity of a patient to provide informed consent.

In the final analysis, there does not appear to be any valid reason to withhold analgesia from patients with acute pain in order to obtain consent. Indeed, such withholding might *compromise* consent. Patients with acute pain should receive analgesia in a timely fashion. Unless they demonstrate obvious incapacity (such as morphine-induced delirium) to make decisions about their care, their consent for treatment should be considered legitimate. That said, this has not been challenged in the courts.

Withdrawal of consent

Case 6.6 "Stop The Test!"

A 58-year-old woman, Ms T, agrees to undergo a colonoscopy by Dr E. During the procedure, despite moderate sedation, she suddenly experiences pain and cries out, "Stop! I can't take this anymore!"

Should the physician continue the examination?

The doctrine of consent gives the patient the definitive right to accept or refuse medical interventions. It includes the stipulation that patients can withdraw consent at any time, even during a medical procedure. This circumstance was addressed in 1993 by the Supreme Court of Canada in the case of *Ciarlariello v Schacter*[55].

Mrs Giovanna Ciarlariello was an Italian-speaking cleaner, who in 1980 at age 49 appeared to have a sentinel bleed from a cerebral aneurysm. To locate the source of her bleeding, a cerebral angiogram was recommended. Informed consent was obtained by radiologists and an intern at adjoining hospitals. Her family was included in the discussion, with a daughter signing the consent form as Mrs Ciarlariello had a limited understanding of English. During a second angiogram, the patient complained of discomfort and hyperventilated. When she calmed down, she said, "Enough, no more, stop the test." After temporarily stopping the test, the physicians, noting an improvement in her condition, recommended completing the procedure. The patient appeared to agree. Unfortunately, during the final dye injection the patient was rendered quadriplegic and later died.

Her estate sued the physicians, arguing, among other things, that it was wrong to continue with the angiogram when the patient had withdrawn her consent.

Halt unless serious harm

At issue in this case was the importance of continuing a procedure, when a patient withdraws their consent during the administration of that procedure. In general, *if consent is withdrawn, the procedure should be halted unless doing so might seriously harm the patient.* In this case, however, the patient agreed, after a period of recovery, to continuation of the test. The court felt her renewed consent was valid because (1) she had previously consented to the same procedure, (2) the risks had not changed, and (3) the patient appeared to understand what was being asked of her in the procedure room.

Onus borne by clinician

If a patient appears to withdraw consent during a test but the procedure is continued, the onus is borne by the clinician to ensure that the patient has understood what is happening. In particular, the clinician may have to demonstrate later that the patient understood the explanation and instructions given to continue the procedure. If this cannot be done, especially if the material risks to the patient have changed, the test should not be resumed. While the entire consent process does not have to be repeated, new material risks must be divulged, and the patient must have the capacity to understand them. If this capacity is lacking, valid consent to continue the procedure can therefore not be given; it would be prudent to stop unless the patient would be put in danger by halting or interrupting the procedure. (Of course, substitute consent could be obtained so long as it is not used as a vehicle to override what the patient would otherwise have chosen.)

Discussion of Case 6.6

Dr E would be unwise to continue the examination on Ms T. He should stop advancing the colonoscope, try to determine why the patient felt pain, and attempt to relieve it. The patient should have the risks and benefits of continuing the procedure explained. Despite sedation, if Ms T is adamant about stopping and understands the implications, her wish should be respected. In an Ontario case, a physician was found guilty of battery for continuing with a sigmoidoscopy in spite of a patient's cries to stop due to pain. In that case, the patient suffered a perforated bowel after the doctor had been asked to stop[56].

V. Special Circumstances and Limits on Truthtelling

Despite modern trends in medicine—such as the legal requirement for consent—that encourage veracity with patients, there are also legitimate "exceptions" to truthtelling and disclosure in broader clinical practice. These are not so much exceptions, however, as they are "special circumstances" that require tact and care from the healthcare professional in exercising the duty to tell the truth.

Box 6.9

Special circumstances that affect truthtelling:

1. Incapacity/dementia
2. Young children
3. Therapeutic privilege
4. "Bad news"

If a patient lacks the capacity to understand and appreciate all the information that would, under ordinary circumstances, be disclosed, the health professional should attempt to tailor such information to the degree that will help them—whether very young or old—appreciate what they can. Decisions to withhold important information from a child, for example, should incorporate a plan for disclosing this as the child grows older. Of course, cases of mental incapacity are not truly exceptions to consent. They are situations, instead, calling for the involvement of a substitute decision-maker (see Chapter 8).

Advanced malignancies, dementia, HIV seropositivity, and neurological conditions such as multiple sclerosis, some of which are still not very amenable to treatment, all have posed challenges for clinicians around how to disclose in a forthright and compassionate way. The truth can result in "labelling" patients with a stigmatizing condition. This can lead to negative consequences such as excessive worry about the future or the failure to fulfill role expectations such as work attendance and family obligations.

For example, a classic study from the early 1980s, found that patients who were told they had hypertension exhibited decreased emotional well-being and more frequent absence from work [57]. It is, of course, well known that people can take on a sick role. In another study, giving more information to patients with cancer resulted in higher anxiety levels than those not so informed [58]. Labelling can also result in shunning, discrimination, and exile. (Think of how patients diagnosed with leprosy, AIDS, or schizophrenia were and are treated.) Concerns regarding other very bad outcomes of disclosure—complete loss of hope, premature death, or suicide—are largely anecdotal and require closer study. But insensitive truthtelling by a cold, unempathetic clinician can have outcomes as bad as those of deception. The experience can be particularly traumatic for ill-prepared patients in cultures less comfortable with openness about critical illness [59].

Box 6.10

"The hurried telling of bad news in a busy clinic with little explanation and no opportunity for the patient to ask questions can result in unnecessary psychological and emotional pain." [60]

Box 6.11

Suggestions to healthcare professionals and trainees for sharing information:

1. Be prepared by having a plan for disclosure before the interview.
2. Be informed about the patient's situation and know how to get answers to any questions you are not able to answer yourself.
3. Try not to be or appear rushed. The sharing of information, whether good or bad, is best done when you and the patient have time for each other.
4. Sit, don't stand; both parties should be reasonably comfortable. Privacy and a pleasant room are always welcome.
5. Ask if the patient would like anyone else to be present as part of the discussion.
6. If there may be cultural, ethnic, or other barriers to truthtelling, consider asking the patient, "Are you the kind of person who likes to know everything or would you prefer us to speak with someone else?"
7. Be honest and use simple, straightforward language. Help the patient understand the information in their own terms.
8. If translation is required, consider using a professional interpreter who is not a family member, as loved ones may sometimes not convey information correctly for their own reasons.
9. If appropriate, prepare a patient for bad news by using phrases like, "Things have not turned out as well as we'd hoped" or "I have some hard information to share with you."
10. Observe for non-verbal cues as to how well the patient is listening and taking in the information. Acknowledge the patient's emotions.
11. Be available to schedule follow-up sessions as needed, especially if the information is serious or uncertain.

Therapeutic Privilege

The concept of "therapeutic privilege" is sometimes invoked if a health professional deems a patient's psychological and/or physical condition so tenuous that telling them the truth may cause significant harm. For example, a surgeon might opt not to disclose to a patient urgently requiring abdominal surgery that there is a remote chance a temporary ileostomy may be needed, knowing the patient has a morbid fear of stomas and would mentally decompensate or decline life-saving surgery. Such deliberate withholding of material information from a patient must be based on actual information about the *particular* patient and not on abstract concerns about patients in general. There are likely very few circumstances in modern medicine when a physician would be justified in exercising such paternalism. This should be done only as a last resort and with the expectation it will be revisited once the patient's condition stabilizes. Even patients with irrational fears and preoccupations have a right to know the facts so as to make decisions based on these. A skilled communicator will almost always find a way to assuage such fears.

It can be difficult to predict what information a patient will find upsetting or how upsetting that "bad news" will be. Poor truthtelling practices, even if the information conveyed is accurate, can have devastating consequences for patients[61]. Studies have revealed the way in which information is communicated may be just as important as the information itself[62, 63]. Care must be taken that information is given at the right time and in the right place. The news may be terrible but the telling of it need not be[64].

Aiming to please and the use of placebos

Is it ever appropriate to propose a treatment the physician knows may not work or only work by the power of suggestion? Such is the problem of placebos. From the Latin, "I will please," placebos have a long (and not always honourable) history of use in medicine. There is no reason to suppose that everything we do in medicine must be based on a clear scientific rationale. In fact, much of what we do lacks such a rationale. Patients can improve by the power of suggestion, by how their doctors relate to them. Every clinician knows there are times when patients improve after the healthcare professional suggests that they *will* get better (this is true not only for doctors but for nurses or any health professional). This doesn't mean prescribing a pill you know is ineffective, but rather bolstering up the patient in a time of crisis or illness.

If practitioners must always and only tell the "truth," they may be unable to maintain patient hope, the patient's belief that they will get better, in the face of terrible news. Indeed, some patients, against all odds, under the influence of the "less-than-the-full-truth" disclosure, do get better (for a while anyway). Some see hope, by its very nature, as being unrealistic and lying behind quotidian human attempts to overcome the finite and fragile limits of human existence. Others see hope as "a confident yet uncertain expectation of achieving good which to a hoping person is realistically possible and personally significant"[65]. The challenge for the clinician is to avoid overly optimistic prognoses encouraging unrealistic hopes and offers of unwarranted aggressive medical treatment[66] while not forgetting the "value of hope empowerment in supporting patients through their illness"[66].

Case 6.7   A Reflex Response

A patient is brought to the ER in shock; he has suffered a serious abdominal wound in a drive-by shooting and needs urgent surgery. The team knows his chances of recovery are slim. But he is still alert and able to talk. On the way into the OR, he turns to the nurse anaesthetist and says, "I'm going to make it, right?"

Discussion of Case 6.7

We all know the importance of telling the truth, but there are times when it seems better to leave the unvarnished truth unsaid. A time-honoured reflex would be to hold his hand, and say, "Of course, you will make it!" or, "We will do everything we can!" Encouraging him to believe he will get better cannot hurt. If this is paternalism, it seems the defensible kind.

Conclusion

In the final analysis, our processes of truthful communication and informed choice are imperfect and flawed. However, they may be, to echo Winston Churchill, better than every other option available. "Shared decision-making" in medicine may be part fantasy. But as one author has pointed out, at a minimum "it provides a reasonable assurance that a patient . . . has not been deceived or coerced"[67]. True informed consent may be part fiction, but it is a good fiction and may be the best we can do. In the next chapter we will look at problems of privacy and confidentiality.

Cases for Discussion

Case 1: A Shocking Shot

Mr V, an active 80-year-old man with a history of stable coronary artery disease, is admitted to the ICU with a large and serious, but quite survivable, presumed self-inflicted gunshot wound to the side of his face. He had become despondent as the primary caregiver for his spouse with advanced dementia but had never been treated for a psychiatric disorder. Neither a suicide note nor advance directive had been found. At the time of his admission Mr V is neurologically intact but heavily sedated and intubated to protect his airway. He is unable to take part in decision-making. A plastic surgeon, Dr A, seeks consent for the repair of Mr V's facial injury from the appropriate substitute decision-makers, his two grown children.

Mr V's children refuse consent. They say their father has "suffered enough" and must have had good reasons for doing what he did. Moreover, they add, at his age, further intensive treatment would not work. They request all treatment be withdrawn and their father be allowed to die. Dr A subsequently declines to operate because of Mr V's children's refusal of consent. "They're the substitute decision-makers," he says. "If Mr V were my father, I wouldn't want him to live either."

Questions for Discussion

1. What should the response be to the children's refusal of consent?
2. How might one respond to Dr A?

Case 2: A Fractured Hip, A Broken Mind

A 76-year-old reclusive single female, Ms D, is admitted to a large tertiary hospital with a fractured hip. When told surgery is required, she refuses to consent. She explains she does not believe she is in a "real hospital," as people had been rude to her and she had noticed dust on the X-ray machine. Ms D says she doubts she has a hip fracture, as she is not in that much pain. "Just send me home with a wheelchair," she exclaims. "I want to discuss this with an old ladies' organization."

Dr S, the resident, finds her line of reasoning unusual and deems her incapable. He wants her prepped for surgery first thing tomorrow morning. In contrast, the anaesthetist in his pre-operative assessment writes in her chart that he found her "entirely competent" to refuse surgery, specifically highlighting the patient's score of 30/30 on the MMSE (Mini-Mental State Examination) that had been part of his evaluation.

The surgeon, Dr W, is eager to proceed with the surgery. "What's the big hold-up?" he asks Dr S.

Questions for Discussion

1. Is there an ethical problem here?
2. What should Dr S do?

✦ 7 ✦

....

Keeping Secrets

Confidentiality and Privacy in the Electronic Age

Thou art the only one to whom I dare confide my Folly.

George Lyttelton, 1744 [1]

Privacy is dead; get over it.

Anon

Respecting patient information has been a fundamental ethical obligation of physicians ever since the time of Hippocrates. However, the evolution of modern, multidisciplinary medicine—where many trainees, healthcare professionals, and administrative personnel might have access to a patient's chart—and the advances in digital technology—from email and texting to audio and video recordings—are creating new challenges. In this chapter, we will examine issues of confidentiality and privacy as they relate to many of these elements of modern medical practice.

I. Confidentiality and Privacy

Case 7.1   The Shame of It All!

....

Mr X, a 44-year-old civil servant, is admitted to the hospital under Dr Y for an examination under anaesthesia of his rectum. It turns out he has a large foreign object lodged in his rectum: the distal part of a poorly made sex toy. It will require removal in the OR. Excruciatingly embarrassed, Mr X can hardly make eye contact with nurses and other staff. He asks: "Do you have to put this in my chart? Everyone in the whole hospital will know what I did. I just want to die."

Will everyone in the hospital know what Mr X did?
What will you say to him?

In an influential 1982 essay, the physician and bioethicist Mark Siegler suggested that the traditional concept of confidentiality was outdated. In the modern hospital system, where dozens of medical and nonmedical staff may with good justification access a patient's hospital chart, the traditional notion of the physician as keeper of a patient's secrets was judged "decrepit" and outmoded [2].

Siegler's insight is at once obvious and yet perplexing. Although many persons may have access to a patient's chart, protecting private patient information seems as important as ever. Since his paper, we have come to understand that this apparent paradox arises from the false assumption that confidentiality and privacy are identical. They are not. Confidentiality refers to "the obligation of third parties to guard the secrecy of personal information" confided to them [3]. It is part of a healthcare professional's code of ethics. Privacy, on the other hand, refers to "the person or group's entitlement to make decisions regarding the use of the information"—that is, control over how and by whom personal information can be used [3]. It is legislated in law, such as by health information statutes.

The distinction between confidentiality and privacy explains why healthcare professionals can remain assured they are abiding by the Hippocratic obligation to respect the confidentiality of their patients, while simultaneously functioning in a system where dozens of other healthcare providers and ancillary workers can have access to the medical records of patients.

Box 7.1

In healthcare, **confidentiality** is a duty of healthcare professionals to protect, from unauthorized eyes, sensitive or personal information they may have about others.

Discussion of Case 7.1

Mr X's embarrassment and concerns about his problem are completely understandable. While many people in the hospital could potentially look at

continued

his medical record, only those legitimately involved in his care are permitted access; they are all obliged by professional and legal codes to respect his privacy. Moreover, on a more general level of addressing his fears, he should be given reassurance he is not the first patient with such a problem and will certainly not be the last. With compassion and honest communication, Dr Y can support Mr X through this experience, letting him know he is not alone and is not being judged. His privacy and his dignity will always be respected.

Box 7.2

In healthcare, **privacy** is the right of individuals to control the information others have about them. This right can be invoked to prevent the government and other third parties from gaining access to personal health information or/ and to hold them legally responsible if they access/disclose the information improperly.

II. Privacy, Confidentiality, and Trust

Case 7.2 Mum's the Word

Late one night, the surgeon on call, Dr S, is asked to see Kaylee, a 16-year-old girl with right lower quadrant abdominal pain. Her mother is present during the encounter. Kaylee's history and exam are very typical for appendicitis. She reports her menstrual periods are regular, and she adamantly denies being sexually active. Quite self-possessed, she signs the consent form herself.

In the operating room at midnight, the appendix is found to be normal, but there is bleeding mass in her right fallopian tube, almost certainly an ectopic pregnancy. A gynecologist is called in and carries out a right salpingectomy (removal of the fallopian tube).

After the procedure, Dr S goes out to talk with Kaylee's mother in the waiting room.

What should Dr S tell Kaylee's mother?

The right of individuals to have their privacy respected by governments and private enterprise is a long-held fundamental tenet of all liberal democracies[4]. The values of autonomy, liberty, and dignity—all versions of the "respect for persons" principle—underpin the concept of privacy. At the end of 1890 two American Supreme Court justices defined privacy as "the right to be left alone" [5]. In other words, privacy is the right to be free from outside intrusion or interference [6].

In contrast, authoritarian regimes tend to devalue privacy, routinely accessing and misusing the medical records and other personal information of their citizens. In China, for example, privacy has been considered to be of "instrumental," not intrinsic, value [7]. However, revelations of massive privacy breaches by Facebook and the National Security Agency in the US, the latter made public by Edward Snowden, highlight how even democratic societies may allow political, security, and commercial interests to override personal privacy rights [8,9].

In the United States, the right to individual privacy has generally been construed as deriving from the Constitution and, in particular, the Bill of Rights [10]. It is legislated federally by the *Health Insurance Portability and Accountability Act (HIPPA)*. The *Personal Information Protection and Electronic Documents Act (PIPEDA)* of 2000 is the corresponding federal legislation in Canada. Although there is mention of "personal health information," PIPEDA applies to such information strictly as it relates to "commercial activity." Because healthcare is largely administered and managed at a provincial level in Canada, each province and territory codifies the protection of individual healthcare information in the form of health information and privacy acts, such as the *Personal Health Information Protection Act (PHIPA)* in Ontario [11]. In general, provinces must meet or exceed the standards set in the federal act (PIPEDA).

Box 7.3

Provincial health information acts regulate

1. how patients and third parties can access personal health information;
2. the way healthcare information is collected, stored, and used;
3. how custodians/trustees (such as nurses, doctors, social workers, and the like) can collect, disclose, and share patient information;
4. how patients can go about correcting their personal health information; and
5. how breaches of the legislation should be remedied.

Justifications for privacy and confidentiality

Protection of informational privacy can be justified on duty-based and utilitarian grounds. "The confiding of information to the physician for medical purposes gives rise to an expectation that the patient's interest in and control of the information will continue" [12]. This is more than a mere "expectation" on the patient's part, however. The right of patients to have control over their own information is a kind of "promise" made by clinicians and the healthcare system in general to patients.

There is also a consequentialist rationale on the right to privacy. Breaching a patient's confidences would threaten the trust on which healthcare depends. This in turn would lead to negative outcomes such as avoidance of appropriate care by patients with stigmatizing conditions.

Discussion of Case 7.2

There is usually implied consent for a surgeon to discuss surgery with close family after an operation. In this case, however, it appears Kaylee did not want her mother to know she was sexually active. Experienced clinicians will note Dr S made two errors leading to this dilemma. The first was failing to rule out a possible extra-uterine pregnancy prior to the procedure. The second was taking a sexual history from a teenager with a parent present.

These errors notwithstanding, Dr S has an obligation to respect Kaylee's confidentiality. At the same time, she does not want to lie to Kaylee's mother. One reasonable approach to this dilemma would be to speak in general terms with her mother and indicate more information could be provided in the morning. Dr S should see Kaylee alone before then to tell her what was found and to assess her wishes. The situation may become very challenging if she insists her mother not be told the findings. It will then be a question of clarifying to Kaylee the many ramifications of not disclosing to her mother (such as lying, deception, issues with fertility in future, possible appendicitis in the future). A social worker as well as supportive nursing staff will likely be helpful in trying to resolve this situation.

Ultimately, though, if Kaylee insists, Dr S has a duty to respect her confidentiality, as unrealistic and impractical as this might be.

Accessing patient health information

Case 7.3   A Favour, Please

You are the attending physician on an internal medicine service when John, a first-year resident, asks a favour of you. He knows he is not supposed to access his own records through the hospital medical information system. So he asks if you would, with his consent of course, access his recent shoulder MRI report and provide him with a copy.

What would you do?

Although the physical aspect of a patient's chart may belong to a physician or institution, the information in the chart belongs to the patient[3]. Patients have a right to their own medical information. However, they cannot access it willy nilly. They must go through proper channels as determined by the applicable health information and privacy acts. This process is changing, however, as patient portals (which permit patients to access their electronic medical record independently) become increasingly common. This trend represents a major shift in the way all persons can access their personal healthcare information. However, many challenges remain, such as how accurate and inclusive the information will be and who will help patients interpret such information. Undoubtedly, patient portals will give rise to many unanticipated ethical issues in the future.

In addition to determining how patients may access their own healthcare information, health information acts regulate how healthcare professionals may collect, access, and share patient information. In order to facilitate patient care, they allow healthcare providers great latitude in collecting and sharing patient information. Obstacles are minimal and healthcare professionals (at least those in the patient's circle of care) have an almost unlimited freedom to access and share information.

To ensure such access is not abused, governments impose a fiduciary duty on physicians and other healthcare providers to use this access to information responsibly and to act in the best interests of their patients. This means healthcare professionals should access and share health information only of those with whom they have a patient-care relationship. In addition, they should access only information relevant to providing care for the active problem—in other words, on a "need-to-know" basis. Thus, for example, it is neither required nor appropriate to take a detailed sexual history if treating a sprained ankle.

Discussion of Case 7.3

Even with the resident's permission, it is not appropriate for you to access his MRI report. You do not have a patient-care relationship with him. It is a clear breach of privacy regulations, as well as a potential boundary issue. He should obtain the results of his exam from the physician who ordered it or from his own family physician. While such requests may seem harmless, especially if permission is explicitly granted, they are strictly prohibited legally and ethically in most jurisdictions. While this issue may become moot in the future as patient portals become more common, it could become of greater concern as information (genetic, personal) becomes more and more complex. There will always be a need for someone to aid patients in the interpretation of their results.

Healthcare professionals should also be aware that medical information systems are routinely audited, and inappropriate queries by healthcare

continued

personnel will often be identified. There are numerous examples of healthcare professionals who have been disciplined for inappropriately accessing patient information[13-15]. In the absence of a patient-care relationship, looking at a colleague's or relative's health information is considered a breach of privacy and could lead to a disciplinary action. Trainees and physicians *can* access their own healthcare information, but they need to go through proper channels.

Box 7.4

The content of the medical record belongs to the patient; the physical record is the property of the "health custodian"—doctor or institution—and is held for the benefit of the patient.

- Patients may have access to their records in all but a small number of cases and may cordon off all or part of it from the scrutiny of others by a virtual "lock box."
- Access and control by the patient of the chart, or parts of it, may be denied if this might compromise the safety of the patient or third parties. The burden of proving this danger is on the practitioner so claiming.
- Denial of access or control may be subject to legal challenge.[12]

Is the commitment to patient confidentiality absolute?

Although privacy and confidentiality are protected by statute and professional standards in Canada, the privilege afforded such communication is not absolute. Physicians can be compelled to disclose private patient health information, if so ordered by a judge. They should be aware, however, that a "subpoena" is not in and of itself permission to breach patient confidentiality. It is simply a command to attend court. Although a subpoena may instruct a physician to bring a patient's records to court, these can be released only with the patient's express consent or through an explicit court order. When in doubt, physicians should seek advice from independent legal counsel, such as the Canadian Medical Protective Association[16].

Informational protection for Psychiatry?

Greater protection has traditionally been given to psychiatrist–patient communications. A trusting therapeutic relationship is essential for effective psychiatric care, especially for those who may already be struggling with trust issues due to traumatic life experiences. In a position paper on confidentiality and privacy in Psychiatry from 2000, the Canadian Psychiatric Association asserted that "[w]ithout confidentiality there can be no trust; without trust there can be no therapy"[17]. Nonetheless, psychiatrists and other mental health professionals are permitted and can be compelled to give evidence in court anywhere in Canada. The "interests of justice" (as in *Smith v Jones*, discussed later in the chapter) may at times quite legitimately outweigh the benefits of privacy despite the therapeutic relationship.

Informational protection for victims of sexual assault

There is also extra protection of medical information for victims of sexual assault. The fear of having one's personal, psychiatric, and medical information laid bare in a courtroom has made many victims of sexual assault wary of laying charges. Bill C-46 of the Canadian *Criminal Code* (amended in 1996) is aimed at encouraging the reporting of such crimes by restricting access to medical, counselling, therapeutic, and other personal records of complainants in sexual offence prosecutions. Psychiatrists and other healthcare professionals are protected from having to release information from an alleged victim's medical records *unless* the accused can come up with compelling reasons for this. This prevents "fishing expeditions" by defence lawyers looking for some reason to cast aspersions on the trustworthiness or credibility of the plaintiff.

III. New Risks to Privacy

Case 7.4 "Just Email Me, Doc"

Mr A is being investigated for fatigue and malaise. Because he frequently travels for work, he requests you notify him by email of the test results.

Is this acceptable practice?

Electronic communication with patients

Another rapidly evolving area with regard to privacy is electronic communication with patients. While email communication with patients has been around for over 20 years [18], newer forms of engaging with patients, such as texting, videoconferencing, social media, and patient portals are increasingly prevalent. All these raise concerns about physicians' statutory obligations to protect privacy (several of these topics will be addressed at length in Chapter 11).

There are pros and cons to emailing with patients [19]. On the pro side, emailing with patients may

- help minimize trivial or unnecessary appointments;
- be an efficient and simple way to deal with prescription refills, appointment/seasonal reminders, and follow-ups between visits;
- be a good way to provide patients with supplemental resources and information;
- be helpful to patients in remote locations or with mobility issues making clinic visits onerous or impossible; and
- actually increase the time available to spend with patients who *do* need to come in for a visit [19].

On the con side, email communication can

- intrude into personal time, since it may be dealt with during off-hours;
- be quite time-consuming;
- create extra work;
- cause worry over wording and documentation, as it will be part of a patient's permanent record; and
- compromise discussions probably best done in person.

From a privacy and confidentiality point of view, the primary concern with electronic communication is security. On the physician's side, unauthorized individuals may gain access to the emails. It is also all too easy to select the wrong name from a drop-down menu or inadvertently "c.c." uninvolved parties. On the patient's side, it is possible for emails to be read by those who are not the primary recipients, be it children, work colleagues, or others. Many employers retain the right to review all employee communication at the workplace.

People are also apt to forget that many providers of free email services "mine" the content of emails for commercial purposes. Google, for example, made news in mid-2017 when it announced it would cease "scanning" Gmail communications for the purpose of providing personalized advertisements. Not widely appreciated was that Google continues to scan and read personal emails, using the information for other commercial purposes [20].

In addition to commercial intrusions by services like Google, there is also the risk of emails being intercepted by hackers or by official and unofficial government agencies. Emails sent or received in public Wi-Fi hubs, such as coffee shops, airports, and libraries, are especially vulnerable to privacy breaches.

Physicians considering using email communication with patients should consult their hospital and medical organizations (including medicolegal) for guidance in this matter. (A list of some of the factors that should be considered when emailing with patients is included in Box 7.5.)

Discussion of Case 7.4

Mr A's request is not unreasonable, since he frequently travels for work (although it may be his travels that partially contribute to his fatigue and malaise). Nonetheless, prior to agreeing, you should clarify what sort of results and information are appropriate for email communication. He should be made aware of the various threats to his privacy, outlined above. It is generally not appropriate to communicate complicated or life-altering information (such as results of an HIV test) this way. Physicians should consider developing email guidelines to ensure that all parties have a common understanding and expectations.

Box 7.5

Twelve considerations when using email with patients:

1. Set up a professional email address (e.g., DoctorX@organization.com).
2. Clarify who will have access to this account.
3. Clarify what types of information will be sent by email and what will not be.
4. Establish expectations for response times.
5. Obtain written consent for such communication.
6. Advise patients of risks to privacy, regardless of the security of the system.
7. Use a private computer for communication, not one shared with others.
8. Establish how email communication will be integrated into the record.
9. Remember that electronic communications are permanent.
10. Never write anything in an email that you could not support if it was known to the patient or publicly disclosed.
11. Do not write or respond to emails when tired or upset, or after having alcohol.
12. Establish whether it is reasonable to be compensated for providing care to patients in this way.[21]

Text messaging in healthcare

Since its inception in 1992, SMS (that is, Short Messaging Service or text messaging) has become one of the most popular forms of electronic communication worldwide. Over 20 billion text messages a day were estimated to have been sent in 2017. While used at times to communicate directly with patients—often for appointment reminders and confirmation—texting is also used frequently by healthcare providers to communicate among themselves regarding patient-related care issues. Studies suggest that at least 60% of hospital-based physicians use SMS messages daily for matters of patient care [22, 23]. The ease and speed of SMS communication make it an invaluable tool when looking after patients.

As with email, text messaging in medicine poses similar concerns with respect to privacy—message transmission is not always secure, messages are retained by the service provider, security of transmitting devices can be compromised, and human error can occur. Although there are some messaging apps that are secure and encrypt messages, they are not always as convenient, efficient, and as universal as SMS. Policies and guidelines with regard to texting about patient care are very much in flux; compliance with privacy legislation remains unclear and elusive [24].

Many organizations suggest physicians should ensure no patient-identifying information appears in care-related texts. This includes dates of birth, hospital numbers, and even room numbers. There is even debate as to whether using patient initials is sufficient for de-identification [24].

Patients requesting to record their encounters

Case 7.5 For the Record

Ms K, a 60-year-old patient, is in your office to discuss results from a recent CAT scan of her abdomen. It reveals she has a pancreatic mass with metastases to her liver. As you begin explaining the findings, Ms K halts the conversation to ask if she can record it on her smartphone. Her family are going to have lots of questions, she says, and she is fearful she will not remember everything.

Should you permit her to record the conversation?
How would you approach this?

Research into the possible benefits of providing patients with recordings of their clinical encounters dates back to the 1970s [25]. The prevalence of smartphones and the ease of digital recording have reinvigorated the topic, leading to renewed discussions regarding the benefits and ethical implications of such practices [26–28].

Increasingly, patients and their families are requesting to record encounters with their physicians [29]. Patients feel this may enhance their understanding as well as facilitate sharing information with family [26, 30]. The literature appears to bear this out, consistently demonstrating improved recall and understanding by patients, as well as high levels of satisfaction [27, 28].

Box 7.6

Five benefits of patient recording encounters with physicians:

1. improves recall, retention and understanding of medical information;
2. provides patients with a sense of empowerment;
3. facilitates accurate sharing with family and loved ones;
4. possibly improves compliance; and
5. possibly decreases misunderstandings.

However, the recording of patient–physician encounters also raises important professional, ethical, and legal issues. Recordings in public spaces such as the waiting room or hallways can inadvertently capture information about other patients. What might be a funny or witty off-the-cuff remark during a patient encounter may come across very differently over time or in a different context. This is unfortunate, as it can interfere with spontaneity and rapport in a patient encounter. But it is a reality of our times.

In addition, clinicians may feel threatened by the introduction of a recording device, causing the mood of an encounter to shift. For many, the primary concern is that such recordings could be used as evidence in a legal proceeding or posted on social media [31]. In the United Kingdom, there is a trend towards regarding these recordings as a form of note-keeping, without the need for patients to ask permission [29].

While most physicians would expect patients to seek authorization to record an encounter, there are many instances where recordings are done covertly [32]. In a 2015 study from the United Kingdom, 15 per cent of people surveyed admitted to having at some time covertly recorded an office visit [30]. In the United States, the legality of covert recording is determined by state wiretapping and eavesdropping statutes. In most states (39 out of 50), only one party to a conversation (that is, the patient) need consent to the recording. In the remaining 11 states, it is a felony to make covert recordings without both parties' consent, and affected parties may seek damages [33]. Although there are some restrictions, in Canada it is legal to record a conversation covertly if one party consents [34, 35]. Regardless of its legality, however, many physicians feel recording without two-party consent can contribute to an erosion of trust on the part of physicians [32].

If patients insist on making a recording, it is not entirely clear where physicians stand if they demur. Although it can be argued that physicians also have a right to confidentiality, this is not something generally recognized or protected by statute. Confidentiality is a one-way street in physician–patient encounters. As requests for recording patient–physician interactions become more customary, however, physician attitudes appear to be changing. The potential for improved understanding and decreased miscommunication is beginning to be recognized [26, 27, 29, 36]. An ambitious group at one cancer centre in Alberta has created their own smartphone app, endorsed by Alberta Health Services, enabling patients to record conversations with their physicians and other providers during clinic visits.

Similar to emailing with patients, physicians would be prudent to draft policies and guidelines related to audio and video recordings and to make these available to patients.

Box 7.7

Ten suggestions to deal with patient requests to record an office visit:

1. Clarify with patients what they hope to achieve with a recording and see if there is an alternative option (for example, sharing your clinic notes).
2. If you decline, explain why.
3. You may use your discretion to proceed with or terminate the encounter.
4. Ensure the patient understands that recording can occur only in private spaces.
5. Note in the chart that a recording has been made and who was present.
6. If possible, obtain a copy of the recording for the patient record.
7. Consider making a parallel recording of your own, with the patient's consent.
8. Clarify how it will be used and that it will not be disseminated publicly.
9. Use the opportunity to ensure patients are well-informed about their conditions.
10. Establish policy and guidelines for your practice.

Discussion of Case 7.5

Whether or not to permit recording is a personal decision on the part of a physician. Ms K has genuine and legitimate reasons for wanting to record the conversation. Anyone who has delivered information of this sort will know that patients frequently go into shock and cannot retain or process information.

As in many such conflicts, good communication will frequently resolve the dilemma. Inquiring into the reasons for wanting to record and offering alternatives to address these concerns may reassure a patient.

Regardless of whether you permit recording or not, you can offer to write down salient points for the patient to convey to her family. You can also volunteer to call her relatives or suggest Ms K return the following day with family for a discussion in person.

IV. Limits to Confidentiality

Box 7.8

"[T]here may be cases in which reasons connected with the safety of individuals or the public, physical or moral, would be sufficiently cogent to supersede or qualify the obligations prima facie imposed by the confidential relation."

Halls v Mitchell, 1928[37]

While respecting privacy and confidentiality is a primary duty of all healthcare professionals, it is not absolute or without exceptions. There are situations when, whether for the benefit of individuals or society in general, the duty of confidentiality can and should be breached.

Mandatory and Discretionary Disclosure

In most North American jurisdictions, there are a number of circumstances in which it is either mandatory or permitted to disclose private medical information (see Box 7.9). As laws may vary according to location, physicians are advised to become familiar with the regulations in their own jurisdiction.

1. Reportable communicable diseases

All North American jurisdictions have a list of reportable infectious diseases. In most cases, reporting occurs routinely as part of laboratory protocol. For example, a lab will automatically notify the Medical Officer of Health of all positive findings for tuberculosis. In these circumstances, both the patient and contacts will be followed up. In addition, in many jurisdictions such as Ontario, a healthcare

Box 7.9

The following is a general, but not exhaustive, list of circumstances requiring or permitting disclosure of personal information by healthcare providers:

- Certain communicable diseases
- Child abuse and neglect
- Vulnerable adults
- Driving safety
- Flying, train, and marine safety
- Fitness to work
- Gunshot wounds
- "Management of the healthcare system"
- Certain criminal activities

practitioner who merely suspects a reportable infectious condition is required to report this to the Medical Officer of Health [38].

It is commonly asked whether those under active treatment for HIV are obligated to inform potential sexual partners of their status. Although the legal issues are very complex, failing to disclose positive HIV status to one's sexual partners, if there is a "realistic possibility of transmission," is considered a criminal offence in Canada, resulting in a possible charge of aggravated sexual assault [40, 41]. There are some exceptions to this, depending on the type of sexual contact. Much is written and debated on this topic. A good resource for up-to-date information is the Canadian HIV/AIDS Legal Network website: http://www.aidslaw.ca.

Box 7.10

"A physician or registered nurse in the extended class who, while providing professional services to a person, forms the opinion that the person is or may be infected with an agent of a communicable disease shall, as soon as possible after forming the opinion, report thereon to the Medical Officer of Health of the health unit in which the professional services are provided." [39]

2. Child abuse and neglect

In almost all jurisdictions, medical practitioners are required to breach confidentiality and report any information about the *possible* mistreatment or neglect of children. Again, the threshold for reporting is having an *opinion*, based on "reasonable suspicion or belief," that abuse is taking place [42]. Failure to report reasonable suspicions may be punishable by fine [38].

3. Vulnerable adults

Laws to protect vulnerable adults, including the elderly and mentally disabled adults, are not as consistent as for children [43]. In Canada, there are no federal laws mandating the reporting of suspected elder abuse; expectations of physicians vary considerably in different provinces [43]. In Ontario, for example, physicians are mandated to report suspected neglect or physical, financial, sexual, or emotional abuse, if it occurs in a retirement home or long-term care facility. For community-dwelling elderly, there is no such obligation [38]. Even if there are no "elder-specific" laws, practitioners need to be aware that many existing laws (such as Guardianship laws) in various jurisdictions can be applied to protect the rights and interests of vulnerable adults (see Chapter 8) [44]. A physician who suspects abuse of a vulnerable person has an ethical obligation to inquire about what can be done and to notify the appropriate authorities.

4. Driving safety

There can be considerable regional variation in the legal duty of physicians to report patients who pose a risk when driving. In Canada, reporting is mandatory in all provinces other than Alberta, Quebec, and Nova Scotia, where it is discretionary. In British Columbia, a physician must report only if an unfit driver continues to drive after being advised against this [45]. In all jurisdictions, physicians are protected against legal action for breaching confidentiality. If a patient files a complaint with the physician's regulatory college, no disciplinary action will be rendered if the physician made a report in good faith.

Conversely, if a physician fails to report a patient who is not fit to drive, the physician can be found legally responsible in certain jurisdictions. The case of *Toms v Foster* in Ontario involved a 73-year-old man whose vehicle struck a motorcycle, seriously injuring the two riders [46]. Despite knowing for the previous two years that Mr Foster was suffering from weakness of the legs and diminished agility due to cervical spondylosis that could affect his ability to drive safely, his family doctor and neurologist failed to report this to the Registrar of Motor Vehicles. Although they argued that reporting was a matter of discretion, the court made clear that physicians owe the public a duty to report such drivers. In this case, the plaintiff was awarded $616,000 with 20 per cent liability assessed against the GP and 10 per cent against the neurologist.

Box 7.11

"We also think it is clear that the duty of doctors to report is a duty owed to members of the public and not just the patient. It is clearly designed to protect not only the patient but people he might harm if permitted to drive." [46]

The discretionary right of physicians to report unfit drivers in provinces like Alberta has recently come under attack. A tragic incident in 2012, where a driver with a known seizure disorder drove into a school, killing an 11-year-old child and severely injuring two others, prompted a fatality inquiry. The justice who carried out the inquiry noted the reluctance of physicians to report unfit drivers. He advised "mandatory reporting" and recommended backup mechanisms to assist with such reporting, acknowledging the burden such an obligation puts on physicians. Suggested mechanisms included automatic notification when patients are put on certain medications or diagnosed with specific conditions [47].

To report a patient can be very challenging; physicians typically do not relish doing this [48]. Reporting patients as unfit to drive may remove one of the last vestiges of their independence. Such a report can permanently compromise the doctor–patient relationship [48, 49]. That said, regardless of the law, physicians do have an ethical obligation to look out for the safety not only of their patients, but also of the public. The principle of autonomy does not give people the right to run over others.

When reporting unfit drivers, physicians are advised to communicate directly with their patients about this decision. It is a sign of respect for patients to explain the rationale for this decision and the statutory obligations for such reporting. It is also important to communicate with other treating physicians about such concerns.

The situation is further complicated by the lack of clear criteria for identifying unfit drivers. Seizure disorders and other obvious neurological conditions represent fairly straightforward situations. But exactly when a patient's arthritis or cognitive impairment reaches a level where driving is unsafe is by no means straightforward. What about the use of sedatives? Prescription analgesics? Antidepressants? The Canadian Medical Association publishes a comprehensive guide to assessing fitness to drive [50]. There are other tools to aid physicians, such as the "Screen for the Identification of Cognitively Impaired Medically at Risk Drivers" (SIMARD) test, but none are entirely reliable. Healthcare professionals may also want to check out the "Driving and Dementia Toolkit" developed by the Regional Geriatric Program of Eastern Ontario and the Champlain Dementia Network [51].

5. Flying, train, and marine safety

Physicians and optometrists are similarly required by the federal *Aeronautics Act* to report pilots and air traffic controllers if they have conditions that might affect flight safety [52]. In addition, the *Railway Safety Act* requires them to report individuals in positions critical to railway safety who may be unable to perform their duties [53]. Merchant seamen may also be required to undergo medical examinations with mandatory submission of a report by the examining physician [54].

6. Fitness to work

A physician may be asked by an employer to report on a patient's fitness to return to work. The specific medical conditions of the patient do not have to be identified and ought not to be without the patient's consent. More complicated situations arise where a physician acts as a "third party" examiner, such as for an insurance company requesting an independent medical examination of one of their clients. In Canada, the Canadian Medical Protective Association reminds its members to obtain express written consent from patients when carrying out a "third party" assessment and to take care "not to disclose more information than is covered by the patient's authorization".[55]

Even if the examination is done for third-party purposes, any suspicious or unanticipated findings with consequences for the patient's welfare must be disclosed to the patient and, with their consent, to their own family doctor[56]. It is not always clear what to do with a patient who refuses to permit disclosure to the employer of a condition that might constitute a grave danger to others at work. In cases of serious and foreseeable harm to others, especially if imminent, physicians are obliged to breach confidentiality.

Case 7.6 A Pain In The Butt

You are working a shift in the ER one night when 24-year-old Mr J comes in under his own power complaining he has a bullet in his buttocks. He relates a somewhat unlikely story about throwing some bullets into a campfire, causing one to ignite and hit him. Sure enough, when you examine him, there is a small entrance wound in his right buttock. An X-ray shows fragments of a bullet in the pelvic tissues. A police officer loitering around the front desk approaches you to ask if you are treating a patient with a gunshot wound sustained in a crime that evening.

What should you tell the officer?

---

7. Gunshot and stab wounds

In 2005, Ontario introduced the *Mandatory Gunshot Wounds Reporting Act*. Over the subsequent decade, seven more provinces and one territory introduced similar legislation. Some jurisdictions include stab wounds, and some require emergency medical personnel, such as paramedics, to do the reporting[57]. Similar legislation has been introduced in most American states as well.

While these laws differ in various small ways, they are generally consistent in not imposing an obligation to keep the patient at the facility until the police come. Moreover, releasing to the police any information other than that mandated by an act could be considered a breach of confidentiality. For example, there is no requirement to disclose anything the patient may have said regarding how they sustained the injury. It is also important to note that these acts typically do not mandate that *physicians* themselves report gunshot wounds—only that the facility must do so. Frequently a nurse or administrative clerk is designated to make this report. Such laws are an attempt to balance public safety with law enforcement, without making healthcare providers an arm of the law [57]. This duty to report has generated some concern that people so injured may not seek treatment. In fact, experience with other mandatory reporting laws have not shown any significant fall-off in medical attendance of those affected by those laws [58, 59]. Needless to say, healthcare professionals need to be aware of their local laws and regulations as regards this issue.

Discussion of Case 7.6

Regardless of how much you may wish to discuss the case with the police officer, it is not appropriate to do so (unless he has a warrant). You should politely indicate that you are obliged for professional and legal reasons to respect the confidentiality of your patients. You might then check with the charge nurse to ensure that the appropriate notification under the mandatory reporting act has been made.

---

8. "Management of the healthcare system"

Numerous other aspects of medical care may require mandatory notification. Requirements vary from province to province but, in general, physicians must disclose births, stillbirths, and deaths they attend or of which they are aware. Certain deaths—ones that are unexpected, suspicious, or occur in unusual circumstances—require prompt reports to medicolegal death investigators, such as the coroner or the local medical examiner (see Box 7.12) [60]. Healthcare fraud, loss or theft of narcotics, and termination of the employment of a healthcare professional for reasons of incompetence or incapacity must also be disclosed to the proper authorities.

Box 7.12

The following types of death usually require notification of a medical examiner:

- death resulting from violence, negligence, or malpractice;
- death by "unfair means" ("suspicious deaths");
- death related to parturition and childbirth;
- death that are sudden and unexpected;
- death from illness not treated by a legally qualified medical practitioner;
- death from any cause other than disease; and
- death under circumstances that may require investigation.

9. Certain criminal activities

It is sometimes asked whether there is a duty to report *past* crimes committed by a patient. The answer must be an unequivocal "it depends." Doctors, in general, have no duty to disclose crimes their patients may have committed [61]. New legislation in many jurisdictions requires practitioners of medicine—and indeed other members of the public generally—to report those who may be involved with terrorism. There is some concern that the *Patriot Act* in the US allows authorities to seize medical records without a warrant and forbids physicians from disclosing this [62]. No such equivalent legislation applies in Canada. However, a Supreme Court of Canada decision in late 2018 involving protection of confidential sources in the media may have implications for physician–patient confidentiality in a Canadian context. In a case concerned with domestic terrorism, the SCC ruled unanimously that the promise of privacy between a reporter and their sources could be overruled when public safety was at stake [63].

It is a different matter if the concern is about future serious crimes, however, as the following case illustrates.

Smith v Jones

A precedent to breach the duty of confidentiality was set in Canada in *Smith v Jones*. Dr Smith, a psychiatrist, was retained by defence counsel to examine a client who had been charged with aggravated assault of a prostitute [64]. The lawyer indicated to the accused that anything he said during the consultation would be privileged.

During the interview with the psychiatrist, the defendant described in some detail an extreme paraphilia characterized by sexually sadistic fantasies and plans to kidnap, rape, and kill prostitutes. The psychiatrist informed the defence lawyer he believed his client was dangerous and likely to commit future offences unless he received proper treatment. Subsequently entering a plea of guilty to the assault charge, the accused received a minimal jail term.

Upon discovering his concerns about the defendant's past and future dangerousness would not be addressed in the sentencing hearing, the psychiatrist sought to disclose his concerns to the courts, in the interests of public safety. The trial judge ruled the psychiatrist should be mandated to breach confidentiality because of a clear, serious, and imminent threat to an identifiable group of persons. The matter was eventually heard by the Supreme Court of Canada. The justices allowed a public safety exception to the "privileged" relationship between solicitor and client that normally prevents evidence from defence counsel from being used against the defendant. While the exception to privilege in *Smith v Jones* involved solicitor–client confidentiality (since technically Dr. Smith was retained by the plaintiff's legal counsel), it clearly had ramifications for confidentiality as it pertains to physicians and patients [65].

Forty years ago, a jurist sagely observed, "No patient has the moral right to convince his psychiatrist that he is going to commit a crime and then expect him to do nothing because of the principle of confidentiality" [66]. Clearly, a judgment of proportionality must be made here: minor crimes are one thing, but confinement, torture, rape, and murder are another.

V. To Warn and Protect

In cases of patients who are a current or future danger to *others*, there is a widely recognized legal concept of a "duty to warn" which overrides the duty of confidentiality. Although this phrase is frequently used, it is not an actual legal duty in Canada. Rather, the breaching of confidentiality by physicians to protect others is not mandated, but "permitted" by law [11]. Many of the provincial health information acts now include provisions permitting physicians the discretion to breach confidentiality in the interests of individual or public safety.

The most influential case pertaining to this issue was that of *Tarasoff* in the United States. In 1969, Mr Poddar told his university psychologist of his intention to kill a former girlfriend, Tatiana Tarasoff. Concerned, the psychologist and his supervising psychiatrist asked the campus police to detain him but he was released when he appeared rational and promised to stay away from her. Two months later, Mr Poddar, who had not returned for therapy, murdered Ms Tarasoff. Because no one had warned the victim of her peril, the California Supreme Court found the two most responsible parties to be the psychologist and the university. They were considered negligent in failing to warn Ms Tarasoff [67].

The court weighed the importance of protecting Mr Poddar's privacy but concluded that this must take second place to "the public interest in safety from violent assault. The protective privilege ends where the public peril begins." According to this ruling, if there is a real hazard to an individual or the community and no other way of relieving this hazard, the patient–therapist confidentiality rule must yield to the interests of safety.

In another US ruling on *Tarasoff* ("*Tarasoff II*"), the court reaffirmed its view that medical professionals ought to err on the side of public safety when it comes to dangerous patients, despite the possible negative implications for privacy: "The risk that unnecessary warnings may be given is a reasonable price to pay for the lives of possible victims that may be saved" [68]. *Tarasoff II* expanded the onus on therapists from a duty to warn to a duty to protect (such as notifying the police or having the patient apprehended for a psychiatric evaluation). Since *Tarasoff,* many US jurisdictions have introduced variations of so-called Tarasoff statutes which impose either a duty or permit physicians to breach confidentiality in the interests of safety [69].

In a Canadian context, the case of Colin McGregor in 1991 strongly influenced how physicians and the public view confidentiality and protection of the public. Following his separation from his wife, Patricia Allen, McGregor stalked her, eventually shooting her to death with a crossbow. It was subsequently revealed that he had, six weeks earlier, informed his psychiatrist of his intention to murder his wife. His psychiatrist took no action to warn Ms Allen or the authorities, citing the Canadian Medical Association Code of Ethics at that time. This case provoked considerable reflection on the part of Canadian psychiatrists as to their duty and right to breach confidentiality and inform persons at risk [70, 71]. A consensus panel, in part funded by the estate of Ms Allen, made recommendations in 1998 regarding the duty to warn for the medical profession.

The limits to confidentiality outlined here may seem morally reasonable but they are not universal. Regardless of the laws surrounding a duty to warn, there will undoubtedly be ambiguous situations, and each physician will have to decide based on their own moral compass.

Box 7.13

A summary of "Duty to Warn" in Canada:

- It is not a true "duty" but rather permission to breach confidentiality in the interests of protecting an individual or group.
- The threat should be to an identifiable person or group.
- The severity of the threat should be grave bodily harm or death.
- The time frame for the threat should be within the foreseeable future (for example, not in 20 years). [11, 65]

Box 7.14

"Privacy legislation generally allows doctors to disclose an individual's personal health information without consent to avert an imminent risk of serious bodily harm to an identifiable person or group." [72]

Conclusion

Confidentiality is far from a decrepit concept, as Mark Siegler suggested [2]. It remains a core value and component of patient autonomy and respect for persons. The complexity of ethical and legal dilemmas to which it gives rise is a testament to its ongoing relevance and importance. It is defended on many fronts, from regulatory authorities, the courts, legislators, and commissioners for privacy. When confidentiality and privacy are breached, patients' autonomy and their trust in medicine and authorities generally are undermined. They can feel as violated as if their dwelling were burglarized or intimate promises broken. Regardless of the limits and challenges to patient–physician confidentiality, it remains one of the core ethical values for all physicians and is not going away any time soon.

Cases for Discussion

Case 1: False Conviction

You are a family physician working in an inner-city drug rehabilitation clinic one day a week. One of your patients, Mr H, admits to you that he has committed numerous robberies over the years to support his drug use. He even confesses that the police have mistakenly convicted another man for one of his robberies.

Questions for Discussion
1. Does this situation justify breaching patient confidentiality?
2. What would you do?

Case 2: It's A Small World

You are a second-year dermatology resident attending this week's Grand Rounds presented by one of your fellow residents. The patient, identified as Ms J, is described as a 23-year-old drug addict who has had multiple sex partners. A photograph of the lesion on her back is presented on the screen. To your great surprise, you recognize the tattoo and realize Ms J is one of your younger sister's best friends.

Questions for Discussion
1. As Ms J's name has been anonymized, is there a breach of confidentiality in this case?
2. Using ethical principles, discuss why or why not consent needs to be obtained to use patient information for teaching purposes.

The Waning and Waxing Self

Capacity and Incapacity in Medical Care

The policy of the law is that where a person, due to mental illness, lacks the capacity to make a sound and considered decision on treatment, the person should not for that reason be denied access to medical treatment that can improve functioning and alleviate suffering.

Former Chief Justice McLachlin, 2003 [1]

This chapter will examine the healthcare professional's complex responsibilities regarding the care of incapable patients—whether they are elderly, young, or in-between. The duty to provide effective medical care and protect vulnerable individuals from harm must be balanced against respecting the right of competent persons to make their own decisions, even if these are considered "bad" choices. Challenges exist in deciding who needs protection from themselves and how far a clinician and others can go in protecting patients with diminished or impaired capacity.

I. Incapacity and Its Discontents

Case 8.1 "Talk to Me, Not My Daughter!"

Ms Q, an 87-year-old woman from Russia with advanced Parkinson's disease living in a nursing home, is suffering from visual hallucinations. Her cognitive function is otherwise normal. She is assessed by Dr P, a geriatric psychiatrist, who advises a trial of a new antipsychotic medication to help control her distressing symptoms. Dr P explains there is a chance the medication could worsen her Parkinson's symptoms, but Ms Q is keen to try something. After

continued

discussing the recommendation with her attending physician, Dr P orders the medication.

As is common in many nursing homes, relatives are routinely asked about any medication changes. When Ms Q's daughter is contacted, however, she refuses to allow this new drug, expressing concerns about over-medication of her mother. When the psychiatrist returns the next month, he discovers the new antipsychotic has never been given.

Should Ms Q's daughter be making medical decisions for her?

Discussion of Case 8.1

When told why she did not get the medication, Ms Q responds angrily, "What's my daughter got to do with it? It's my decision. If I get side effects, I'll let you know!"

Indeed, she is right to be upset, as she is quite capable of making her own treatment decisions. Ms Q might be old and infirm, but this does not mean she lacks the capacity to make an informed choice about the treatment of her hallucinations. This is not an uncommon phenomenon in nursing homes, where elderly, frail patients are frequently presumed to be lacking decisional capacity.

With Ms Q's permission, Dr P makes a courtesy call to her daughter and explains the reasons for the medication and her mother's capacity to decide for herself. After some discussion, the daughter agrees a trial of medication seems reasonable.

Capacity and competency

Traditionally, the terms "capacity" and "competency" are distinguished based on their use in clinical and legal contexts. Capacity refers to clinical judgments about an individual's ability to understand and process information. Competency refers to a legal judgment. Thus, a patient found lacking in capacity by a physician may be referred to the courts for a competency hearing. This distinction notwithstanding, many experts in the field use these terms interchangeably—and we will do so as well [2, 3].

Box 8.1

Competence is not a diagnosis but an assessment of functional capacity.

Competencies, not competence

The capacity to make decisions is at the foundation of all patient autonomy in medicine. In the past, capacity to make healthcare decisions was often understood as an either/or phenomenon, usually based on an individual's diagnosis (for example, dementia, Down syndrome, schizophrenia). However, decisional capacity is more complex than this. For one, not everyone with the same diagnosis (such as dementia) has the same degree of impairment. Capacity may also wax and wane or be partly reversible with treatment. In addition, not all decisions require the same degree of decisional capacity. The capacity to consent to a flu shot is very different from the capacity to consent to open-heart surgery. Competency to make medical decisions is highly time- and context-specific [4]. For these reasons, mental capacity is best construed as a set of "functional capacities" an individual must possess in order to make specific decisions [4,5].

Box 8.2

....

"The competence to decide is therefore relative to the particular decision to be made." [6]

The presumption of competency (sort of)

An adult person is presumed to be competent to make decisions about care, unless there are reasonable grounds to suspect otherwise. The onus is on others to prove incapacity. This is the precedent in common law and codified in various statutes [3].

The presumption of competency notwithstanding, there is actually a large group of individuals in society for whom, in practice, the converse applies: they are presumed lacking in capacity, unless otherwise demonstrated. This is the case for certain disabled people, for children, for some whose first language is not English, and even for many elderly people living in long-term care homes (as in Case 8.1). In most of these circumstances, there is no malicious intent on the part of those involved, but the assumption of incompetence is frequently based on stereotypes of and prejudice towards these groups. Furthermore, it can be difficult for those without considerable resources (intellectual, financial, and social) to challenge these assumptions and to demonstrate their competency to make their own decisions [3,7].

Causes and prevalence of incapacity

One of the main tasks for healthcare professionals in dealing with cognitive incapacity is the heterogeneity of the etiologies and degrees of incompetence. Incapacity may be due to dementia of the Alzheimer's variety or other neurologic conditions (such as Huntington's or Parkinson's). It may be a result of cerebrovascular disease, trauma (acute or chronic), hydrocephalus, infections (such as HIV, Creutzfeldt-Jakob disease, neurosyphilis), kidney failure, liver disease, hypothyroidism, and more. Incapacity may be related to drug use or acute illness. It may be secondary to mental illness (schizophrenia, bipolar disorder, depression), or immaturity (that is, children). It may be congenital (Down syndrome). Loss of capacity may be temporary or permanent, reversible with medications or made worse with them. It may be progressive or stable, and it may wax and wane daily.

Surveys have shown that incapacity is extremely common but frequently unrecognized in acute-care hospitalized adult patients [8]. The authors of one study estimated that, overall, 40 per cent of hospitalized patients lacked "decisional capacity" as it related to their treatment. More important, however, was the finding that of 50 patients who underwent specific cognitive testing and were deemed lacking in decisional capacity, only 12 (24 per cent) were identified by the clinical team as lacking in capacity [9]. Other studies have similarly confirmed that decisional capacity is frequently not recognized by physicians [10]. While doctors may overestimate the actual functional capacity of their patients, they may also underestimate the enabling measures (such as decision aids, or translators) that could help patients to be more capable and self-directing.

II. Assessing Capacity

The goal of most capacity assessments is to establish whether an individual is capable of making decisions, whether financial, medical, legal, or other. In the context of healthcare, such assessments usually deal with whether a person is capable of making a specific decision about their own medical treatment.

Case 8.2   A Questionable Consent

Mr G is a 44-year-old man with a long history of less than optimally treated schizophrenia. He presents to the emergency room with a comminuted fracture of his left arm. His injury and the surgery proposed to correct it are explained to him by the orthopaedic resident on duty. Willing to have surgery, Mr G provides consent to the resident, but is evasive in explaining how the injury happened. The surgery resident wonders if the patient's mental disorder obstructs him from giving valid consent. He pages the resident on call for Psychiatry to see the patient.

Should the on-call psychiatry resident see Mr G before his surgery?

Box 8.3

....

The two key questions for determining an individual's decision-making capacity:

1. Can the person understand the information that is relevant to making a decision about treatment?
2. Can the person appreciate the reasonably foreseeable consequences of their decision?

Most assessments of capacity take place informally in the context of a discussion with a patient. When a patient engages in a normal conversation with a physician about treatment and asks appropriate questions, then capacity is tacitly assumed. If, on the other hand, a patient appears excessively confused by the information, or asks strange or inappropriate questions, or declines treatment for apparently frivolous or cavalier reasons, then doubts about their decisional capacity may be raised and, due to this, a formal capacity assessment may be quite appropriate. The healthcare professional proposing the treatment should do this assessment, although, in complex or contested cases, others may need to be consulted.

It should be noted, however, that just because a patient declines a recommended treatment does not mean they are incapable or in need of a capacity assessment. Respecting an individual's autonomy means accepting their decisions, even if we think it is not in their best interests or may even result in death (see Chapter 4).

Tools to assess capacity

In a 2011 review of the topic, Sessums identified 19 instruments or tools for assessing capacity [10]. The very presence of such a large number of instruments reflects the challenges of assessing capacity.

When discussing the assessment of capacity, a few issues stand out:

1. Most instruments used to assess capacity assess cognitive ability and not necessarily specific decision-making capacity. These are distinct abilities [11].
2. Competency is a set of functional capacities and dependent on the specific issues at hand. No instrument is going to be able to cover every possible situation.
3. Capacity to make decisions is a complex, multi-dimensional phenomenon. Some subjectivity on the part of the assessor will be difficult to eliminate entirely.

4. The gold standard for validating these instruments is an expert or forensic psychiatrist. However, an old study from 1997 demonstrated a
   rate of agreement among five expert physicians to be no better than
   chance [2, 12].

Discussion of Case 8.2

It is usually refusals of treatment which trigger capacity assessments. In theory,
however, all patients with possible impairments of decision-making capacity
should have their capacity assessed, whether or not they disagree or agree
to a proposed treatment. But Mr G's mental disorder is not the most pressing
issue. What matters is whether he understands and appreciates the decision,
and whether his decision is freely made. If so, then his consent should be considered valid. The surgical resident's assessment of capacity in this case should
suffice, given the surgery service is the one proposing the treatment.

A request for a psychiatric consultation would be reasonable if the resident is uncertain about the patient's current ability to reason. Although the
surgery resident may be erring on the side of caution, it is better than blithely
assuming the patient is capable. Moreover, having Psychiatry see the patient
pre-operatively may facilitate post-operative management.

As it turns out, Mr G is delusional but not as regards the surgeons (whom
he feels are on his side) or the nature of his injury. Despite his psychiatric disorder, he is able to understand information about the surgery, weigh the risks
and benefits, and appreciate the foreseeable consequences of his decision. He
is considered competent to give consent for surgery.

III. Capacity and Consent

Capacity has been called "the gateway to medical decision-making." [13] cannot make informed or reliable decisions. Some findings that might call for a closer scrutiny of
an individual's capacity are

- confused or irrational thinking,
- inability to retain information,
- fluctuation in alertness, and
- obvious influence of drugs or alcohol.

Numerous authors have pointed out that in order for a person's decision to
be considered capable, there are four questions to ask. These are listed in Box 8.4.

> **Box 8.4**
>
> When assessing decision-making capacity, consider the following [2, 4, 5]:
>
> 1. Does the patient manifest a preference?
> 2. Is the patient capable of a factual understanding of the situation?
> 3. Does the patient appreciate the facts presented?
> 4. Can the patient use the information presented in a rational fashion to reach a decision?

Understanding, appreciation, and reasoning

Complexity of medical information, anxiety and stress due to illness, fear, the gulf in knowledge between physician and patient, and poor communication skills on the part of the physician, all have an impact on a person's apparent capacity. Less easy to assess are those patients able to recite the facts but whose reasoning is so clouded by strong emotions or delusions that they cannot truly appreciate the meaning of the facts in relation to themselves. Such impairment of mental faculties may be very subtle and require careful consideration. Some questions that may help in assessing a patient's understanding and appreciation are listed in Box 8.5.

> **Box 8.5**
>
> Questions to help in assessing understanding and appreciation:
>
> 1. What is your understanding of the problem right now?
> 2. What treatment has been proposed?
> 3. Are there any other options for you?
> 4. What is your understanding of the risks and benefits of treatment?
> 5. What might happen if you are not treated?
> 6. Why have you decided to proceed (or not to proceed) with treatment?
> 7. Do you feel hopeless? Or that you are being punished? Or that someone is trying to harm you? [2, 14, 15]

IV. Treating and Protecting the Vulnerable

Up to this point we have discussed issues that arise when competent adults lose their decision-making capacity. But there is also a significant population of individuals who have always been deemed lacking in decisional capacity because of a mental disability. Though they may be capable of participating in some medical decisions, they will frequently require medical decisions to be made for them over the long term. This group includes persons with congenital disabilities (such as Down syndrome) and acquired disabilities (for example, head injury).

Advance directives

Incapacity is sometimes considered to be an exception to the requirement of obtaining consent from a patient as regards medical treatment (see Chapter 6). Of course, it is not: incapacity requires the healthcare professional to search for an appropriate person—a substitute decision-maker—to speak on behalf of the incapable person. Living wills and advance directives are a recommended way for competent patients to try to ensure their future medical care will follow their preferences. These are discussed more fully in Chapter 15. A well-thought-out advance directive that has been thoroughly discussed with family may make it easier for families to let their ailing relative die "naturally," without technological encumbrances [16].

Who is the patient?

"The past," Karl Marx wrote, "weighs like a nightmare on the brain of the living" [17]. Indeed it can, especially for those brains transfixed by the past. The influence of the past on the present is all too often the new contested territory between families and healthcare professionals. The battle to refuse care having been won, the struggle has now become, for some, one of obtaining whatever care the patient wants or, purportedly, would have wanted. Many of us are re-born as we age—or at least we come to lead lives we could not have predicted. It is our families who often have the hardest time adapting to the "new self" and accepting "natural" limits to care. Not surprisingly, sick patients and their surrogates may misinterpret their condition and their future, seeing them in a rosier fashion than they actually are [18]. This may impair realistic assessments of the usefulness of aggressive care. Here is one such case.

In 1998 Mr Sawatzky was a 79-year-old resident of a nursing home with advanced Parkinson's disease and multiple other co-morbidities including previous strokes. These had resulted in severe cognitive impairment, limited communication, and difficulty swallowing. Despite a tracheostomy to protect his airway, he experienced repeated episodes of pneumonia. After one such bout, the treating physician decided Mr Sawatzky's condition was deteriorating such that he would not benefit from "calling a code" [19]. Previous attempts to write a No CPR order had been met with resistance from Mrs Sawatzky, who some clinicians felt had an unrealistic understanding of her husband's capabilities and limitations. The physician wrote the order in Mr Sawatzky's chart but did not discuss it with his wife.

Several months earlier, Mrs Sawatzky had refused consent for the tracheostomy, which led to the public trustee taking over as the substitute decision-maker for her husband. The public trustee was contacted by the physician about the No CPR order but declined to be involved, seeing this as having to do with "non-treatment" rather than active treatment. When Mrs Sawatzky eventually discovered such an order had been written, she sought and received a court ruling to block this [19].

In hindsight, there are aspects of this case's management that may have predicted the trip to court. First, there was a communication problem that was not resolved before the No CPR order was written. Second, why did the doctor think Mr Sawatzky could benefit from a tracheostomy then and *not* from CPR now? Did Mrs Sawatzky appreciate that the tracheostomy tube could prevent problems and maintain comfort whereas performing CPR would do neither? Third, it appears the No CPR order was written without input from other clinicians. Fourth, the order was not communicated to Mrs Sawatzky in a respectful way—she found out only after the fact, a circumstance that may have made the order appear untrustworthy. Had these issues been addressed, it is *possible* this trip to court could have been avoided. But there would have to be agreement that the question as to "*who* should make the decision?" should be replaced by "*how* will the decision be made?" This would require efforts on both sides to "talk it out" [20].

As it turned out, Mr Sawatzky was transferred to another institution where, presumably, his wife's wishes were accommodated.

V. Substitute and Assisted Decision-Making

The process of substitute decision-making for individuals who lack decisional capacity is highly variable depending on the circumstances of incapacity as well as the jurisdiction. In Ontario, for example, issues around consent and capacity are often dealt with by the Consent and Capacity Board. In other provinces, the courts or the office of the public guardian may deal with these issues. Who has decisional authority in a given situation can be very confusing, and healthcare providers should clarify the process in their own locations.

Substitute decision-makers

Regardless of jurisdiction, however, any citizen of sound mind has a right to designate a substitute decision-maker (SDM) who can make healthcare decisions on their behalf in the event they are not capable of doing so at some point in the future. An SDM is usually (although not necessarily) a close family member and may be stipulated in an advance directive (or Power of Attorney for Personal Care, depending on the jurisdiction) or be based on a hierarchy of relatives (see Box 8.6). Other terms frequently used synonymously with SDM are "agent," "surrogate," "healthcare representative," "proxy," and "attorney for personal care."

Box 8.6

A hierarchy of substitute decision-makers. In some jurisdictions family SDMs are preceded by court- or board-appointed patient representatives.

1. Spouse or adult interdependent partner (for example, common-law spouse, etc.)
2. Adult son or daughter (eldest, regardless of gender)*
3. Father or mother
4. Adult brother or sister (eldest, regardless of gender)*
5. Grandfather or grandmother
6. Adult grandson or granddaughter (eldest, regardless of gender)*
7. Adult uncle or aunt (eldest, regardless of gender)*
8. Adult nephew or niece (eldest, regardless of gender)*

*In some jurisdictions equally ranked family members (for example, siblings) must make decisions by consensus or, where they cannot agree, have disputes resolved by a public guardian or, in Ontario by the Consent and Capacity Board (CCB).

Case 8.3   Whose Life Is It Anyway?

Mrs F, a 78-year-old widow, had been living an active and full life before sustaining a subarachnoid hemorrhage as a result of a motor vehicle accident and lapsing into a coma. She is now intubated and ventilated in the ICU. She has an advance directive specifying her son, an evangelical minister, as her substitute decision-maker. Despite her son's religious affiliation, or perhaps because of it, she has instructed not to be kept alive "artificially if she will be unable to tend to her garden or enjoy walks in the forest." After six days in the ICU without improvement, her CAT brain scan and EEG are repeated, indicating severe brain injury with little chance of functional recovery.

When her physicians broach the topic of discontinuing life-sustaining measures, Mrs F's son adamantly refuses to consider any such actions. In fact, he insists that they implement tube feedings. Even when confronted with her express wishes in her advance directive, he rebuffs the ICU physicians, insisting, "She made me her substitute decision-maker, so I'll make the decisions as I see fit!"

What should the ICU physicians do?

Despite the authority given them, an SDM does not have *carte blanche* when making healthcare decisions for an individual. The SDM should be instructed to act in accordance with known wishes expressed by a patient when capable, or, in the absence of clear guidance from a patient, should make decisions consistent with the values and beliefs of the individual. If these wishes are not known, an SDM should act in the best interests of the patient. Physicians have an added duty to ensure an SDM is acting in accordance with these principles of substitute decision-making.

Discussion of Case 8.3

The legal and moral answer to this dilemma is quite straightforward. As her substitute decision-maker, Mrs F's son is obligated to act in accordance with her wishes, as expressed in her advance directive. It is clear that Mrs F would not want to be kept alive on life-support in this situation.

Although an advance directive is a valuable instrument, there can be considerable confusion if not carefully planned and executed. Mrs F may have made her wishes clear in her advance directive, but she presumably failed to adequately inform and instruct her son about her wishes and ensure that he would abide by them. For whatever reason—sometimes children are so attached to their parent they cannot "let go"—the son was letting his own needs take precedence over what his mother would have wanted.

The way out of this dilemma, as with many such cases, is usually with good communication and empathy. Compassionate discussion with her son about his mother's prognosis, as well as her previously expressed wishes, may solve the problem. Involving nurses, representatives from pastoral care, an ethics consultant, social workers, or a patient/family ombudsman office, may help the son recognize his duty as a substitute decision-maker. If, however, he continues to insist on aggressive care, it might be necessary for the ICU physicians and hospital counsel to pursue a legal remedy (such as, in Ontario, the Consent and Capacity Board or, in most jurisdictions, the courts). While this is always a distasteful option, the healthcare professionals' fiduciary duty is to Mrs F.

Assisting in decision-making

Just as we should not regard capacity as an "either/or" phenomenon, neither should we likewise regard the matter of substitute decision-making. Clearly, there is a role for a more nuanced approach to help patients with diminished or limited capacity in making healthcare decisions.

Several provinces have taken such initiatives by introducing categories of assisted decision-making. In addition to a *substitute decision-maker* or guardian, Alberta, for example, allows patients to designate someone as a *supported decision-maker* or as a *co-decision-maker*. A *supported decision-maker* is allowed access to the person's medical records and can help explain treatments. A *co-decision-maker* can help an adult with moderate impairment to make a decision. For example, someone with moderate dementia, who still retains some degree of decision-making capacity, may benefit from a co-decision-maker to help with significant decisions, such as whether to undergo surgery or change medications. Frequently this will be a spouse or child who has a close relationship with the person involved.

VI. Mental Illness and the Right to Refuse

Mental illness represents a unique challenge when it comes to decisional capacity. While some patients with mental illness may have profoundly disordered thought processes and clearly not be competent to make decisions, others may have an exceptional ability to retain, understand, and rationally manipulate information, but nonetheless lack insight into or appreciation of their situation (that is, anosognosia). Situations involving the latter type of individual represent some of the most challenging ethical dilemmas in medicine, as they exemplify the tension inherent in balancing respect for autonomy and protecting persons from harm.

Case 8.4 An Odiferous Condition

Ms M, a 56-year-old single woman who lives alone, presents to the emergency room complaining of a foul odour she cannot seem to escape. Complaining it follows her everywhere, she is convinced there is something wrong with her nose. When the ER physician, Dr S, enters the cubicle, the smell is overwhelming. She sees an obvious visible deformity beneath Ms M's clothing on her right chest. Examination reveals a 10 by 15 cm ulcerated mass in her right breast, the obvious source of the problem.

When asked about the breast mass, Ms M downplays it, reporting that it appeared a few weeks before, but denying it bothers her. It's the odour she can't stand. It is obvious she is in profound denial about a large, infected breast cancer. When her condition is explained to her, she expresses disbelief, declaring it's just a bruise and will get better on its own. She thanks Dr S, telling her she would like to go home.

How should the case of Ms M be managed?

The right to refuse

Respect for autonomy means healthcare professionals must respect the right of competent patients to refuse treatment, even when this does not appear to be in their best interests [21] (see Chapter 4). If a patient with a mental illness refuses treatment, this choice must be respected—as long as the patient is competent when they express it. And the presumption in law is that an adult is competent unless there is evidence to the contrary.

However, the professional duty of care for patients with reduced capacity is clear. One legal authority wrote some time ago: "As a general rule it may be accepted that a higher duty of care to avoid acts of negligence is owed to a person of unsound mind, than to a person of full capacity. The extent that the duty is increased must depend on the circumstances of the case and the nature of the incapacity" [22]. We take this to mean clinicians have to exercise particular caution in the care of patients who have impaired capacity and are unable to comprehend, and so authorize, the consequences of their decisions.

Discussion of Case 8.4

It is obvious Ms M does not appreciate the gravity of her situation. Believing the patient is clearly a risk to herself, Dr S consults the psychiatry service as well as the surgery and oncology services. Ms M is admitted against her wishes under a mental health admission certificate, on the basis of suffering from an as-yet-to-be-determined mental disorder and at significant risk of suffering substantial physical deterioration if not treated. When subsequent workup and evaluation confirm a large stage 3 breast cancer, she is advised to have surgery and chemotherapy. She appears to understand the recommendations, but remains ambivalent about undergoing treatment.

When the doctor asks Ms M directly for her consent, she initially hesitates, but then finally agrees to surgery and chemotherapy.

Allowing psychotic patients to refuse psychiatric treatment based on their prior wishes means patients who may pose a grave danger to others can be committed to an institution but not be treated, which in turn may result in their prolonged incarceration in a psychiatric facility. This "made no sense to psychiatrists," the American psychiatrist Paul Appelbaum has written [23]. These ideas, applied in practice, effectively turn psychiatrists into jailers. As well, allowing such patients greater freedom to refuse treatment may lead to more frequent use of restraints or solitary confinement, increased rates of assaults, and a greater deterioration in the clinical status of the untreated psychotic patient.

Respecting a psychiatric patient's prior wishes to refuse treatment may seem, in principle, no different than not transfusing a Jehovah's Witness patient dying from blood loss. But the logic behind treating psychotic patients is not simply to protect them as well as others, but also to try to restore their autonomy. Most psychotic patients are not a danger to others. Construing the "right to refuse" in this way, however, will potentially put psychotic patients who refuse medication at a much greater risk of suffering or serious harm, whether by accident, suicide, illness, or altercations with police.

Intelligence without insight: the case of *Starson v Swayze*

Another case illustrating the strong judicial protection of autonomy and presumption of capacity is the story of Scott Schutzman. Having changed his name to simply Starson (no first name), he insisted on being referred to as "Professor Starson" (although not actually a professor). Described variously as a brilliant autodidact in physics and as a troubled individual with bipolar or schizoaffective disorder, Starson had been in and out of psychiatric hospitals for over 25 years because of his propensity to make death threats and appear menacing to others.

In the late 1990s he was admitted involuntarily to a psychiatric facility in Ontario after uttering death threats during an altercation with a landlord and found "not guilty by reason of mental defect." When he refused antipsychotic medications, complaining they interfered with his ability to pursue physics (they "dulled his mind and reduced his creativity"), his psychiatrists felt he lacked decisional capacity and sought judicial leave to treat him against his will. This was taken to the Supreme Court of Canada, which ultimately found in favour of Starson (six votes to three) and against the judgments of lower-level tribunals.

At the heart of this case was the issue of whether Starson was competent to refuse treatment. Central to finding someone capable is the requirement that the person acknowledge their illness and how treatment will impact them (the "appreciation" test discussed above). Although Starson persistently denied that he suffered from a mental illness, he did admit that he had some "mental problems" and was "different." The Supreme Court found his admission that he was "different" was sufficient evidence he was capable. It was not necessary that he acknowledge he had a serious mental illness. While denial of illness on its own is not evidence of incapacity, it should be taken into account along with other symptoms a patient may exhibit (such as delusional thinking, hallucinations, and threatening behaviours).

The Supreme Court's view that self-admission of "difference" is sufficient acknowledgement of a mental disorder is a very low bar indeed. Denial of mental illness is common in those with disorders of the mind. "Roughly half of patients with active psychotic illness are thought to have anosognosia—no insight into their disease" [24]. How could a refusal of treatment based on Starson's view of his situation be considered informed? As one legal scholar commented, "If you do not believe you are ill, it would never make sense to take these powerful brain-altering medications" [25]. A robust dissent by then Chief Justice McLachlin argued that "[o]ne cannot appreciate the benefits of treatment unless one understands and appreciates the need for treatment" [1].

Only after further significant deterioration was Starson eventually treated with the approval of his mother, his SDM. He was readmitted several times as an involuntary patient, each time refusing medications. Since 2013, Starson has been living in the community after being conditionally discharged from the criminal justice system. The conditions of his discharge require that he remain on his anti-psychotic medications and check in weekly with his psychiatric team. According to news reports, he remains grandiosely delusional and still denies any psychiatric illness [26].

Starson illustrates the sometimes-tragic consequences inherent in trying to balance respect for autonomy with the state's obligation to protect vulnerable persons who cannot protect themselves. Patients may end up "warehoused" because they do not receive treatment for their conditions. Or they eventually deteriorate, until finally there is legal justification to intervene.

Empirical studies from the United States suggest that only a small percentage of patients refuse their psychiatric medications (less than 10 per cent on most wards, but up to 75 per cent on forensic units, where the patients may be trying to avoid being jailed) [2]. One reason the numbers remain small is that difficult patients who refuse treatment may be discharged early to "roam the streets," even though they are "just as ill" as before [2]. When denied appropriate treatment, the homeless and psychiatrically ill often face a harsh and cruel reality [27]—one which does not provide much protection for this vulnerable population [28]. This is hardly a triumph of autonomy; it is, more the triumph of *anomie*.

Limits on the right to refuse?

It is not yet clear what this Canadian judicial recognition of an involuntary patient's right of treatment refusal will mean in the long term. In the United States, although committed patients may refuse their treatment, most get it anyway [29]. Their refusals are usually overridden by review boards or courts that accept the physician's view of appropriateness.

In Canada, there is federal legislation allowing the courts to order treatment of the mentally unfit accused so that they may come to trial [30]. Thus, there are other social interests—such as the administration of justice—that limit a patient's right to refuse treatment in specific circumstances. Finally, "community treatment orders" are a less restrictive therapeutic option for patients with a persistent and serious mental disorder [31]. Such orders allow patients to remain in the community so long as they take their medications. This kind of mandatory outpatient treatment order is now found in many jurisdictions [32].

VII. Children's Right to Refuse

Children represent a unique category in the discussion of decisional capacity. Their capacity to make decisions is based primarily on their degree of maturity. Moreover, where children are involved, there is an intrinsic sense that the stakes are higher and the duty to ensure that their best interests are followed seems even more critical. This may be because adults view minors as inherently more vulnerable—in the "baseball game of life," it seems more heartbreaking if there is disruption in the first few innings.

The "mature minor" doctrine

There is no formal age of consent in Canada except in Quebec, where under the Civil Code the age of consent is 14 years [33]. In all other provinces and territories, the ability of a child to consent is determined by their maturity, not chronological age. Age still plays a role, however. Depending on the specific jurisdiction, a person under 18 or 19 (the so-called "age of majority") is considered a minor, and generally presumed *not* capable of consenting, unless deemed mature enough to do so by a physician or other healthcare worker [34]. Within the context of common law, this is referred to as the "mature minor doctrine" [3]. The question as to whether confidentiality applies to mature minors remains unclear, since it often falls under other legislative initiatives and jurisdictions [35].

The general approach in practice, when obtaining consent to treat adolescent children, is to assume they are capable. As with adults, they must have the emotional maturity and intelligence to understand the nature and purpose of the proposed treatment and appreciate the reasonably foreseeable consequences of such treatment. (Indeed, even young children may have the wherewithal to make very complex medical decisions [36].) Such determinations are usually made informally and on a case-by-case basis [37].

The 1985 British case of *Gillick v West Norfolk* is frequently cited as the seminal case in common law establishing children's rights to make medical decisions for themselves. In this case involving the prescription of birth control to girls under 16 years of age, the United Kingdom's House of Lords asserted, "As a matter of Law the parental right to determine whether or not their minor child below the age of sixteen will have medical treatment terminates if and when the child achieves sufficient understanding and intelligence to understand fully what is proposed" [38].

Box 8.7

The mature minor doctrine: A mature minor is a person under the age of majority (18 or 19), who has been assessed and deemed as having the intelligence and maturity to appreciate the nature, risks, benefits, consequences, and alternatives of a proposed treatment, including the ethical, emotional, and physical aspects of the disease.

Minors and refusal of life-sustaining treatment

If the mature minor doctrine means children can consent to medical treatment that is commensurate with their level of maturity, then it would follow they should also be able to refuse medical treatment. This latter situation poses unique problems. When these cases have come to courts in Canada, outcomes have been inconsistent. Most of these cases tend to involve adolescents who are Jehovah's Witnesses (JW) refusing blood products. (Healthcare professionals should not assume, however, that all JW members would not want blood products—some do despite church doctrine [39]. Clinicians should speak to any JW patient on their own to assess their adherence to this doctrine.)

A 1985 Ontario case involving a 12-year-old girl with acute myeloid leukemia who refused blood transfusions on religious grounds was argued in the Ontario Provincial Court. Although there were many factors influencing the case, the court ultimately ruled that she could decline blood products, as she had "wisdom and maturity well beyond her years" and possessed "a well-thought-out, firm and clear religious belief." In the eyes of the court, the hospital's proposed treatment dealt with the disease in a physical sense only and failed "to address her emotional needs and religious beliefs." She died two weeks later [40, 41].

Another case dealing with an adolescent's refusal of blood products took place in New Brunswick, Canada, in 1994. Joshua Walker, a 15-year-old Jehovah's Witness with acute leukemia, was also allowed to refuse life-sustaining transfusions. The Court of Appeal found him to be competent and therefore able to be the author of his own actions. In his case, the chemotherapy was modified, and he was able to successfully complete treatment without need for transfusions [42, 43].

After 1996, the courts in Canada appeared less accepting of adolescents refusing treatment for life-and-death matters [44]. The 2002 case of Bethany Hughes, a 16-year-old Jehovah's Witness in Alberta, is a case in point. Suffering from acute myelogenous leukemia, she refused blood transfusions on the basis of her religious beliefs. Although she was deemed a mature minor based on her level of maturity and understanding, the court found her decision to be "non-voluntary," as she was considered to be under the "undue influence" of her JW mother [45]. The judge was not alone in this sentiment, as several authors have pointed out the coercive elements involved in the Jehovah's Witnesses' refusal of blood products [39, 46]. Despite receiving multiple transfusions against her will, Bethany Hughes died from her disease in 2002.

While the issue remains incompletely resolved, a ruling of the Supreme Court of Canada in 2009 seems to have it both ways. In another Jehovah's Witness case involving blood transfusion, the SCC acknowledged that adolescents with mature judgment should be allowed to make decisions about their healthcare but, at the same time, that there is a role for the state to retain "an overarching power to determine whether allowing the child to exercise his or her autonomy in a given situation actually accords with his or her best interests" [3, 47].

The case of Makayla Sault

Makayla Sault was an 11-year-old Indigenous girl diagnosed in 2014 with acute lymphoblastic leukemia, a form of childhood cancer which, in her situation, had an approximately 70 per cent chance of cure. She underwent an initial 11-week course of induction chemotherapy that left her debilitated and in the ICU for part of that time.

During her recovery from this first course of chemotherapy, she wrote a letter to her doctors explaining she had experienced a vision of Jesus telling her she was cured [48]. With the prospect of two more years of similar treatment, she begged her parents to let her stop the chemotherapy. She declared she did not want to die in a hospital on chemotherapy, which she described as "killing" her. Instead, she wanted to pursue traditional Indigenous approaches to healing. Remarkably poised and self-possessed, Makayla appeared in videos and on TV several times making her case. Her parents, both pastors, supported her choice.

The local children's services agency was notified with the general expectation that they would intervene and apprehend her. They ultimately opted to respect the decision of Makayla and her family. They concluded that Makayla was not a child in need of protection—her parents were not felt to be manipulating her nor were they mistreating her—and that the decision to pursue traditional Indigenous healing was within her rights as an Indigenous citizen [49, 50]. In the wake of the Truth and Reconciliation Commission's inquiry into residential schools in Canada, there was also undoubtedly some degree of political expediency in their decision. The optics of a government-run institution once again removing an Indigenous child from her home was, to say the least, distasteful.

But there is more to Makayla's story. She made a very compelling argument for being allowed to refuse further treatment. Despite her initial assertion about being cured, she later acknowledged she would probably die without treatment. But she asserted she was not afraid to die; her belief in Jesus allowed her to accept her eventual fate as his plan. Much of the time she seemed more composed, mature, and insightful than the adults around her. Moreover, the thought of treating her with extremely toxic chemotherapy for a prolonged period, and with no guarantee of success—against her, her family's, and her community's will—well, that was not an easy decision [51].

Makayla's story, unfortunately, did not have a happy ending. After discontinuing chemotherapy, she and her family sought "nutritional counselling" at a controversial clinic in Florida. Approximately nine months after stopping chemotherapy, Makayla died from a stroke related to her leukemia [52]. Her family claimed this was a result of the chemotherapy she had received the year before [53].

One very similar final case functions as a postscript to Makayla's story. Another 11-year-old Indigenous girl from the same area, JJ (who cannot otherwise be identified), diagnosed with the same disease, was started on chemotherapy about six months after Makayla was treated in 2014. About 10 days after the start of her treatment, she also chose to discontinue chemotherapy, with her family taking her to the same Florida clinic Makayla had visited. The children's services agency that had ruled in the Makayla case reached a similar decision in JJ's case and affirmed its respect for Indigenous rights to pursue traditional healing.

In contrast to Makayla's case, the physicians involved asked the court to intervene in this case, but it declined [54]. Interestingly, however, about five months after declining to intervene, the court issued a "clarification" statement, affirming that the best interests of the child remain paramount, while simultaneously upholding the right of Indigenous peoples to use traditional medicine [55, 56]. It was also revealed that JJ had restarted treatment with chemotherapy the month before, about two months after Makayla had died from her disease. It appears JJ successfully completed her treatment and remains in remission.

Conclusion

Capacity is an essential element of autonomy [13]. Without mental capacity, there really is no autonomous choice. At the heart of all discussion involving capacity and choice is the attempt to balance respect for the individual's right to govern their own life with the obligations of healthcare workers to help them avoid foreseeable harm. This is not an easy balance to maintain. Protecting people with diminished capacity, whether due to dementia, congenital disorders, mental maladies, or immaturity, while simultaneously respecting their right to choose, highlights a constant tension, an essential challenge for healthcare professionals. It challenges all of us to be tolerant, respectful, and open-minded. In the next chapter we will explore the issue of what it means to help patients.

Cases for Discussion

Case 1: A Refusal to Eat

Ms C is a 58-year-old woman with an unremarkable medical history who was apparently well until she stopped eating approximately three weeks ago. She had worked as an accountant until the birth of her children, now 21 and 25 years old. Both parents are deceased, her father having died in a farming accident when she was a child and her mother in her late 50s due to a rapidly progressive dementia. Ms C has repeatedly said she does not want to die as her mother did, in a nursing home, incontinent, lacking in dignity. "Better to die with your boots on," she has told her family.

Ms C is now quite ill. She is dehydrated and her electrolytes are out of whack. She seems unconcerned but looks pale and seems withdrawn. She

continued

explains she would like to eat but cannot, due to an upset digestive system. She plays with her food and says she'll maybe eat tomorrow if her stomach feels better. "I need to cleanse out my intestines and liver," she says to the nurse looking after her. She says she's done this before and does not believe she will die. She refuses any artificial hydration and nutrition, specifically, an IV and nasogastric tube. She wants to go home. Her husband is not much help. "She's stubborn, all right. She'll do whatever she needs to do," he asserts, and shrugs in an offhand way. "I think we'd best go home," he adds.

Questions for Discussion
1. Why might Ms C be refusing nutrition?
2. Do you think she is an autonomous person?
3. If you feel Ms C is not competent, would you go along with her husband's decision to take her home?

Case 2: A Refusal Of Medication

Mr M, a 26-year-old male living with his parents in a small agricultural town, was diagnosed with paranoid schizophrenia a number of years ago. He is often aggressive, and does not trust his parents or doctor. He says the prescribed medicines make him "mad." Mr M stopped taking them two months ago and resists all attempts by his parents to take him to see his psychiatrist. While on medication he was able to work, but now he has spent the last six weeks wandering around the town and returning home to sleep when he feels tired. His mother is worried he will be assaulted or jailed if he becomes aggressive. She confides her fears to her son's doctor, and is advised to give him an antipsychotic mixed in his coffee. She takes this advice, with the result her son quiets down and starts working again. Every time Mr M's parents bring up the subject of his treatment he shouts he will run away from them if he is forced to take pills again. His mother continues her deception, concealing his medicines in his coffee or other food.

Questions for Discussion
1. Is Mr M's refusal of pills a capable one?
2. Was his doctor's advice appropriate?
3. Can you foresee any problems with the mother's actions?
4. Does this kind of situation occur elsewhere?

♦ 9 ♦

Helping and Not Harming

Beneficence and Nonmaleficence

Regard your patients as human beings, while never forgetting they are your patients.

Michael Balint, 1959 [1]

Beneficence is the commitment of healthcare professionals to the well-being of their patients. Once a practitioner takes on an individual as a patient, that person is owed a special duty of care. For that duty to be fulfilled, the clinician is expected to meet the standard of a competent practitioner's care and skill in similar circumstances. However, beneficence in medicine involves more than competence in caring for one's own patients. It also entails commitments to respecting the values of patients and to professionalism (explored in Chapter 10). Beneficence requires knowing what it means to help and to harm patients, when to offer to help or "rescue" others, and when not to do so.

I. The Principles of Beneficence and Nonmaleficence

The Oath of Hippocrates directs physicians to use their skills to benefit patients and keep them from harm. The principles of nonmaleficence and beneficence are the oldest and most important guiding tenets of medicine. Codes of ethics for healthcare professionals frequently begin with the instruction to "[c]onsider first the well-being of the patient"[2] or some such similar sentiment.

Beneficence means doing good, showing active kindness, or assisting others in need. For the medical professions, helping others is not an option but a role-mandated requirement. Doctors never muse to themselves, "Hmm . . . shall I help my next patient get better or not?" The principle of "nonmaleficence" or "do no harm" expects health professionals to refrain from doing evil or making anyone ill[3]. At a minimum, by their interventions—meant to make people better or to prevent harms and setbacks to patient interests—health professionals try not to make patients worse off than they were before their interventions.

Case 9.1 No Surgery Wanted

You are a surgeon with an 81-year-old female patient, Ms R, who has just been diagnosed with pancreatic cancer, a malignancy usually leading to death within a year of diagnosis. Surgery is the only option that might prolong her life, but involves a risk of significant adverse effects (post-operative sepsis, delirium) and a risk of death from the surgery itself (intraoperative cardiac arrest, hemorrhage). Informed of the diagnosis and treatment options, Ms R explains she has always been terrified of surgery and adds that she feels she has lived a full life. She declines the surgery.

Should you accept Ms R's refusal of surgery?
What if Ms R was 35 years old with two young children, not yet school-aged?

The quality of care

In exercising the duty of beneficence, medical professionals are expected to offer only *proportionate* treatment—treatment where the likely good outweighs the risk of harm. But doing good for a patient often entails causing a degree of harm. A surgeon causes injury to remove a diseased organ; chemotherapy causes nausea, vomiting, and hair loss; CAT scans involve exposure to radiation. While we often presume we can make our decision by weighing the pros and cons of a given treatment, the truth is that the matter is more complex than just putting pros on one side of a scale and cons on the other. Each individual evaluates the benefits and harms of a given treatment with their own internal gauge. For some, loss of hair from chemo is a minor issue; for others, it is a life-changing event.

At the end of the day, the principle of beneficence is about working with patients to help them decide how they wish to proceed. Together, physicians (along with other professionals) take into account not only patient preferences but also quality-of-life issues for the patient. These are the issues that capability theorists, such as Sen and Nussbaum, prioritize, such as maintaining one's independence, the ability to relate to others, the capacity for happiness and satisfaction, and the capacity to maintain dignity and hope.

Box 9.1

....

While not exhaustive, the following list includes the major issues that the principle of beneficence requires healthcare professionals to consider:

- the patient's pain and suffering, both physical and mental;
- the standard of care, its attendant risks and benefits;
- the possibility of death and disability;
- the possibility of restoration of health and functional status;
- the patient's quality of life as seen from the patient's perspective; and
- the patient's expectations regarding treatment.

The patient's views

Just how these outcomes should be weighed against quality-of-life factors will depend ultimately on a patient's personal values. What these are should be actively elicited from the patient, rather than presumed by the healthcare provider (and family members). It is this subjective quality of well-being that makes beneficence dependent on the principle of autonomy (see Box 9.2). Objectives for the health-care professional—increasing a patient's "disease-free survival," for example—may be meaningless to the patient if they mean more isolation, dependence, disability, or suffering. We ought to be humble about these matters—the patient is usually the best judge of which choice is best, of which option best suits their needs.

Box 9.2

....

In deciding what is beneficent, healthcare professionals must take into account whether the proposed medical intervention is not only likely to improve the person's condition, but also consistent with the person's values, beliefs, and expressed wishes regarding their condition.

Doing nothing is sometimes better

Sometimes, when the possibility of harm is high and the likelihood of benefit low, it is better to recommend the patient do nothing, recalling the adage, "Don't just do something; stand there!" (Some have called this the "zero option"[4].) Judging when one should "just stand there" can be difficult, often because of uncertainty and the lack of evidence for outcomes. As well, physicians are used to "intervening."

Doctors are often less "risk averse" than patients when it comes to procedures and drugs. (This may in part account for the overprescription of opiate drugs by physicians, underestimating the risks of addiction and death.)

Doing nothing is, in fact, a choice involving risks of its own; this should not be confused with nonmaleficence. For example, watchful waiting is an acceptable option in early-stage prostate cancer but carries the risk that, despite proper vigilance, the patient's cancer may advance to an incurable stage. Some are prepared to take this risk in order to avoid the more immediate risks of active surgical treatment.

Discussion of Case 9.1

Although the only possibly "curative option" for Ms R is surgery, how likely is a cure with surgery? What are the chances that, following surgery, she would have a reasonable quality of life? The answers to these questions should be sought whether the patient is 81 or 35 years old.

The discussion should ultimately target what would be accomplished by the proposed surgery and whether such goals are consistent with the patient's preferences. For example, Ms R's surgeon might consider it a "success" to extend her expected lifespan of eight to twelve months by an additional four or six months. The patient might not—especially if the surgery is expected to be burdensome and healing prolonged. Given the surgery is unlikely to be curative, Ms R ought to be asked what she would like to achieve in whatever time that is left to her. The experienced and careful clinician will be able to recognize when surgery should be attempted and when it should not. It is fair to say that patients who have lived a full life may not seek all possible life-prolonging measures as younger patients might do. On the other hand, one must guard against ageist assumptions (on the part of the healthcare professional, family, and even the patient) that might deny an elderly patient beneficial care.

We can, at times, in medicine strive too hard to rescue patients. The task then is to restrain the *furor therapeuticus*, "the dangers of which every experienced medical teacher should and does warn his students"[5].

Case 9.2   A Rush of Blood to the Head

It is the last month of Dr F's residency training program. On one of his last half-days, he is happy to see on his list two of his favourite patients, Mr and Ms D, a lovely Eastern European couple, both in their mid-80s. They appreciate his diligence. On this day, he is surprised to hear bruits over both of Ms D's carotid arteries (the main blood vessels to the brain). Dr F sends her for neck Dopplers (an ultrasound) to check on her circulation. These reveal a 90 per cent carotid artery blockage bilaterally.

Ms D is then referred to a surgeon who recommends an endarterectomy but cautions her that, with or without surgery, she is at high risk of having a major stroke.

"Well, I certainly don't want that, Doctor!"

Later, she questions Dr F, expressing her ambivalence about the proposed intervention. The resident tells her that of course she doesn't have to go ahead with the procedure, but points out there aren't many options for her.

Ms D agrees to the surgery, which is successful: blood now flows through her carotid arteries. She is sent home from hospital two days later. On her third day at home, Ms D suddenly collapses and cannot be revived. A post-mortem reveals she died of a massive cerebral hemorrhage.

Did Dr F do anything wrong? Did the surgeon?

The practical dilemma for clinicians is to know when to go out of their way to save a person at risk (such as a person at risk of renal or respiratory failure) and when to avoid attempting a "heroic" rescue, as this action would be disproportionate to the duty (such as trying to "rescue" a patient imminently dying, already "in the article of death," *in punto di morte*). The danger is they can go overboard for their patients by doing too much or, alternatively, abandon them to their fate by doing too little. Good practitioners learn by experience how to devise a fine balance between these two extremes.

Discussion of Case 9.2

The resident is distraught over this outcome. In trying to be a good and thorough clinician, he feels he sent this patient to her doom. "If only I hadn't checked her circulation," he would say to anyone who would listen, "she never would have gotten on this medical roller coaster and she'd still be alive today!" The surgeon, too, feels bad about the patient's death, but is more philosophical: "This happens now and again."

Mr D is, of course, devastated, by his wife's outcome—one that was hardly predictable (although this does happen in one in 400 cases of endarterectomies due to the new flow of blood rushing through old arteries). However,

continued

he is surprisingly sanguine, saying Mrs D had a "good life," and thanks the medical team for doing all they could.

The resident should be reassured that just as it is hubris to believe he can save everyone, so it is prideful to think that he, as a medical professional, is always responsible for deaths of patients under his care. Some people just have "poor physiology," others have plain bad luck, and others die because of untreatable or aggressive disease.

Nothing "wrong" was done in this case, but such unwanted outcomes remind us that the urge to use medical and surgical interventions is a two-edged sword. The only way to manage the uncertainties and the dangers of modern medical interventions is through shared decision-making. That process was followed in this case. Ms D had agreed to the surgery, albeit with understandable hesitation.

Box 9.3

Furor therapeuticus: therapeutic zeal that can sometimes cause clinicians to try to do "too much" good.[5]

II. A Duty to Attend?

The "duty to rescue" is one encapsulation of the healthcare professional's "duty to attend." This is the obligation to proportionately serve the needs of patients— better to call it the duty to *offer help* to patients in harm's way. People can take it or leave it—it is their right, in our democratic society, to reject or accept medical assistance. Healthcare professionals are also not obliged to roam around looking for people to help (although they might do so in emergencies such as in the aftermath of terrorist bombings, earthquakes, or floods). Usually, clinicians wait for patients to come to them by ambulance, with family assistance, or by walking into their office, clinic, or emergency unit.

However, some patients can have mental or physical disorders—depression, delirium, raging infections, multi-organ failure—that impair their ability to act autonomously[6]. The end result is that they are vulnerable and may need a helping hand. The principle of beneficence implies a limited duty to rescue (or at least offer to rescue) such individuals under an acceptable version of paternalism—a weak paternalism[7] (see Chapter 8).

A doctor's duty

It is generally understood that the healthcare professional is the one to decide whether to attend to a person. Physicians are not obliged to take care of every person that comes to their doors: important factors are the MD's skills, attitudes, and training, as well as their roles and duties. For example, an obstetrician cannot decide at the last moment not to go the aid of the next patient scheduled for delivery. A doctor who specializes in delivering babies might, however, be of less help in caring for an acutely psychotic patient in an emergency. A casualty officer in an emergency room must see *all* who attend while they are on shift (obviously with help, as needed, from other doctors, allied healthcare professionals, and trainees). By contrast, a physician in independent office practice can decide whom to see and when to see them. But must such a doctor, if working in a rural area, see all patients within a 10-mile radius of their office if no other doctor is available? Within 100 miles? Limits must and can be set. Physicians cannot look after everyone. They can limit their practices in ways they see fit and avoid any suggestions of patient abandonment.

Case 9.3   Is There a Doctor in the House?

You are on a long-awaited vacation, flying to Mexico, celebrating with several friends your successful completion of medical school. Now others can call you "Doctor." A half hour into the flight, just as you are settling into your seat to read your favourite author, an announcement comes over the loudspeaker, "Is there a doctor on board the plane?"

How would, and should, you respond? Must you respond?

Discussion of Case 9.3

Must a physician respond in emergencies? The answer is yes—and no. Properly trained clinicians should offer to help without having to think twice, assuming there is no evident danger to them in doing so. On the other hand, strangers in distress are not your patients; as such, you do not owe them a duty of care—from a legal point of view, anyway. Professionally, there are ethical expectations of assistance in such circumstances [8]. If you do help, at least in the United Kingdom and in North America, there are "Good Samaritan" laws

continued

legally protecting those who provide assistance to others who are injured or ill. No doctor has ever been sued for helping in such settings.

Quebec and many European Union countries, by contrast, require not only physicians, but also any citizens passing by an emergency or an accident, to stop and provide or call for medical aid. European civil law imposes certain duties of social assistance on its citizens, as opposed to Anglo-American jurisprudence that frees citizens from social encumbrances, so that "it is only a matter of individuals in English law to decide not to intervene" [9].

It is expected that physicians, wherever they work, will carry out their work and exercise their professional roles responsibly and carefully. Whether a trainee or a professional in practice, there are role-mandated duties of care and responsibility. In an emergency department, making decisions about who is really ill and needs urgent care and attention, for example, is a challenging but teachable skill; ignoring patients or not taking them seriously is a recipe for potential disaster for both the patient and the healthcare professional.

III. Risks to the Professional

Healthcare professionals cannot avoid taking on some risk associated with their careers. There are low-grade risks, such as a family doctor getting the common cold from a young patient. There are more serious perils for surgeons, such as contracting HIV or hepatitis C infections.

There can also be situations—epidemics, wars, and disasters—that exceed the dangers of ordinary professional civil life. Performing CPR in an airplane or catching a cold from a patient is one thing, contracting Ebola or SARS quite another. Is exposing oneself to such increased hazards ethically required or simply allowable?

Healthcare professionals are not required to sacrifice themselves or their families in emergencies or otherwise. A patient waving a gun in the ER is a job for the police, not the medics. Physicians are also not required, but may selflessly volunteer, to work in unsafe environments, for example, improperly equipped ERs or hospitals facing terrorist bombardment or lethal gas weapons.

However, as a last resort, most jurisdictions *do* have the legal authority to require qualified healthcare professionals to render aid during medical emergencies—if they are so qualified [10]. Although the freedom of a physician to decline work in natural disasters and pandemics may be limited by statute, most members of the profession typically put aside their own self-interest and do whatever they can to help out in such situations.

Perfection not expected

Wherever they work, healthcare professionals must bring a "reasonable degree" of skill and care that could be expected of "a normal, prudent practitioner of the same experience and standing"[11]. They are expected (or may be required) to take "reasonable precautions" to look after their own safety, the safety of trainees under their supervision, and the safety of their patients[12, 13].

It is understood that clinicians will follow "approved practice" or what a "substantial" number of practitioners would do[14].

Box 9.4

A legal standard of care for all healthcare practitioners:
"A doctor is not guilty of negligence if he (sic) has acted in accordance with a practice accepted as proper by a responsible body of medical men (sic). [A] doctor is not guilty of negligence merely because there is a body of opinion that takes a contrary view." [15]

The courts recognize that the appropriate exercise of medical beneficence must allow for different diagnostic and therapeutic interventions, the choice among which may be determined by professional judgment and patient consent. Nonetheless, choices of clinicians following the profession's "standard of care" can be and have been found negligent if common practice would be judged as egregiously unsafe in the eyes of an ordinary person[16].

Box 9.5

"[T]here are certain situations where the standard practice *itself* may be found to be negligent. However, this will only be where the standard practice is *fraught with obvious risks* such that anyone is capable of finding it negligent." [italics added]

Ter Neuzen v Korn, 1995[16]

Standard practice has, therefore, been found wanting and physicians liable if that practice harms patients. For example, the opioid crisis may lead to legal and professional charges against MDs who presumed they were "safely" prescribing narcotics in following the recommendations of others. So far, those doctors who have been convicted have not followed safe prescribing procedures and were found wantonly reckless and indifferent to a patient's life. That is not to say the ordinary prescribing habits of these dangerous drugs is liability or risk free for physicians. It should be remembered, as well, that patients cannot give legitimate consent to negligent practice, so their consent is no bar to findings of professional misconduct. The perilous prescription of opioids was, unfortunately, aided and abetted by pharmaceutical companies that misrepresented to the public and the profession the truly hazardous nature of narcotics such as oxycodone and fentanyl[17].

Box 9.6

"Prescription opioid therapy is associated with substantial known risks . . . By . . . availing themselves of best practices . . . liability potential can be mitigated [by physicians]—a strategy that will also serve to reduce prescription opioid-related morbidity and mortality."[17]

IV. Endangering One's Self

Some people are difficult to help. They seem to put themselves deliberately in harm's way—as if stepping into the path of an oncoming bus—and challenge the professional as to when and whether to intervene. Here is an example.

Case 9.4   No Fools Allowed

Ms E is an 84-year-old patient who is as fiercely independent as she can be—she's outlasted several husbands and considers most men incompetent fools. An inveterate smoker, she likes nothing better than lying in bed in silken pyjamas, imbibing her single malt scotch, reading magazines, and smoking cigarette after cigarette. To make a house call on this patient is like taking a trip back in time to some smoky 1950s lounge bar. The patient also hates most aspects of aging—she cannot stand the way it has gradually stripped away her dignity, her smooth complexion, her muscle strength, her stamina, her joie de vivre, and now her memory.

Most frustratingly, Ms E is finding it hard to cope with the requirements of living on her own. Bills are accumulating, papers and magazines are in piles everywhere, the bathrooms are filthy, food is rotting in the fridge, stale air hangs like a thick haze about her house, and cigarette burns have punctured her bedroom carpet, her sheets, and even her usually immaculate pyjamas. Will she accept any help or consider moving? No way! Ms E is, in her own view, "perfectly fine."

What should her primary care provider do?

What can be done about the refusal of care by an individual failing at home? There may be legislation allowing clinicians to rescue and institutionalize "free-ranging," seriously-at-risk vulnerable adults. This can provide an administrative solution to patient "intransigence"[18]. Such laws vary in different jurisdictions and so medical professionals should confirm their possible legal options.

Taking these protective steps does deprive people of their independence, in some cases at a time in their life when much has already ebbed away. Whom are we going to institutionalize against their will? All people who don't bathe regularly? (Hardly—unless there is evidence of a broader failure of self-care.) The inveterate hoarder? (Maybe—if they are at risk of dying under a mountain of garbage.) A gun-toting angry reclusive? (Possibly—although not "ebbing away," they may be a threat to the lives of others.) A healthcare professional must make judgments about how grave and imminent the dangers are in order to justify the revocation of a patient's liberty.

Discussion of Case 9.4

Obviously, an evaluation of Ms E's capacity to make a decision about her place of residence needs to be made. As well, an overall assessment of her mental status is called for. How imminent are the risks to her well-being? Can supports be put in place that would minimize these risks and allow her to stay in her home? Are there any family members available to help? The goal is to seek the least restrictive alternative that will protect her, while preserving her liberty. Ms E is not such a direct threat to others that she can be removed from the house by the force of law, but her physician does worry about her smoking in bed.

Many avenues are explored but the patient's fierce independence slows the process down considerably. Everyone bends over backwards to try to accommodate her. She agrees to have help but then does not let them in the house; she agrees not to smoke in bed but new burn marks are later found; her driver's licence is revoked but she is seen driving anyway. She is just capable enough to barely cope. Then, one day Ms E fails to answer the door. The police

continued

are called, break in, and find her lying at the bottom of the stairs with a broken arm and hip, barely conscious. She cannot resist being carried away. She is admitted to hospital and later discharged to a nursing home. Resistance is, at this point, futile.

There was something inevitable about her ultimate fate. It is unlikely any other course of action would have had a better outcome. What Ms E needed was something money couldn't buy: someone to care for her. In such cases, there is only so much that healthcare professionals can do.

The suicidal and the reckless

Those living in a democratic system have the right to live as they see fit, within limits, not necessarily as others would want. As long as their actions affect only themselves and they are capable, they can live recklessly and make poor choices. There is one limit to this allowance for personal choice that seems fairly well settled: patients who are actively suicidal are treated as ill and incapable, and may be hospitalized without their consent.

However, some put autonomy above all and have argued, for example, that an act of suicide is just another option. Like deliberately stepping in front of an oncoming train, suicide is just an option that people can "select" and, if that is their "choice," then we ought not interfere with it. We disagree—we think healthcare professionals have a standing obligation to try to prevent deliberate self-harm and would distinguish these cases from legitimate refusals of care. (The evolving area of medically assisted dying on the basis of psychiatric illness represents a unique challenge to this view and is discussed further in Chapter 16.) In the latter cases, either the patient has an advanced illness and has had the opportunity of multiple consultations or the patient's refusal of care derives from deep religious or cultural reasons. In more ethically troubling cases, ignoring patient self-harm would be akin to allowing a person to be hit by an oncoming bus or not preventing them from jumping off a bridge. Not all acts of deliberate self-harm are the same.

Case 9.5   An Acceptable Request?[19]

In 2008 Ms W, a 26-year-old former charity shop worker, called an ambulance after taking a lethal dose of antifreeze. Although she said she wanted to die, she did not want to do so alone or in pain. According to newspaper reports, she had an "untreatable personality disorder" and had attempted suicide by swallowing antifreeze on nine previous occasions in less than a year. Each time, she had accepted dialysis treatment to flush the toxic solution from her system. This time, however, she produced a suicide note declining dialysis.

The consultant, Dr H, who would have treated her antifreeze ingestion, sought legal advice from hospital counsel. The counsel's opinion was that treating Ms W was illegal, as it would contravene her express wishes not to be rescued. As a result of this legal opinion, Dr H concluded that he could not intervene. Ms W died the following day. Questioned about his decision to withhold dialysis, he explained, "I would have been breaking the law, and I wasn't worried about her suing me, but I think she would have asked, 'What do I have to do to tell you what my wishes are?'[20]"

Did Dr H do the right thing in following the dictates of Ms W's suicide note?

Many religions and jurisdictions do not see deliberate fatal self-harm (suicide) as a legitimate and authentic option. But there has been a long history, since Socrates and the Stoics, of viewing suicide as a noble and thoughtful gesture by an autonomous agent in the face of undignified circumstances. This is now increasingly considered an acceptable rational choice in states of severe and intractable suffering, whether mental or physical. There is currently considerable debate as to whether directives to limit care and to hasten a patient's death can be made in advance of an illness such as dementia[20].

Discussion of Case 9.5

While Dr H's fidelity to a suicidal patient's wishes may seem admirable, we think his actions are unfortunate for two reasons. First, it makes lawyers into arbitrators as regards appropriate care (see Chapter 1 on the legal and the moral). This, we think, treads on the professional responsibility of doctors. Second, it fails to distinguish legitimate requests for premature death in the context of irreversible illness and untreatable suffering from illegitimate requests occasioned by reversible illness and incapacity.

A note declining life-sustaining care, in the context of an emergency caused by the patient in a self-induced crisis, should not be considered an acceptable request based on autonomy. Suicide attempts are made for many reasons—sometimes in the context of a mind unbalanced by a serious mental malady, sometimes for what seem to others as trivial reasons, sometimes in a

continued

moment of despair, or at other times for well-considered purposes. A suicide attempt can be a cry for help—not a competent refusal of care or an understandable reaction to impossibly difficult life circumstances. "Only 10 to 14 per cent of persons commit suicide over the decade following a failed attempt, suggesting that in most suicidal persons, the desire to die is transient"[21]. There is a professional debate whether physicians should ever abide by suicide notes, no matter how capable the patient appears to be.

Can suicide ever be a rational choice? It can be, but it is not a choice to which healthcare professionals should readily assent, especially if the patient is in crisis. It would be more appropriate, at least initially, not to abide by the suicide note and do what is needed to save Ms W's life. Once stabilized, the depth and authenticity of her wish to die could be explored more fully. If living wills privilege the wishes of one's prior self, which prior self ought the clinicians have heeded in this case: the self who wanted to be rescued and dialyzed nine times previously, or the self now refusing dialysis on the tenth overdose?

Where were the people who knew her best: her family physician or psychiatrist, for example? Were all forms of treatment for her "personality disorder" really tried? One can only hope that these other avenues were explored. If they were, it might make the non-treatment of Ms W more acceptable. In the end, there is only so much you can do for some patients.

Professional liability

> ### Box 9.7
>
> "Suicide should be considered the response of someone, whether suffering from mental disease or not, who is unable to find a solution to a relational crisis."[22]

In looking after and assessing their depressed patients, clinicians sometimes worry about being held liable if they miss the seriousness of a patient's wish to die. In general, such fears have been unwarranted[23]. Where the courts or the professional regulatory colleges have found a professional liable, the circumstances have usually involved a failure to follow appropriate clinical practice, such as neglecting to look over available medical records for evidence of past attempts at suicide or failing to see or to re-examine a patient before discharge[24]. Such rulings have also considered the harmful outcomes as "foreseeable," had the professional taken into consideration all the relevant factors (for example, having a gun at home). This is clearly the crux of the matter, since predictions of patient suicide are far from certain.

As long as healthcare professionals perform comprehensive and careful assessments of their patients, they are unlikely to be held liable if one of their patients dies by suicide[25]. Prognostic error, in this area of medicine as with other areas, is unavoidable. As long as clinicians have exercised "due skill and diligence" in their assessments, they have met the professional standard of care.

V. Parental Refusals of Treatment

The care of young children is another area where the principle of best interests comes to the fore as a guiding principle. Recommended treatment ought to reflect the course of action that will provide the most benefit and cause the least harm to the juvenile patient. Infants and very young children cannot express wishes to direct their own care, although they clearly have interests that must be protected. Children may also have very strong *preferences* that should not be ignored. The striking difference in medical decisions related to young children, as opposed to adults, is that healthcare professionals usually cannot have independent recourse to the young patient's wishes.

The interests of a young child seem to be inextricable from those of the family—it may be difficult, if not impossible, to determine what the child wants or needs, other than through the filtering lens of the parents. Parents bring important cultural, religious, and ethnic beliefs and customs that may influence how they and their offspring view the various medical options.

But may parents, for example, refuse what seems to be the best medical therapy for their child? Is this ever acceptable? The brief answer to this question is *sometimes*—but only under certain conditions: decisions made by parents for their young children need to conform to a best-interests standard of judgment as the first and most important consideration.

Discretionary therapy

Medical therapy is sometimes considered "discretionary" if not required to save a child's life or prevent serious injury or disability. In such circumstances, parents have some leeway to take the physician's recommendation under advisement. Whether or not to give antibiotics to a child with an ear infection is one example. (This should not trivialize such decisions, as even common illnesses such as otitis media can be grave.)

Parents are allowed to enrol their children in hockey leagues or other contact sports, despite increasing data indicating some children are seriously injured
or die every year in such activities. Refusal by parents of "ordinary care," such
as childhood immunization, is allowed in many jurisdictions, if the refusal is
an "informed" one. (While parents in most jurisdictions[26] are allowed to refuse
vaccination—despite there being no credible evidence supporting refusal[27]—this
decision may have an impact on other aspects of the child's life such as the child's
eligibility for school.) Clinicians should make attempts to educate parents and
voice their professional opinion as to what they think is in the child's interest[28]—
in a culturally sensitive way, of course.

In general, physicians are permitted to intervene only if parental refusal of
treatment seriously imperils the health of the child. (We have seen already that
all healthcare professionals have a duty to report cases of suspected child abuse;
see Chapter 7.) Doctors in Ontario, for example, are required to report vaccine-
refusing parents to public health authorities who can then order the parents to
attend an educational session about vaccination.

Child welfare authorities may be called in for assistance in situations
of lesser gravity—for example, when healthcare professionals see evidence
of poor parenting skills—to help parents cope with the responsibilities of
raising children. The focus is usually on the child's best interests, as well
as respecting their nascent autonomy and avoiding removing them from the
family.

Caution must be exercised here, however. (See Chapter 17 on cultural factors.)
The extent of the abuse and suffering caused by the coerced removal of Indigenous children from their families and communities is only now being recognized
and has left a legacy of distrust of those who would impose their values on other
communities[29].

Refusing treatment: Cultural respect vs child safety

Where medical therapy will, on best medical evidence, prevent death or serious
injury to the child, the parental power to refuse treatment is reduced. In Canada,
the United Kingdom, and most US states, legislation obliges parents to provide
their children with the "necessaries [or the necessities] of life." (The precise language varies depending on the locale.) If parents, whether by design or through
neglect, mistreat their children or do not provide them with the necessities of
life,[30] the children can be removed by the child welfare authorities for the needed
treatment to be given[31, 32]. Although cultural factors are important here and must
be respected, the rights and welfare of the child—to obtain needed and necessary
care, to have an open future, to be free from abuse and abandonment—cannot
be ignored.

In true emergency situations, healthcare professionals should not wait for formal judicial approval before instituting emergency care. "Consent to medical care is not required in case of emergency if the life of the person is in danger or his integrity is threatened and his consent cannot be obtained in due time"[33].

Children cannot be martyrs

The limits to parental authority were at issue in 1923 in the leading US case, *Prince v Massachusetts*. In that case, a Jehovah's Witness was charged with violating child labour laws in allowing her nine-year-old niece to sell religious pamphlets on the street.

Box 9.8

"The right to practice religion freely does not include liberty to expose the community or the child to communicable disease or the latter to ill health or death . . . Parents may be free to become martyrs themselves. But it does not follow that they are free . . . to make martyrs of their children before they have reached the age of full and legal discretion when they can make that choice for themselves."

Prince v Massachusetts, 1923 34

This much-cited decision serves as the basis for limiting the right of parents to refuse treatment for their children and has informed legal and ethical judgments since then. Thus, while adult Jehovah's Witnesses may refuse necessary blood transfusions for themselves, they may not do so for their children. In January 1995, the Supreme Court of Canada unanimously upheld the judgments of lower courts that a Jehovah's Witness couple had no right to refuse a blood transfusion for their infant.

Box 9.9

"A parent may not deny a child—even for religious reasons—medical treatment judged necessary by a medical professional and for which there exists no legitimate alternative."[35]

B.(R) v CAS of Metropolitan Toronto, 1995

When parents refuse life-saving therapy, precedents exist in many juris-dictions to allow the authorities to apprehend the child and provide the needed treatment. In several US jurisdictions, however, parents of critically ill children have not been prosecuted despite the death of their children on account of their refusal of treatment on "religious grounds"[36]. For example, the use of prayer by a Christian Science practitioner, in place of accepted medical care, is allowed in 34 US states[37]. In half of these states, however, a court can order the treatment of a child regardless of the parent's views.

The Stephen Dawson case is a well-known Canadian case that raised the issue of parental refusal in a complex and secular way.

The Dawson case: parents not free to expose child to risk of permanent injury

Stephen Dawson was severely mentally and physically disabled since contracting meningitis as an infant. When he was of five months old, a shunt had been in-serted to drain off excess cerebrospinal fluid. Blind, partly deaf, and incontinent, he could not feed himself, walk, stand, or talk. Stephen suffered seizures and, to his parents, seemed to be in pain. At age 7, when his shunt became blocked again, his parents finally refused consent for remedial surgery on the grounds it would be better to allow him to die than to prolong a life of suffering. Stephen was ap-prehended by the child welfare society and the British Columbia Supreme Court authorized surgery[38].

The court accepted medical evidence from pediatricians that Stephen's life was not entirely gloomy—he was happy despite his disabilities. The judge did not believe that Stephen would be better off dead: "This would mean regarding the life of the handicapped child as not only less valuable than the life of a normal child, but so much less valuable that it is not worth preserving." Troubled by the seemingly "imponderable" quality-of-life issue, the court was also worried that without surgery an even worse fate might await Stephen. Without the shunt he might continue to live, but with more pain and disability. In allowing the surgery the court followed the longstanding UK judicial precedent that "it has always been the principle of the Court not to risk the incurring of damage to children which it cannot repair"[39].

While parents "are not obliged to provide the best and most modern med-ical care for a child, they must provide a recognized treatment that is available"[40]. A treatment less likely to succeed, that goes against the core cultural values of a family and child, and so leads to more suffering on the child's part, may be within the child's and parent's discretion to refuse.

Experimental treatment not mandatory

In 1989, the parents of a seven-month-old child with biliary atresia refused authorization for liver transplantation. At that time, only 65 per cent of the children who received this treatment lived at least five years. Representatives of Saskatchewan's Ministry of Social Services sought legal authorization for the treatment on the grounds that not doing the surgery might constitute child abuse.

However, at trial, a majority of the doctors who testified defended the rejection of surgery as a reasonable option because of its long-term uncertain outcome and the burdens it would impose upon the child. Although recognizing that it might save the child's life, the provincial court judge refused to order transplantation, agreeing that the parents' refusal was "completely within the bounds of current medical practice." The parents' rejection of treatment was not a rejection "of the values society expects of thoughtful caring parents" but based on their concern for the child's best interests[41].

There is thus some discretion allowed in deciding that parental rejection of standard treatment is appropriate if that choice is seen as defensible by a reasonable body of medical opinion. In general, where the treatment is complicated, the right (or best possible) decision should be made consensually by parents and healthcare providers and should take into account not only technical factors but also the cultural, psychological, and emotional aspects of the child's situation (see Chapter 17).

VI. Parental Requests for Treatment

What about the opposite situation: does the principle of beneficence allow parents to *choose* whatever therapy they wish for their dependent children? The answer is, in general, yes, but only if the therapy is medically appropriate and consistent with the best interests principle. The leading Canadian legal case suggesting there are limits to parental choice is *E (Mrs) v Eve*[42]. As Eve's mental age was that of a very young child, the ethical principles behind this decision would be applicable to the care of young children generally.

E (Mrs) v Eve

Eve was a 24-year-old cognitively impaired woman cared for by her parents. The parents, who felt that she (and they) would not be able to cope with a pregnancy, requested she be sterilized for contraceptive purposes. Eve was considered by the courts too handicapped to give consent and unable to express her wishes regarding sterilization. The Supreme Court of Canada believed the parents were requesting the sterilization for the convenience of themselves and not for the benefit of the patient. The court considered the state's obligation to protect those citizens who are incapable of protecting themselves—under the *"parens patriae"* doctrine. This doctrine empowers the court to "act in the stead of a parent for the protection of a child"[43].

Made in Canada eugenics

Canada, like many countries, at one time explored eugenics in a misguided notion to improve and "benefit" society. As with all such attempts, this ultimately metamorphosed into an endeavour to cleanse society of individuals with perceived undesirable traits. It was mostly in Alberta and British Columbia where laws involving forced sterilization of the so-called "mentally defective" were implemented and acted upon. Over the 44 years following the passing of the *Sexual Sterilization Act* in Alberta in 1928, an estimated 3000 individuals were sterilized. Throughout this dark period of that province's history until the Act was finally repealed in 1972, First Nations, Inuit, and Métis people, as well as women and children with developmental delay, were disproportionately selected and sterilized[44-47].

On the *Eve* decision

In a unanimous decision the Supreme Court of Canada declared that "sterilization should never be authorized for non-therapeutic purposes under the *parens patriae* jurisdiction." As a result of the *Eve* decision, the courts require that sterilization—indeed any medical procedure—can be performed on persons incapable of consent only for medically necessary reasons.

After *Eve*

In the aftermath of *Eve*, non-therapeutic interventions, especially ones that are irreversible and pose some risk of harm, should not be carried out on children (or other dependents) merely because the parents authorize them.

Just how far to extend the *Eve* decision is unclear. Is circumcision of the male neonate permissible? (It is at the present—the risks are small, it is an important ritual for various religious and social traditions, and it is defended by some on medical grounds, although there is much debate about the evidence for this.) What about bone marrow donation by one young sibling to another? (Probably it is—if the best interests standard takes into account psychological benefit to the sibling without illness. See Chapter 14.)

Cosmetic surgery for a child with Down syndrome? (Suspect—is it of direct benefit to the child or done for the parents? Is it important the child look like others?) What about cochlear implants for a deaf child who can sign? (Dubious—if the child does not wish it and seems happy and well adjusted to Deaf culture[48].) Enrolling a child in a research trial? (Sometimes acceptable; see Chapter 18.)

The principle behind *Eve* is not easy to apply as the next case demonstrates.

Case 9.6 The Pillow Angel

A six-year-old girl, Annie L, has a severe and untreatable neurological disorder that has left her profoundly impaired, with the mental life and physical abilities of a three-month-old child. She is looked after by her parents at home. They inquire as to the possibility of ceasing Annie's physical maturation—specifically, they would like her bone growth halted and her sexual maturation prevented by surgery to avoid menstruation and pregnancy. They argue she will never benefit from or understand her sexual development and that a smaller size will make her easier to care for—she will be a "pillow angel." As such, Annie will be less likely to develop pressure sores and feeding problems or to require institutionalization. Keeping her small would make looking after her easier and more comfortable for all [49].

Is the parents' request for such treatment of Annie a legitimate one?
Which do you think is better—to stunt Annie's growth or not?

Discussion of Case 9.6

This real-life case elicited a storm of public controversy. The argument was made that it was in Annie's "best interests" to be kept small and immature so others could look after her more easily. On the other hand, it appeared this child would be undergoing intensive medical treatment, with its attendant risks, for the convenience of her parents. The case suggests that the lives of the disabled are tolerated only if they conform to the needs and tolerances of the fully abled.

continued

The proposed solution seems a modern version of Procrustes' "one-size-fits-all" bed in ancient Greek mythology. Welcoming strangers into his home, Procrustes offered them food and a place to sleep. Once on the special bed, however, the poor stranger was tortured: stretched if too short or his legs chopped off if too tall. The message to the disabled would seem to be, "You're welcome to stay but only on condition you are easy to look after and not overly demanding."

This case is less a condemnation of the child's parents than a sad commentary as to how little support society provides for children with special needs and their families.

That said, these parents did an incredible job looking after an irreversibly seriously disabled child—a task emotionally, physically, and financially burdensome, which many would shun. She *would* be much better off at home, cared for and loved, than in an institution. Here is where an *ethics of caring* might take precedence over an *ethics of rights*: one infringes on the right to be free of intrusive interventions; the other champions the right of families to care for their dependents in realistic ways[50].

Resist the clearly harmful

It should go without saying that one should never comply with a parental request for therapy that promises clear harm and no benefit to a child. Such is the case with all forms of female circumcision[51]; in its traditional form it is mutilating, always harmful, medically unjustifiable, and certainly illegal under North American and European child abuse laws[52]. This is where respect for other cultural traditions must give way to looking after a child's best interests. Of course, imaginative solutions are possible. Recently, for example, "genital nicking" has been proposed as a compromise intervention[53].

In other cases of questionable—but less clearly harmful—requests for therapy, the wise healthcare professional should discuss with the parents the reasons for their requests, rather than dismissing them out of hand. It would also be important to include the child's views, if possible. It is professionally prudent and respectful of parental authority (and also respectful of the child) to try to understand their perspectives and attempt to negotiate a mutually acceptable solution. This may involve looking at other options—less hazardous and more readily correctable ones first—that will try to meet the needs and concerns of all involved. Particularly contentious disputes can be helpfully addressed by mediation and multidisciplinary teams designed to examine the ethical, cultural, and medical facets of the problem[54].

Conclusion

Beneficence and nonmaleficence are key principles informing medical care today. Relevant to all healthcare professionals, they speak to the expectations the public has of medicine and the codes of conduct by which health professionals measure their own performance and those of their peers. Differences of opinion as to harm and benefit should encourage communication and a search for common ground. The next chapter will cover some evolving issues of what it means to be a modern healthcare professional.

Cases for Discussion

Case 1: Come Back Later

Mr A visits his family doctor, Dr L, for a persistent cough and weight loss. His last visit to the clinic was 15 years ago. He is now 71 years old and somewhat of a recluse, living alone in a small apartment, venturing out only to buy a few food items. Dr L thinks he looks unwell and orders blood tests and a chest X-ray.

"You don't think it's anything serious, do you, Doc?" he asks. His family doctor responds there could well be a problem and encourages him to get the tests done. Instead, Mr A goes straight home. He phones Dr L the next week, however, saying he feels no better. He agrees to do the tests and make a follow-up appointment but then doesn't come back.

Concerned, Dr L decides to make a house call. He knocks on Mr A's apartment door, but there is no answer. He knocks again but is met with silence. When he calls out, "Mr A, is that you?", he hears a shuffling sound on the other side of the door. "Mr A, how are you? It's Dr L—from the clinic. May I come in?"

"Not now!" Mr A replies through the closed door. "I'll come to your office when I'm feeling better."

Questions for Discussion
1. What factors should Dr L consider in deciding whether or not to agree to Mr A's request to be left alone?
2. Would it be permissible to breach his confidentiality by speaking to his neighbours or his superintendent about him?

Case 2: Risky Business

Ms R is a 70-year-old widow, hospitalized with cognitive impairment and advanced Parkinson's disease. No longer able to swallow without aspirating her food, a gastrostomy feeding tube has been placed with consent from her 40-year-old son, her only relative. On several occasions, however, he is found secretly feeding his mother by mouth. Moreover, after a weekend visit to her home, she returns to hospital with bruises sustained in falls when he went out and left her alone unsupervised.

Questions for Discussion
1. What is the ethical problem here?
2. Is this necessarily elder abuse?

Conduct Becoming

Medical Professionalism

In all dealings with patients, the interest and advantage of their health should alone influence the physician's conduct towards them.

Robert Saundby, 1907[1]

It may seem somehow anachronistic to write about professionalism in medicine at a time of seeming "post-professionalism"[2]. Information is only a click away on the Internet, with the result that everyone is an "expert" these days. Knowledge, of course, is a necessary component of being a professional, but attitude and judgment are as important, if not more crucial. A constellation of knowledge, skills, and attitudes establishes the core competencies of any healthcare professional[3].

I. Maintaining the Connection

Medical professionals can be distracted from their work by all sorts of factors—everything from the desire for money and fame to family issues and personal preferences. However, trustworthy healthcare professionals, when buoyed by the appropriate commitments and aptitudes, even if feeling under siege, are like those unsinkable kids' bath toys—push them under the water as hard as you like; they always bounce back up.

Case 10.1 An Unexpected Death

Melinda R is a 19-year-old woman admitted to an urban hospital for routine gallbladder surgery. Her discharge is delayed as her bowels are sluggish and her incision hurts more than she expected. On Friday, three days after surgery,

continued

although still in some discomfort, Melinda begs to be discharged home, a two-hour drive away. She does not want to spend the weekend in hospital. Her surgeon, Dr T, authorizes the discharge despite not having seen her or her parents that day. Busy in the OR, she reasons the nurses would have alerted her to any concerns. Melinda is advised by the discharge nurse to go to her local hospital if she develops any troubles. Dr T arranges to see her in follow-up in her clinic in a week's time.

On the drive home with her parents, Melinda suddenly feels short of breath. Once home, she is overcome by fatigue. Feeling quite ill, she retires to her bed. Several hours later, she collapses on the way to the toilet. Her parents call 911. Although the paramedics arrive within minutes, she cannot be revived.

Distraught and overwhelmed with grief, her parents call Dr T. "If our daughter was so sick," they angrily exclaim, "how could you have let her go home?"

How should the surgeon respond?

Discussion of Case 10.1

The unexpected death of a patient, so close to discharge, should be seen as an "ethical emergency." Dr T (and the hospital representatives) should offer to meet with the family as soon as feasible and answer, as well as they can, whatever questions the family may have. A laconic response by the surgeon or the hospital could turn this situation into an ethical disaster. The wrong response would be to say, "These things happen . . ."

Complete transparency, honesty, empathy, and avoidance of any sense of defensiveness are critical for discussions with the grieving family. The surgeon and other staff also need to be appropriately self-aware: What can they learn from this event? What are the critical things that could have been done differently?

As it turns out, autopsy results later reveal that Melinda died from "DIC" (disseminated intravascular coagulation), a syndrome characterized by multiple blood clots, extensive bleeding, shock, and cardiopulmonary failure. Usually acute and unpredictable, DIC carries a high mortality, even for hospitalized patients. The abnormalities in clotting might, or might not, have been revealed prior to her discharge if routine bloodwork had been done. Her surgeon might, or might not, have recognized her condition if she had been examined before discharge.

Thus, even with the best efforts, Melinda's death might not have been foreseen or preventable. But this is not the message the family needs to hear.

What they need to hear is something like this from Dr T: "We (myself, the team, the hospital) are truly sorry for your loss and understand your anger and grief. We can only imagine how hard this must be for you. We will meet with you until we get answers that satisfy us all. We will review all our procedures and practices to see what we could have done better and what we can do to prevent such events in the future. Please accept our sincerest apologies and regrets for this terrible outcome."

Such an apology is not an admission of fault or liability: it is simply an acknowledgement that all wish a different outcome had transpired and that those in charge will take responsibility for exploring what occurred (see Chapter 12)[4]. Timely heartfelt expressions of regret and sorrow, being taken seriously, and appropriate follow-up corrective action—not defensiveness and silence—are what families want and need from healthcare professionals in times of crisis and loss. Behind this episode is one of the most common reasons for complaints and lawsuits against doctors: a failure to communicate[5].

II. A New Professionalism

The perception that medicine was failing in the public's eyes as a trustworthy enterprise devoted to patients led to a series of ethical initiatives. "Medical Professionalism in the New Millennium: A Physician Charter" was launched in 2002 by various Internal Medicine societies for physicians to "promote an action agenda for the profession of medicine that is universal in scope and purpose"[6].

This charter for a "new professionalism" is based on the ethical principles that, as we have already seen in Chapters 2 and 3, underpin the practice of medicine, namely, the primacy of patient welfare, patient autonomy, and "social justice." According to the charter, physician obligations include a series of commitments that, together, would help reset medicine's moral compass (see Box 10.1). The charter's principles could (and should) apply to any of the healthcare professions.

Box 10.1

Medical professionals shall exhibit or strive for the following:

- professional competence,
- honesty and respecting the confidences of patients,

continued

- interprofessional respect and politeness,
- appropriate relations with patients and other staff,
- improvement of the quality of care,
- advocacy for fair access to care,
- keeping up with scientific knowledge,
- maintenance of trust by managing conflicts of interest, and
- adherence to professional responsibilities such as regulating members and setting standards.

CanMEDS

There has been remarkable uptake of The Physician Charter in the years since its introduction[7]. A similarly influential pan-Canadian report for providing "high-quality safe patient care" (Canadian Medical Education Directions for Specialists or "CanMEDS")[8] was released in 2005 and updated in 2015. It has also found widespread professional support[9]. We have tried in this book to iterate the themes and principles found in these documents.

Professionalism starts at the patient's bedside.

Professional manners

Peabody wrote almost a century ago, "The secret of caring is caring about the patient"[10]. Such caring requires attitudes such as civility, tolerance, patience, competence, and accountability—simply recognizing and putting the interests of patients first and foremost. This is the everyday meaning of professionalism.

Box 10.2

"Patients clearly and rightly feel doctors* should heed minimum standards of courtesy, should acknowledge their patients' human distress, just like anyone else."[11]

*We should expect "minimum standards" of politeness from all staff—and not only to patients and families but also to each other and to healthcare trainees as well.

Politeness and kindness are attitudes that reveal one's commitment to patients. Rudeness and just plain bad manners—behavioural outbursts such as screaming at staff or patients, not respecting a patient's privacy, leaving a patient in distress, failing to apologize for lateness, not saying please or thank you, not returning messages, neglecting to provide explanations to patients for clinical manoeuvres, and just not listening—can lead to staff or trainee grievances, patient or family disappointments, and complaints to the regulatory authorities.

Case 10.2 Show A Little Respect!

Dr N's life at the hospital seems a little crazier than usual. In addition to her outpatient clinics getting busier than ever, she has agreed to head up the department's interprofessional Grand Rounds schedule. Flattered when asked by the department head, who praised her work habits and youthful energy, she is now finding this a thankless task. Dr N has to pester her physician colleagues to present—most eventually do, if sometimes reluctantly.

"Now, if only they would listen at Rounds," she mutters to herself.

These take place over lunchtime and she can't help but notice that some of her colleagues seem more interested in the food than listening to their colleagues. They spend most of the rounds talking and being preoccupied by their cell phones.

What, if anything, is wrong with this picture?
What, if anything, should Dr N do?

Sometimes thought to be unimportant, how others are treated in everyday life can loom large in a hospital. Rudeness and incivilities generally can have a profound effect upon morale, leading to impaired performance and medical errors[12].

Discussion of Case 10.2

An unhappy and unsafe work environment—a toxic one—can start with "trivial" events such as doctors not paying attention to others. The culture of tolerated ordinary rudeness needs to be addressed. Dr N could start by speaking to some sympathetic colleagues. Have they noticed the problem? Has there been deterioration in the environment? The tone needs to be reset, and it starts at the top[13].

Dr N should speak to her departmental chief to figure out the best way to handle this.

Interprofessional education and work is the wave of the present and the future of medicine[14]. Fostering a culture of respect among all healthcare providers means that all members of the team listen to one another and the skills of all are maximized. Failing to hear other team members can have a negative impact on the quality of care. Better, safer outcomes for patients and greater patient satisfaction are more likely when the contributions of all are acknowledged and utilized.

There is general agreement that healthcare professionals should be sensitive to the impact of how they present themselves to a patient. Their appearance should not be distracting or create the impression they do not take their work (or the patient) seriously. Studies have traditionally suggested patients prefer certain attire on the part of their care providers. Studies from the United Kingdom[15], a South Carolina veteran's hospital[16] Hawai'i[17], and Korea[18] have all shown, for example, that patients have a preference for doctors who wear white coats. Of note, these studies have not shown that physician appearance has a negative impact on patient care. A recent US study looked at physicians with body art—tattoos and piercings. It found, interestingly, that while patients may not like the body art, this did not significantly affect their clinical care or their perceptions of the competence of the care provider[19]. This suggests patients are more concerned about being *cared for* than the appearance of who cares for them. The attire of health professionals, in other words, may not always appeal to patients but should not elicit concerns unless accompanied by a poor quality of care.

Physicians display indifference and not caring through their interpersonal behaviours. In one study, surgeons were more likely to have a malpractice history if, in their tone of voice, they conveyed to patients a lack of empathy and understanding and failed to register concern or anxiety[20]. Other desirable behaviours to make the patient feel prioritized include making eye contact, talking with a friendly smile or the appropriate gravitas, sitting at the patient's bedside—all ways to lessen the patient–professional distance in an age of technology and anomie. Firmly shaking hands may be preferred by many patients—though not in all cultures—as a sign of mutual respect[21]. These are small but mighty gestures that can cement the connection between clinician and patient and are all more important than the care provider's appearance.

Professionalism vs "doing your job"

While it may be hard to define, almost anyone who has ever been a patient recognizes what is a professional caring attitude and what is not. Compare the clinician who begins her interview with a patient by saying, "We have only 10 minutes today and so can deal with only one concern," to one who unhurriedly starts the conversation by asking, "Tell me how things have been for you lately." Or compare the hospital official who says, "The care your relative received in hospital was entirely appropriate. What happened after her discharge is in the hands of the coroner," to one who says, "The care your relative received in hospital was entirely appropriate. While we can't be responsible for what happens after her discharge, we can understand your concern. We will work with the coroner's office in an urgent way to see if this terrible outcome was in any way related to her care here."

Something important is present in the attitude of the practitioners who do go beyond the minimum in caring for patients. They care about what is done and how it is done, and they respond to patients in ways that are respectful, compassionate, and humane. They commit to focusing on the unique needs of patients and are not distracted by their own issues[22]. True healthcare professionals do not allow their own interests to come before or to interfere with their commitment to their patients' interests. One issue of great concern to many in the profession and the public is that of conflicts of interest.

III. Conflicts of Interest

> ### Box 10.3
>
> A conflict of interest is any situation in which a healthcare professional's primary commitment to the patient is unduly influenced by other interests (such as financial rewards or academic prestige).

Trust is the crux

Conflicts of interest are pervasive and inevitable in medical practice. The very fact, for example, that many physicians are paid on a fee-for-service model represents a conflict of interest. The more service they provide, the more they get paid. For this reason and many others, the courts have long recognized a fiduciary duty on the part of physicians to act in the best interests of patients[23].

Medicine's ability to help and to heal requires an atmosphere of trust, of which the courts remind us time and again. A Canadian Supreme Court judgment explained that "the essence of a fiduciary relationship . . . is that one party exercises power on behalf of another and pledges . . . to act in the best interests of the other"[24]. This much-cited judgment states the crux of professionalism and of ethics in medicine.

Trust is threatened when a healthcare professional strays, or appears to stray, from their role-mandated duties due to conflicts of interest. A healthcare professional even mentioning monetary concerns can set the patient–clinician relationship off in the wrong direction.

Box 10.4

"The relationship of physicians* with patients is of a fiduciary nature. Hence, activities that might affect that relationship by altering physicians' clinical behaviour are not acceptable."[25]

*And any regulated health professional, we would say.

Case 10.3   Who's Helping Whom?

An 84-year-old single female, Ms P, in the early stages of a dementing illness, attends her dentist of many years, Dr F. In the course of the visit he mentions that he has fallen on hard times financially and might have to close his clinic. Ms P, who is quite well-off, asks, "Is there anything I can do to help?" Quite fond of the dentist, she generously offers him $50,000—as a loan or a gift, Ms P doesn't really care. She lives alone and her nearest relatives, living some distance away, visit infrequently.

Should Dr F accept Ms P's offer?

Discussion of Case 10.3

As difficult as his circumstances might be, if Dr F accepts Ms P's largesse, it would be an egregious violation of professionalism. Ms P is vulnerable on two counts: she has been his client for many years and the money offered trades in on misusing this professional relationship for his benefit. Ms P is also vulnerable on account of her medical condition and her social isolation. Is her early dementia affecting her judgment, for example? Of course, it is wrong and unprofessional of him to even have this conversation in the first place with Ms P. Dr F should apologize for raising the issue with her, thank Ms P for her kind offer, and seek other ways of managing his difficulties.

Conflicts of interest can occur when the health professional's primary commitment—acting in the best interests of the patient—is influenced by other interests of the clinician (such as the professional's own financial well-being, as in Case 10.5) or of some third party, such as the state, a pharmaceutical company, or even the hospital (which these days may be interested in profit-making ventures, too). This can threaten to overwhelm, or be seen to overwhelm, the trustworthiness of the health professional[26].

For example, is it acceptable for professionals to send patients to a pharmacy or to a testing facility located in the same facility in which they work? (This should be fine, as long as it is a public institution and the physician receives no financial kickbacks, such as gifts or reduced overhead, from the facility.) What if a clinician sends his patients to his spouse who happens to be a physiotherapist? (Quite possibly not acceptable, as it could be considered a kind of self-referral, unless there were no other options.) What if a physician sells exorbitantly expensive unproven drugs to desperately ill patients or takes money from patients? (A no-brainer: go straight to jail or to the discipline committee of the regulatory authorities if caught[27].)

A difficult area for many physicians that can create all sorts of conflicts of interests is their relationship with the pharmaceutical industry—"Big Pharma," as it is known.

IV. Professionals and Industry

Case 10.4   Supping with the Devil

You have a particular interest in hypertension and are willing to try new drugs for your patients with resistant hypertension. One such drug, "Syperia," is released following a large international drug trial showing it to be at least as safe and as effective as the leading drugs for this condition. A pharmaceutical representative asks you to take part in a phase IV research trial (undertaken after a drug has been approved for use). All you have to do is switch patients to Syperia and assess their response to treatment every three months. For every patient you enrol, you will receive $100 per year; you will also receive an extra $100 at the study's completion for your efforts.

Should you agree to participate in this research?
What are your concerns, if any?

Discussion of Case 10.4

This type of "study" is purported to assess the effectiveness of a new drug in "real-life" patients. Sometimes called a "seeding" trial, this may be an attempt to influence practitioner prescribing patterns[28], a practice that has attracted

continued

widespread condemnation[29]. Would you, in taking part, be doing so for your patients' interests or for your own? Are you going to tell your patients about the impetus for the trial and your financial benefit? Even if you convince yourself you are prescribing the drug for the benefit of your patients, many people would not see it that way (a perceived conflict of interest can be as deleterious to trust as an actual conflict). Notice it is not the amount of money that is at issue but the perceived lack of independent judgment—"a conflict of interest"—that triggers concern[30].

Box 10.5

Clinicians can partially manage and mitigate conflicts of interests with industry by

- disclosing their recompense from pharmaceutical industry to their patients,
- ensuring patients understand the research to which they are consenting,
- ensuring that patients and their families appreciate what the research entails,
- accepting only reasonable compensation for work actually done and avoiding gifts from industry, and
- carrying out only bona fide research that has been vetted by a trustworthy research ethics review board and passes the credibility test: will it contribute more to the fund of usable knowledge or more to someone's wallet? How will others see your relationship with industry?[31]

"He who sups with the devil," goes the proverbial saying, "should use a long spoon." Concerns about health professionals' relationships with the pharmaceutical industry have led to formal strategies to make the spoon longer and the meal taken at a more open table. In the United States, the federal Open Payments Program, required by the *Affordable Care Act*, has been collecting information since 2014 about the payments drug and device manufacturers make to physicians and teaching hospitals for perks such as travel, research, gifts, speaking fees, and meals, as well as ownership interests that physicians or their immediate family members have in these companies[32]. The assumption is that transparency will lessen the risk of inappropriate relations developing between physicians and the pharmaceutical industry[33].

Dollars for Docs, sponsored by Pro Publica[34], is another US site offering a searchable repository of information on industry payments to doctors[35].

Similarly, in Canada, the Canadian Medical Association has supported guidelines for physicians' relations with private industry[36]. Gifts from the pharmaceutical industry above $10 in value are to be reported. This includes just about anything physicians might receive from industry, including stock options, research grants, consulting fees, travel to and from medical conferences, and even knickknacks.

Not unreasonably, there is a widespread impression by the public that prescribers are still "on the take" from the pharmaceutical industry[37]. One of the most profitable industries, it ranks second among all spending on lobbying efforts by private business in the United States[38]. Indeed, tens of billions of dollars are spent yearly by pharmaceutical companies on physician-directed gifts, ads, and various other promotional efforts to influence their prescribing patterns[39]. The stakes are smaller in Canada, but the situation is not substantially different[40].

This promotion by industry may encourage the early adoption of beneficial drugs. The downside, however, is that prescribers may prematurely turn to unproven, expensive, or even deadly drugs.

Case 10.5   Drug Redux

You decide to join the Phase IV Syperia trial, confident you are immune to any untoward influence of the study on your practice. There are many alternatives for refractory hypertension, but the new drug's apparent lack of side effects and once-daily dosing may make it a valuable alternative for your patients. You see the rep from the pharmaceutical company before your clinic, accept drug samples for use with your patients, decline the $100 offer, but agree to attend an educational dinner at a pleasant restaurant with a speaker on resistant hypertension, sponsored by the same company.

Are you doing anything unprofessional in accepting this invitation?

Discussion of Case 10.5

Doctors have, until recently, routinely seen biopharmaceutical representatives. Many found they got useful, if biased, educational information from them; many also liked having samples to "offer" their patients. Many would additionally attend drug dinners sponsored by industry. Rarely are such educational sessions now simply promotions for new drugs; speakers have their independence and attendees are not stupid.

continued

On the other hand, whom are we kidding? The pharmaceutical companies aren't stupid either. Studies have shown time and again that clinicians and
trainees who accept certain interactions with industry are more likely to prescribe their drugs [41]. The information supplied by industry to the profession
(and in the United States to the public by direct-to-consumer advertising) is not
reliable [42]. As well, the most heavily promoted drugs often add little in the way
of therapeutic benefit [43]. According to a recent study, there was a significant
association between physicians receiving a meal promoting one of four brand-
name drugs and higher rates of prescribing the promoted drug compared with
alternative generic drugs in the same class [44].

Box 10.6

"The receipt of industry-sponsored meals, even just a single meal, was associated with an increase in the rate of prescribing the brand-name drug that was
being promoted." [44]

Physicians are, in short, a "cheap date" for the pharmaceutical companies.

Faced with such formidable and influential resources, clinicians should periodically and assiduously monitor their drug prescribing patterns to ensure their
true independence from the industry. Comparing their prescribing habits with the
recommendations in evidence-based guidelines will help ensure their integrity
and also lessen their reliance on industry for their education. Forming a critical
appraisal reading group with other prescribers could be another check on possible
industry influence. (See Chapter 18 for more on research ethics.)

Conflicts of interest can put the healthcare professionals' interests before those
of the patients. They constitute violations and crossings of appropriate boundaries
now recognized as not infrequent occurrences in medicine. Professional relationships can suffer and patients can be harmed when appropriate therapeutic boundaries are not recognized and respected.

V. Boundaries Large and Small

Transgressions of professional boundaries fall into two categories: violations and
crossings [45]. "Crossings" are minor infractions of a boundary. These are deviations from expected professional behaviours, such as accepting small tokens of

appreciation from patients or attending a social function held by a patient. This can sometimes be appropriate, so long as the therapeutic relationship—which defines the distance needed for objective decisions about healthcare—is not undermined. Thus, crossing a boundary, such as consoling a patient after a "bad" experience by sharing a personal (but not *too* personal) story—for example, "I, too, had an episode of delirium after my surgery. The experience was awful."—may be acceptable if used to demonstrate the professional empathizes with the patient's experience.

"Violations," on the other hand, are more serious boundary transgressions that compromise the professional encounter, such as having a sexual encounter with a patient. Boundary violations also go beyond the sexual to include other forms of personal and inappropriate infringements on the therapeutic relationship. Entering into a business relationship with a patient can also be a type of boundary violation, depending on the specifics of the case. For example, hiring a patient to work as a nanny or domestic help would not be appropriate. Developing a new type of stoma appliance with a patient might be acceptable but the patient's care ought to be transferred to another care provider. A violation undermines the patient-centred therapeutic nature of a clinician–patient encounter that puts the patient's best interests first, and replaces it with a situation where the healthcare professional's needs may displace the patient's.

Box 10.7

"A physician owes his or her patient the classic duties associated with a fiduciary relationship—'loyalty, good faith, and avoidance of conflict of duty and self-interest'" [46].

Any sexual involvement with a patient has always been considered a misuse of the healthcare professional's power and authority: "it is the doctor's breach of fiduciary trust, not the patient's consent, which is the central issue regarding sexual misconduct" [46]. There is some leeway with respect to relations with former patients for physicians and other regulated healthcare professionals (usually a year or two after the last clinical professional encounter). However, psychotherapists must adhere to more stringent standards because of the deeply personal and intimate types of shared information. Thus, sexual relations with former or current patients are forbidden in most, if not all, codes of ethics for any health professionals engaged in psychotherapy [47]. In such circumstances it is the healthcare professional, not the patient, who will be held responsible for boundary violations. The consent of the patient is no bar to allegations and findings of professional misconduct.

Case 10.6 An Uncomfortable Revelation

You are a primary care clinician seeing a new patient, Ms G, for the first time. In taking her history, you ask about her most recent medical care. She tells you she has been without a primary care practitioner for some time. Reluctantly, she states she did not feel comfortable seeing her former doctor, Dr E, as he had made, on more than one occasion, sexually explicit remarks to her, even asking her out on a "date." Ms G has told no one else about this. Dr E's interactions with her left her feeling soiled and guilty—as if she had somehow encouraged him.

What should you do?

Discussion of Case 10.6

In most jurisdictions, members of a regulated healthcare profession, such as nurses, dentists, optometrists, radiation technologists, pharmacists, and psychologists, have an ethical and professional obligation to report the sexual abuse of patients. For example, the Canadian Medical Association (CMA) advises doctors to report if they have "reasonable grounds, obtained in the course of practising the profession, to believe that another member of the same or a different professional regulatory College has sexually abused a patient" [47]. Failure to report could itself be considered professional misconduct. Thus, they advise physicians take "every reasonable step to ensure that such behaviour is reported to the appropriate authorities" [48].

In this case, knowing what to do about Dr E shouldn't be hard. His interactions with his former patient clearly constitute sexual misconduct. You should report him as the CMA recommends. It is preferable for the allegations to be submitted with Ms G's consent. However, if she prefers not to register a complaint, you may inform the regulatory College of the purported offender without naming her. Note that, without direct evidence from a patient, the courts and other oversight authorities may reduce any assessed penalties or, in the absence of corroborative information, not be able to pursue the matter at all. The medical profession is, of course, along with other professions, increasingly sensitized to the importance of this matter to society as a whole.

Going too far

As well as obvious violations related to sexual impropriety, the helping professions also come with more subtle dangers. In wanting to heal patients, we sometimes go beyond the boundaries of acceptable medical care.

Receiving gifts from patients can encroach upon the appropriate distance between clinician and patient. Gifts of a small nature are usually acceptable so long as they remain simply totemic representations of the therapeutic encounter; small gifts can be, for example, respectful and courteous "thank you's" from patients and are not necessarily wrong [49]. However, even seemingly trivial gifts, if driven by the wrong motives (for example, to seek a "special" relationship with the doctor), may degrade the professional relationship and undermine the quality of care provided [50].

What about "gift giving" *by* healthcare professionals *to* patients? The existing literature mostly deals with transactions such as giving patients bus fare to go home or providing money to buy needed drugs they cannot afford. While frowned upon, giving money to or doing favours for patients is nowhere considered un-ethical *per se* by regulatory authorities. (Providing patients with free samples of needed drugs is usually considered a good thing.) What about more significant "gifts" donated by a clinician to their patient?

Box 10.8

"It is common for helping professionals to feel responsible for meeting their clients' every need . . . it can be difficult indeed to sort out the differences between a 'healthy' giving, born of our deepest desires to love, and an 'un-healthy' giving, springing from unfulfilled psychological needs—for approval, for achievement, to appear more saintly than we really are." [51]

Can a practitioner ever do too much for their patients? The answer is yes: clinicians can indeed go too far in trying to aid patients. (And, unlike Case 9.2, not on account of a *furor therapeuticus*, but due to an improper boundary crossing.) The next case, based on real events from Newfoundland, received much publicity.

Case 10.7 Too Far From Away

A 33-year-old physician, Dr T, was in a Newfoundland jail awaiting extradi-tion for the murder of her ex-boyfriend in Pennsylvania. Apparently estranged from her family, she had no one to put up the $60,000 for her bail set by the Newfoundland and Labrador court. In desperation, she called her psychiatrist, pleading with him to help her. Concerned about her mood, he cancelled a half-day of patients to attend her bail hearing and provided the surety for

continued

the bail [52], allowing Dr T to be released from jail. Tragically, she subsequently drowned her infant son and died by suicide.

Was the psychiatrist's action a breach of professionalism?

Discussion of Case 10.7

Unfortunately, fate is unkind to many patients, dealing them blows of ill fortune and harm. It is not usually the job of healthcare providers to assist patients in avoiding all the harms and stressors that nonmedical ill fortune—from stock market crashes to job losses—hands them. Healthcare practitioners may help patients cope with the outcomes or impact of such events on their lives, but they do not, in general, seek to intervene in the private lives of their patients to prevent such bad events from occurring.

The psychiatrist's action in providing surety for Dr T's bail went far beyond what is reasonable or expected professional behaviour. He was either naïve or extremely misguided about this patient. In any case, the psychiatrist's action was a serious and unprofessional boundary violation.

Other observers would agree the psychiatrist's actions were serious—but also entirely forgivable. His motivation seemed therapeutic and not obviously self-serving. At worst, he may have been motivated by an overwhelming desire to rescue Dr T—a mistake in judgment, certainly, but not a crime deserving of punishment. That he sought no supporting peer opinion suggests he acted impulsively and thought little about the implications of his actions. Psychiatrists, in particular, must be careful not to allow their boundaries to become blurred: to go too far in trying to rescue a patient undermines the requisite therapeutic space needed for patient independence and healing to take place [53].

Requests for favours from patients

When faced with an unusual or inappropriate request from a patient, the astute clinician should ask for the opinion of others, such as their peers, professional insurers, or professional and regulatory authorities. This advice can help ensure that your actions do not go beyond the normal clinical interventions made by professionals. Unusual or personal favours for patients can have pernicious results for the therapeutic encounter and can damage the reputation of healthcare professionals and medicine generally [54].

Bottom line: clinicians must exercise prudent judgments of proportionality in doing the right thing. The further removed an action is from the profession's approved practice (the standard of practice of your peers), the more careful your reasoning regarding it must be.

VI. Fitness to Practise Medicine

Healthcare professionals learn over time and with experience how to make judgments regarding the appropriateness of patient requests. This requires the professional to keep up to date with the ever-evolving standards of care. Maintenance of competency and fitness to practise medicine are of concern to all of the health professions. The question is this: who decides whether a health practitioner is competent and fit to practise? Internet sites providing ratings of physicians are one form of patient-driven scrutiny doctors are now facing.

Case 10.8   An Unfair Rating

Dr S is a relatively new general internist with a growing practice in a mid-sized city. One day, a colleague alerts her to some negative reviews found on a physician-rating site. When she checks it out, she finds most of the reviews are very positive. However, the two most recent reviews are extremely negative.

   Both contributors rate her bedside manner as exceedingly unprofessional. One reviewer disparages her by saying she couldn't diagnose a common cold if her life depended on it. While she has some suspicions as to who may have rated her, she is not certain. She can see no validity in their complaints.

How should Dr S respond to these comments?

Rate my doc

Over the past decade, there has been a proliferation of online physician-rating platforms [55]. Most of these ventures are specific to the United States, where the business side of medicine is much more salient, and patients are primarily regarded as customers. Several have expanded to Canada and beyond. Two of the most popular and well-known sites are RateMD and WebMD. They are but a small part of the larger online trend enabling the public to rate and rank all forms of goods and services.

   One might have reservations about whether the service provided by a physician should be evaluated in the same way as the service of a restaurant or an electrician. Seen from a patient's perspective, however, the ability to read reviews about a physician may represent a genuine form of empowerment. And there is no question there are many physicians who would benefit from some feedback about parking charges, booking appointments, leaving messages, timeliness, friendliness of office staff, and bedside manners [56].

The evaluation of physicians and their services on such sites may be problematic, however, for a number of reasons:

1. Given the vast knowledge gap between patients and physicians, patients may not be equipped to realistically assess the quality of treatment they receive [57].
2. It is very difficult to know whether there is any correlation between a physician's ratings and actual quality of care [58].
3. Given that physicians are often the bearer of bad news or unpopular advice (such as dealing with obesity, smoking or progression of cancer), patients may be resentful and inclined to "shoot the messenger."
4. There is a risk that physicians' treatments might become oriented towards garnering positive reviews as opposed to providing the best and most appropriate care. Popularity should not be confused with professionalism.

For these reasons and more, many physicians are wary of these sites [59].

Discussion of Case 10.8

Both patients may be projecting frustration and anger with their own illnesses onto Dr S. It is nonetheless valuable for her, as for all physicians, to take a moment and reflect as to whether there may be some truth in patients' comments. She could talk to her peers or, perhaps, to other patients. Even a nasty, vindictive person can still have a valid reason for concern.

If certain patient complaints about some conditions, such as inordinate wait times or rude staff members, are legitimate, and if other conditions (like astronomical parking charges) are not fixed in cement, the doctor should take action. As well, providing patients with a mechanism to give feedback, such as anonymous patient satisfaction forms in the clinic or the comment section of a clinic website, empowers patients and demonstrates a commitment to improve one's practice.

Finally, it is well within Dr S's rights to have these comments removed. Most physician-rating sites have a mechanism whereby physicians can flag or respond to erroneous and libellous comments. It is important to set the record straight. It also illustrates why it is important for physicians to monitor their online reputations.

If, at the end of the day, Dr S cannot honestly see any validity in their complaints, she should probably just forget about them. You cannot love or be loved by every patient in your practice [60].

Physician-rating sites derive part of their impetus from mistrust of the peer regulatory authorities by patients and families. How effective these regulatory authorities are, for example, in screening out dangerous or unfit doctors by self-reporting has been much disputed[61]. The failure to identify poorly performing doctors has resulted in the loss of professional self-regulation almost everywhere outside Canada[62]. The Internet and new social media have led members of the public to take this matter into their own hands, "patient no longer," as the saying goes. However, these sceptical views do not take into account the very serious and almost universal nature of revalidation ("maintenance of competency" or "recertification"—the terms vary[63]) efforts made by the health professions themselves and their regulatory colleges[64]. No one benefits or wants incompetent practitioners at the wheel. As we said much earlier in this book (see the Introduction), most physicians do not go to work wondering whom they can harm today. The idea that they might harm patients is anathema to clinicians and a powerful internal mechanism to keep up their skills and knowledge.

Fitness to practise

It is not just keeping up with medical knowledge that makes one fit for practice. Health professionals, like anyone else, can suffer illnesses and conditions that can affect their ability to practise medicine. It is generally agreed that where a healthcare professional has a condition that might affect the safety of their patients and that may worsen over time, it is incumbent upon the individual to be knowledgeable about their condition, to be vigilant in monitoring it, to seek care from appropriate medical practitioners, and to accept recommendations regarding proper care and treatment.

For example, professionals carrying infections such as hepatitis B or C, or HIV—diseases that are transmissible and serious—are required in most jurisdictions to inform their regulatory organizations, which may then mandate medical monitoring and set limits on their practices. Further information is available through state and provincial licensing bodies and, in Canada, from the Canadian Medical Protective Association[65].

The same rules of self-disclosure to medical licensing authorities would apply to any health professional with a condition—depression, early cognitive impairment, degenerative neurological conditions, or physical disorders—that may impact their fitness to practise. All jurisdictions now require self-disclosure of potential or past impairments for purposes of public protection. Such disclosure would be expected at times of licensure enrolment and/or at renewal. However, this must be balanced against the professional's right to privacy[66]. Regulatory authorities typically assess impaired professionals, make recommendations regarding their eligibility for practice, and offer them confidential help. Healthcare professionals are not obliged to disclose their own health status to their patients unless required to do so by regulatory authorities.

Physicians (and nurses) in Canada are permitted, and indeed encouraged, to report to the appropriate local authorities colleagues whom they suspect to be unfit to practise because of illness or addiction. After several rather horrendous cases[67], the United Kingdom has enacted far-reaching legislation making it mandatory to report unfit healthcare professionals while protecting the "whistle-blowers"[68]. Canada had a similar and only slightly less tragic episode with the deaths of 12 infants undergoing cardiac surgery in Winnipeg in 1994[69].

Whatever the legal or regulatory status of such reporting, there would seem to be strong ethical reasons to report colleagues who constitute—by reasons of incompetence, inexperience, illness, or criminal activity—a danger to patients. Traditionally, healthcare professionals have been reluctant to discuss the mistakes of their colleagues or to "blow the whistle" on an incapacitated co-worker. This may be out of misguided loyalty or fear of repercussions for themselves[70]. It is a form of professional protectiveness that cannot be justified.

Conclusion

It is said that Hippocrates refused to attend to the sick of the Persian Empire[71]—at that time at war with Greece—despite being offered a considerable recompense by the Persian emperor. This could be taken as a tale with a favourable moral: a good clinician is not swayed to treat patients by the lure of money.

A less generous interpretation would be that Hippocrates refused to treat patients in need because of a morally irrelevant reason—they were not Greek citizens. This would not be in the true spirit of medical professionalism; clinicians should be motivated by the needs of those before them, wherever they come from.

There are so many distractions to doing the right thing in medicine that it is easy to forget the moral underpinnings of healthcare. A new and invigorated professionalism suggests we must be more vigilant than ever when it comes to the clinical failings of our colleagues and, indeed, of ourselves. But there is more to being a professional than knowing the rules and duties attending to one's work.

In the next chapter we will look at how the new digital media promises much and scares many in healthcare.

Cases for Discussion

Case 1: A Case of Self-referral

Dr R, an orthopaedic surgeon at a community hospital, attempts to refer his 55-year-old patient, Ms F, who had undergone a total shoulder arthroplasty, to his privately owned physiotherapy facility. She responds she would prefer a referral to a competitor's clinic where she had a previous good experience with the physiotherapists[72].

Dr R tells Ms F she will receive better care at his facility, as he will be present to follow up with her on a more consistent basis. Furthermore, he suggests that his "team," the physiotherapists working at the clinic, are more capable of following his instructions and requirements. The physician, however, is not familiar with the other clinic and so has no basis for suggesting this, nor does he provide Ms F with alternative options to his own facility for receiving therapeutic care.

Questions for Discussion

1. Has Dr R fulfilled his legal and moral duties by referring Ms F to his clinic?
2. What must he disclose to Ms F about his physiotherapy arrangements?
3. If you were a trainee in physiotherapy or physical medicine, would you have any responsibilities to discuss the arrangements and the alternatives with the patient?

Case 2: To The Max!

A general internist, Dr Max Y ("Dr Max" to his patients), has been in practice for more years than he cares to remember. The "senior statesman" in his group practice, he is well liked by his patients, many of whom he has seen for years and gotten to know quite well. From time to time patients ask for reassurance he will not be retiring. He jokingly tells them he will be "working to the max. Don't worry! I'll be here until they have to carry me out!"

But worry they do—especially the nurses in the clinic where he works. Now in his mid-70s, he just doesn't seem as sharp as he used to be. Two weeks ago he ordered the wrong dose of epinephrine for a young patient. As a result, the patient developed palpitations and had to go to the ER.

And just this week he gave meperidine (Demerol) IM, an old drug he had always used with good effect for acute pain, to Ms M, a 55-year-old patient who had pleaded with Dr Max "to do something" for her bad migraine. Unfortunately, he had forgotten her psychiatrist had recently prescribed Nardil, an equally old MAOI antidepressant. This drug should never be taken with Demerol due to the risk of a hypertensive crisis. Indeed, after the Demerol injection, Ms M complained she had a splitting headache and had "never felt so bad."

continued

Questions for Discussion

1. Why might Dr Max be making these mistakes?
2. How should Dr Max respond to these events?
3. Given the context of these events, which one of the following statements is the next most appropriate step?
   a. Dr Max should be encouraged to resign from the clinic.
   b. Dr Max must be reported to the appropriate authorities.
   c. Dr Max must take extra caution in carrying out his duties.
   d. Dr Max should see his own family doctor.

The End of Forgetting

Ethical and Professional Issues with Social Media

The facility to communicate immediately, widely, and interactively with patients and the public via digital technologies is transforming medicine. Nowhere is this more evident than at the intersection of social media and medical practice. However, new technologies have also provided novel twists and turns, new dimensions, and urgency to enduring ethical topics such as consent, privacy, and confidentiality. In this chapter we will look at the ethical and professional issues raised by social media.

Case 11.1   To Friend or Not to Friend

Dr B is a young physician recently out of residency who has set up practice in a large city. Within a couple of months, he starts to receive messages on his personal Facebook page, asking whether he wishes to "friend" certain people, many of whom are his patients and with whom he has no social connection. These are not actual friend requests, but rather "friend suggestions." He does receive a friend request from a patient, Mr C, with whom he shares a passion for various sports.

Why do you think Dr B is getting these "friend suggestions" from patients? Should he accept the friend request from Mr C?

I. Friends, Boundaries, and Privacy in the Age of Social Media

Social media and social networking sites represent a complex group of digital technologies and websites that facilitate the creation and sharing of information. Because of their versatility, ubiquity, and ease for sharing information, social media platforms have rapidly become mainstream for many healthcare professionals.

From a professional perspective, social media can be used for disseminating medical information [1], promoting health and healthy lifestyles, facilitating discussion between patients with similar issues, linking like-minded health professionals, recruiting subjects for research, and more. For some, this is now a necessary element of a modern medical practice [2, 3].

When it comes to social media, the primary ethical challenges for physicians (and other healthcare workers) are issues of confidentiality, privacy, and professionalism. Most professional associations and licensing bodies have developed resources and guidelines for physicians and other health professionals around using social media professionally [3-9]. These resources emphasize that the standards of professionalism and ethics are no different whether dealing with patients online or in person. Physicians, trainees, and allied healthcare professionals using social media must be cognizant of laws and regulations dealing with privacy, confidentiality, defamation, copyright, plagiarism, and physician advertising [9, 10].

Facebook and friends

At the current time, Facebook is the dominant social media platform throughout the world [11]. It can be used to provide updates about a medical practice, as well as provide educational resources to patients and families. The opportunities for health promotion and communicating collectively with patients are extraordinary.

Relations with patients on social media

Integrating social media into a medical practice poses challenges to the traditional physician–patient boundaries. Regardless of privacy settings, Facebook will sometimes prompt users to consider "friending" people who have merely been viewing their page or profile.

The frequency of "friend" requests from patients to physicians is difficult to measure and available data about this is limited [11, 12]. It is also complicated by pre-existing Facebook friends who may request to become patients [13]. Healthcare professionals should be aware that being "friends" with patients on social media blurs professional boundaries. Almost all legal, professional, and regulating organizations advise against this [3, 4, 6-8].

Online boundaries

The primary boundary issue for healthcare professionals on social media is excessive self-disclosure. Revealing too much of themselves to patients can undermine the therapeutic relationship as well as their fiduciary duty to act in the best interests of their patients [8, 14, 15].

Discussion of Case 11.1

Dr B is likely receiving notifications about possible friends because patients are searching him online and landing on his personal Facebook page. Even if he has set his privacy settings appropriately, people searching him will likely still be able to see part of his profile, who his friends are, and photos in which he is tagged.

Despite a congenial relationship with Mr C, Dr B should respectfully decline the friend request. Even if they have numerous interests and friends in common, it is important to maintain an "appropriate therapeutic distance" and not blur the physician–patient relationship. Dr B can let Mr C know in so declining he is simply following professional guidelines.

Box 11.1

Friend requests on social media can

- create a dual relationship with patients,
- blur the physician–patient boundary, and
- compromise patient privacy and confidentiality.

Can preceptors and trainees be "friends"?

Most educators feel it is generally not appropriate for preceptors to become social network friends with current trainees or learners. There is a significant power discrepancy [16, 17] and it is important to maintain an appropriate supervisory distance. Moreover, trainees may feel it is impossible to decline requests by preceptors for fear it will negatively affect their training. That said, as some trainees become more senior, a very collegial and personal relationship may develop quite naturally with preceptors, allowing for some social media interactions. But care should always be taken such circumstances.

Case 11.2   More Than Just a Friend

Dr P is a middle-aged urologist in a large metropolitan city. One day he receives a private message from Mr K, an acquaintance from his mosque who is also a Facebook friend. The message reads, "Hello Dr P, I really hate to bug you, but my family doctor retired last year and I've not found a new one. I'm having increasing problems with frequent urinating, especially at night. Any chance you could prescribe something? Perhaps I could see you in your office about my problem?"

Is it acceptable for Dr P to engage with Mr K online about his medical problem? Is it appropriate to give him advice? To write a prescription? To take Mr K on as a patient?

Discussion of Case 11.2

While Mr K's request may seem reasonable, Dr P ought not dispense any specific advice over Facebook's messaging app. It is likely not secure nor private. It is also not conducive to taking an adequate history, let alone physical exam. By giving medical advice he also risks entering into a doctor–patient relationship, without having seen or assessed his acquaintance.

It is appropriate for Dr P to validate Mr K's concerns ("Sounds like you're really having a rough time"), but also to advise him to attend a primary care physician or an urgent care clinic.

If Dr P does eventually enter into a physician–patient relationship with Mr K, then he should discontinue their Facebook friendship. While the issue may not always be black and white, being friends on Facebook raises boundary issues. It is advisable to keep one's professional and personal spheres separate on social media.

Box 11.2

Five techniques for separating the "personal" and "professional" online:

1. Create a professional social media profile that is distinct from a personal one.
2. Ensure that your personal social media is discreet and not easily found by patients searching for you online.
3. Always use the highest level of privacy/security for personal social media sites.
4. Consider a Facebook "business" page or LinkedIn as the interface with the public.
5. Create guidelines and policy for use of social media in your practice [1, 17, 18].

II. The Personal and the Private

Regardless of how well a clinician delineates their professional and personal social media presences, it is easy for the lines to become blurred. Consider the following case.

Case 11.3   My Personal Life Is My Business!

During a post-graduate session on professionalism, a surgical resident comments that he was reprimanded by his program director for some "dodgy" Facebook posts he made while on holiday in Mexico with some buddies.
  "What I post on my personal social media is my business," he asserts, and then asks, "Why should I be held to a higher standard than other professionals?"

Is the resident right? Are medical professionals held to a higher standard? Is he right from an ethical perspective?

Physicians are entitled to a private life. What they do in that sphere should not, in general, be an issue in their professional lives. In days past, a physician who got drunk at a wedding, took off his shirt and danced on a table might have a few awkward queries to answer for in the following weeks. Eventually such an incident would be consigned to the dustbin of embarrassing life moments and, if not entirely forgotten, would fade into obscurity with time.

However, in the era of social media, images, videos, and audio from such an event might quickly appear on various platforms and remain indefinitely present online. Patients searching for this clinician online might find the first thing they encounter is a video entitled "table-dance at a wedding." In the brave new world of social media, the private sphere is shrinking. The implications for healthcare professionals can be quite severe [19-22].

Box 11.3

In the age of the Internet and social media:
"It's often said that we live in a permissive era, one with infinite second chances. But the truth is that for a great many people, the permanent memory bank of the Web increasingly means there are no second chances—no opportunities to escape a scarlet letter in your digital past. Now the worst thing you've done is often the first thing everyone knows about you".

Jeffery Rosen, 2010 [23]

Discussion of Case 11.3

The surgical resident has a cause for concern. His personal life should be private. However, social media is akin to a room with a large front window facing the street, with privacy settings like the curtains drawn across the window to block passersby from looking in [24].

Is the resident at fault if he leaves the curtain slightly open, enough so people can peek in and observe him doing something unprofessional? Shouldn't they have the decency to walk by without looking in, even if the curtain is open?

This type of restraint is not the reality of the digital age. There are few obstacles to copying, modifying, and disseminating personal information. Comments made in one circumstance can be taken out of context. Unprofessional behaviour in one sphere can easily bleed into another sphere. Hence, the expression "privacy is dead" (see Chapter 7). We are mistaken if we think our online personal lives are not potentially accessible by the general public.

The resident is also mistaken if he believes this lack of privacy affects only physicians. There are countless examples of ostensibly private social media posts impacting people's employment, education, divorce negotiations, and more [25]. One need only peruse the news for the latest social media scandal.

Privacy settings in social media

Anyone who has tried to sort out social media privacy settings will attest to the fact that they can be confusing and hard to use [26–28]. Because social media is so many things to so many people (that is, business use, personal use, group use), privacy is rarely clear-cut—which makes creating widely accepted privacy settings extremely challenging. Moreover, despite repeated concerns about privacy settings, most users of social media are still quite undiscerning when it comes to making friends online. According to a 2016 study, over 50 per cent of Facebook and Instagram users accepted a friend or follower request from a complete stranger [29].

In addition, many users of social media do not appreciate the implications of the business model on which social networking sites are based. Almost all social media generates revenue by advertising to users, based on data collected about them from their social media use: "When it comes to social media, users are not the customer; users are the product" [30–33]. Social media sites, as well as some of their advertisers, can often collect vast amounts of user information and then use it for commercial or political purposes. The Facebook-Cambridge Analytica scandal in 2018 is a case in point [34, 35]. Although some sites, such as Facebook, are attempting to be more transparent about their collection and use of user data, collecting users' personal data remains the *modus operandi* for attracting advertisers to their platforms [36, 37].

One might suppose a review of such policies would have a sobering effect on users, but Aljohani has documented that the vast majority of social media users do not believe the following factual statements regarding Facebook's privacy policy are actually true:

Facebook can

1. collect and use all the information they receive about you to suggest advertisements for you;
2. track your web surfing anytime you're logged into the site;
3. use your public information, such as your profile picture, in ads, without asking you first, and without any compensation to you; and
4. collect information about your device locations, including specific geographic locations through GPS, Bluetooth, or Wi-Fi Signals. [29]

Box 11.4

....

"Don't make the mistake of thinking you're Facebook's customer, you're not—you're the product. . . . Its customers are the advertisers." [38]

Regardless of what privacy settings are used, personal posts, comments, images, and videos appearing in ostensibly private spaces are not really private. In the first place, they can and will be used for commercial purposes by the social networking sites. Secondly, they can easily be copied and disseminated, either inadvertently or with malicious intention, and impact the professional sphere. A personal space is not the same as a private space [10, 14, 39]. In the age of social media, healthcare professionals are naïve if they believe that online personal space is truly private.

Consider some of the following examples:

1. A nurse makes a strident comment on his personal Facebook page opposing a safe drug injection site near the hospital where he works. A screenshot of the post subsequently appears in a local newspaper with the headline, "Nurse Opposed to Treating Patients with Addiction."
2. A friend posts and tags a picture of you celebrating with him over beers at a sports event. A patient comments about it in clinic the next day. He is a friend of a friend and saw it when your name was tagged.
3. After a particularly tough day, an internal medicine resident posts an entry on her Facebook page about a medical error she observed at work

that day. A social worker from the ward, who is friends with the resident, sees it and notifies the patient.

4. While on a break in the ER, a physician posts a comment on her personal Facebook page about how tired she is, having had a little too much to drink at a wedding the night before. Unbeknownst to her, she has neglected to properly set her privacy settings. A patient she is assessing in the ER comments, "Hey Doc, hope you're not too hungover to treat me."

5. In a fit of frustration, a resident writes a disparaging comment about a colleague on his Facebook page. The next day he regrets this and deletes it, but it has already been copied and reposted.

6. A medical student is perplexed he was not matched to a residency program, despite being a strong student and having done ample electives and research in his area of interest. Frustrated and dejected, he contacts a program director to ask why he wasn't accepted. In response, the program director sends him a link to a Facebook page of a friend of the student's; there is a picture of him clearly very inebriated, in a state of partial undress, making an obscene gesture at the camera.

These examples highlight the fact that despite attempts to keep our personal and professional online identities separate, our online presence can be very complex, with the personal and professional easily intertwined.

Box 11.5

When it comes to our use of social media, there is a persistent tendency to confuse the notion of a personal space with a private space.

III. Patients Using Social Media

Case 11.4 A Google Dilemma

Ms V, a nurse with the transplant team, is aiding in the process of preparing Mr C for a liver transplant. The patient has progressive end-stage liver disease, secondary to longstanding alcohol abuse. He has been compliant with the workup so far and appears very motivated to have a transplant. He has assured Ms V and the transplant team that he is in recovery, sober for the past eight months, and attending 12-step meetings.

Mr C, who is very gregarious, is involved in the local art and theatre scene. Somewhat curious about his work, Ms V Googles him and lands on his personal Facebook page. His privacy settings permit general viewing. While perusing some of his entries, Ms V sees several recent photos of Mr C celebrating with family and friends. In many of these photos, he is holding what look like alcoholic beverages. Although she cannot be sure, it certainly appears as if he is "lit up" in several of the photos. Checking the dates of the photos, she finds they have been posted in the past month.

Was it wrong for Ms V to Google Mr C? To check out his personal Facebook page? What should Ms V do, given she suspects Mr C is still drinking?

Although healthcare professionals are privy to some of the most intimate aspects of a patient's life, this does not mean they have a right to access all aspects of the patient's life. The information they access should be relevant only to the care they are providing. This has implications when searching for a patient's information online. Without an invitation from the patient, checking out a patient's Facebook page or other social media simply for interest or voyeuristic reasons is inappropriate. Several organizations and guidelines have pointed out that patients have an expectation of online privacy from physicians, even if the information is not, strictly speaking, private [5, 40]. As noted already (Case 11.1 above), looking up someone on Facebook may put you on their "suggested friends" list.

There may be some situations when searching a patient's social media might be reasonable, such as if there are concerns a patient may be suicidal or homicidal [4, 41]. It might even be justified if one is suspicious of fraudulent medical activity [42] or one needs to urgently track down a patient who did not provide up-to-date contact information [43].

However, such instances are likely few and far between. Anytime professionals play detective, they should question their own motives. First, searching online to substantiate patients' statements can undermine trust, which is central to the healthcare relationship. Second, patients are entitled to a reasonable expectation of privacy [40]. And third, information found online is ripe for misinterpretation.

Discussion of Case 11.4

While Ms V's actions are not born of suspicion or mistrust, she does inadvertently stumble onto information suggesting that Mr C is not being honest and compliant with his preparation for transplantation. This fairly innocent

continued

boundary violation places her in a difficult situation. With whom does her primary commitment lie?

This scenario is not unique to social media. Ms V could just as easily have encountered Mr C having a drink in a restaurant. However, the facility of social media to record and disseminate information takes the possibility of inadvertent discovery of information to a whole new level [44].

Now that the cat is out of the bag, Ms V should discuss the situation with the transplant team. While she should be concerned about potentially spreading aspersions about Mr C, she does have an obligation, both to other potential transplant recipients, as well as donors, to ensure the responsible use of donated livers. It is also possible that her impression is a misunderstanding. Thus, she ought to tell her colleagues the circumstances under which she came upon the information. This may help if Mr C ever makes a complaint about her to a regulatory authority. Finally, Ms V and other team members should meet with Mr C to discuss her findings on Facebook so he can have an opportunity to respond. It would also be appropriate for her to apologize to him and explain the circumstances under which she discovered this information.

IV. Photographs and Patient Privacy

It should be no surprise that one of the primary concerns of engaging with patients over social media is the risk to *patient* privacy. Regulated healthcare professionals have not only an ethical, but also a statutory obligation to protect patient privacy (see Chapter 7). Those who compromise the privacy and confidentiality of patients online are not only breaching an ethical obligation, but a legal one as well, and may be subject to both disciplinary actions as well as civil penalties. While every healthcare provider knows never to disclose identifying personal patient information, whether online or elsewhere, the issues can become quite complicated when it comes to social media [2, 45].

Case 11.5   Whose Wound Is It Anyway?

You are a family medicine resident on rotation in the ER. You are seeing a homeless and self-neglecting man with a huge infected wound on his right thigh crawling with maggots. The attending physician tells him she would like to show it to the surgeon on call. She snaps a photo of the lesion with her phone and sends it to the surgeon for advice. She also copies you on the message.

The next week, while reading some medical blogs online, you see a picture of the same wound on a blog called "Nightdoc in the ER." It is, in fact, the very same picture you received from the physician in the hospital. And the author is clearly the physician with whom you worked the week before.

Is there anything wrong in taking a photo in this circumstance? Sharing the photo on a blog? Blogging about the case?

Clinical photography and online posting

Nowhere is the impact of digital technology on patient privacy more evident than in the area of digital clinical photography. Any healthcare professional can take a high-quality photo or video with a smartphone and distribute it worldwide in a matter of seconds. There are many ways in which patient privacy can unwittingly be compromised as a result:

- There may be patient-identifying information not readily apparent on a small phone screen: tattoos, birthmarks, or unique features.
- There may be location-identifying information such as other patients, staff, a sign, a hospital label or logo visible in the background.
- Many photos are geotagged with precise location and time information that can be accessed by those in the know.
- Personal photo libraries, whether on a phone or in the cloud, can be hacked.
- If the photo is posted online, someone local may recognize the scenery and location.

An example of unintentional disclosure of patient information occurred in 2012, when a patient's personal information was inadvertently linked to her breast augmentation photo when posted on a surgeon's website. Although she had provided written consent that the photo could be used anonymously for the purposes of advertising, teaching, and case reports, there was a clear specification she would remain anonymous. Although the photo included only her torso, her name was easily visible when the cursor hovered over it: a small, but costly mistake[46]. Numerous other examples exist[47].

Another area where digital medical photography and social media frequently intersect is in the realm of medical missions to developing countries, during which participants typically have intense, life-altering experiences. Quite understandably, they may want to share those experiences, both medical and social, with friends and colleagues via social media. Yet there are frequently significant questions with regard to appropriate consent and removal of identifying information about individual patients [48]. When doing humanitarian work and donating one's time and skills to less fortunate populations, there is a tendency by some participants to take licence with the usual ethical obligations for consent and privacy [49].

Clinical photography and consent

Any discussion of clinical photography would be incomplete without a discussion of consent. As we have already discussed the nature of consent in Chapters 5 and 6, our discussion here need only be brief.

1. The digital nature of such photos means they are easily reproducible and distributable. Patients should be told how photos will be used and stored.
2. At a minimum, patients should provide express oral consent for any clinical photography. In most instances, it would be prudent to obtain written authorization from the patient (that is, express written consent). Many institutions provide a specific digital photography consent form for this reason.
3. If a patient photo is for promotional or other commercial uses, then written authorization is mandatory [47].

One challenge with clinical photography deals with ownership of an image. While a clinician who takes a photo may think of it as theirs, patients see it as their image and rightly want control over how it will be used. There are numerous examples of digital photography being used for various purposes without proper consent from the subject in the photograph. If and when patients make a complaint, the findings tend to go consistently against physicians.

Discussion of Case 11.5

This case illustrates a number of ethical pitfalls associated with digital and social media. In this scenario, the physician who took the picture and posted it did not obtain appropriate consent, did not ensure protection of the patient's privacy, and distributed it in a cavalier fashion to the resident working with her. What she did may not be illegal, but is very ethically dubious.

Taking the photo and sending it to the surgeon is reasonable, if done securely and with the consent of the patient. However, this indigent patient is highly vulnerable—too sick, too confused, and too intimidated to voice any objections to the ER physician. The physician should explain to him the importance of photographing the wound in its present state. She should reassure him that, other than showing it to the surgeon on call, she will keep it private. Later, when the patient is recovering on the ward, the physician could initiate a longer discussion about the photo and explain how else she would like to use it. Assuming the patient agrees, it would be advisable for the physician to obtain express written consent[47]. This approach demonstrates the respect due to all persons.

V. Internet Etiquette and Telling Others' Stories

One of the main attractions of social media is the opportunity to share stories and experiences with others. Medical professionals are not immune to this inclination, with countless medical- and health-related blogs authored by physicians. Concern over patient privacy has always been front and centre of the debate about this form of social media[50, 51].

Blogging or writing about one's patients without their consent is a recurring issue for physicians—whether it be case reports in medical journals or memoir books by physicians. The following is a case in point.

Case 11.6 A Soldier's Story

Dr Kevin Patterson, a Canadian surgeon-novelist who had recently finished a tour of duty, wrote a story in 2007 about the death of a Canadian soldier he had treated. The article, describing in explicit and gruesome detail the soldier's final hours, was published within weeks of his death on the website of a widely circulated US magazine[52]. The identity of the deceased soldier was not concealed. The Department of National Defence viewed this as a breach of confidentiality for which Dr Patterson faced court martial[53].

Was Patterson wrong to write about the soldier's death?

Discussion of Case 11.6

According to the magazine, the soldier's family did not object to publication of the story and, in fact, expressed gratitude for Dr Patterson's heroic efforts to save their loved one. But the surgeon's claim that family approved the publication did not absolve him of his duty to protect the soldier's identity. Although he had the best of intentions—to honour the death of the soldier and publicize the sacrifices made by the troops—the breach of confidentiality had a negative

continued

impact on other family members and friends of the deceased. The posting of the article on the Internet so soon after the soldier's demise no doubt contributed to his family's distress.

The duty of confidentiality *should* persist after a person's death. The length of time that must elapse before personal information can be *legally* released without prior patient or family consent varies from place to place; in some countries, there may be no posthumous protection; in others, such as Canada, more than a century must elapse before it can be released.

Although Dr Patterson was exonerated by the Department of National Defence, he was found guilty by his provincial regulating body of professional misconduct for breaching patient confidentiality. The penalties imposed included a formal written reprimand, a fine of $5000, and an agreement to donate $7000 to charity [54]. He reassured the governing body that "any future writings based on medical scenarios . . . would not include the identities of patients or any information that could identify patients" [55].

Opinions about the propriety of such writing vary and are determined primarily on the basis of whether patient anonymity can be ensured. However, there are many ways patient anonymity can be inadvertently compromised. The standard usually applied is not whether a stranger could identify the patient, but rather whether the patient or a family member could recognize themselves in the story [56].

While writers of medical blogs, books, and case reports might argue their mission is to edify and enlighten the public and their colleagues about a unique illness or circumstance, the matter can look quite different from the perspective of the patient. Is the patient's story being exploited for the purposes of self-promotion of the writer? It is hard to deny that, on some level, a patient's story is being co-opted and exploited for the personal benefit of the writer. And from a legal perspective, personal health information belongs to the patient, not the physician [56].

Regardless of where you come down on this issue, it is not black and white. Even physicians who write about their patients on a regular basis admit to conflicted feelings on the subject [57–59]. We (the authors), too, have experienced this conflict in our teaching and our writing. Over the past several decades, the community standards around patient vignettes have changed dramatically in the direction of increasing respect for patient privacy. Many of the cases in this book are entirely fictional, but are based on real dilemmas the authors have encountered or been privy to. Others are either in the public domain (by way of being reported in the media or featured in well-known court cases) or have received

> **Box 11.6**
>
> ....
>
> "There is a consensus in Canadian law that personal health information is 'fundamentally one's own' and that individuals should, in most circumstances, be the ones deciding how the information should be used."[56]

patient or family consent. In any case we have changed the names and altered the case circumstances to address this issue. As for "appropriating" the stories of others, perhaps we stand guilty as charged—but so too are all writers from Cervantes onwards.

Telling patients' stories, of course, is not unique to social media. Physicians have been writing about their patients for millennia, with their work usually published in obscure and arcane places such as medical journals and textbooks. The Internet, social media, and online journalism have democratized the process, making potential voyeurs of us all. We can access with ease events half a world away—events which, until the advent of digital media, would have been hidden away and never scrutinized by the general public. Digital media makes the ethical challenges raised by such writings all the more acute.

Social media guidelines

Prior to setting up an online professional social media presence, physicians would be well advised to have in place formal guidelines and policies on the use of social media in a practice/clinic. Even if a physician is not considering a professional social media presence, such guidelines and policies are still a good idea. As illustrated above, policies can help when it comes to explaining boundaries to patients. They are also valuable to help ensure that office staff, trainees, and other professionals working in healthcare are aware of expectations vis-à-vis engagement with social media.

Conclusion

In this chapter we have discussed a number of ethical issues related to social media. Many of the ethical questions raised are not new, but social media gives them a new dimension and an intensified degree of urgency. Privacy and confidentiality are the Achilles heels of medicine. For this reason, they warrant special and detailed attention, particularly with regard to ever-changing technologies.

Box 11.7

Some guidelines and cautions for online posting:

1. Ensure that comments posted online are subject to the same strictures as any communications.
2. Remember that the standards for medical professionalism online are the same as those for offline.
3. Be professional, respectful, and civilized at all times.
4. Keep your personal and professional online identities separate.
5. Know the terms and conditions of your social networking sites.
6. Use the strictest privacy settings for your personal online identities.
7. Be aware that the identity of anonymous participants can almost always be ascertained.
8. Regard all information on the Internet as essentially public, regardless of privacy settings.
9. Remember that anything posted online can be very difficult, if not impossible, to remove.
10. Consider waiting 12 to 24 hours before posting to ensure this is what you really want to say.
11. Avoid potential, perceived, or real conflicts of interest.
12. Be aware that commercial enterprises are increasingly exploiting social media.
13. Be honest about who you are when participating in online group discussions.
14. Avoid excessive self-disclosure.
15. Avoid friending or following patients online.
16. Restrict patient information to that which is relevant to their care.
17. Keep medical advice general when discussing issues online.
18. Never post identifying patient information online without express written consent.
19. Ensure that patients and their significant others are not able to recognize themselves in any online writing or photos that you post.
20. Be aware that there are many ways to inadvertently disclose patient identification.
21. Don't forget that patients frequently search out their physicians and may see what you post.
22. Keep your own social media and web presence up to date.

Cases for Discussion

Case 1: It's A Virtual World

Dr D has recently completed his medical training and is ready to go into independent practice. He and several colleagues are unhappy with being a "doc in a box" with the usual ten-minutes-per-patient-visit routine. They decide to set up a "virtual clinic" that will combine the power of modern computing with the ability to interact online with sick patients at home. Patients will be able to book appointments online and have access to advice by email. Fees will be charged for online advice or assessments and be paid through PayPal. Access to the patient's hospital files, research participation, and genetic testing will be incorporated into the patient's electronic medical record.

Question for Discussion

1. What are the pros and cons for patients and for healthcare professionals of such a virtual clinical arrangement?

Case 2: The Pose That Pauses

You enjoy trawling the Internet and come upon a site that links persons in the community with health professionals. One part of this site is devoted to graduate-level trainees and newly minted health practitioners acting as mentors by providing hints and insights into medical culture to younger, would-be medical students.

As you scroll through the site, you recognize a physician assistant who has posted a number of pictures of himself establishing a central venous line in a patient. In one photo he holds a syringe at a man's neck with the caption, "When you can't start a line in a junkie's arm, go for the neck."

Question for Discussion

1. What, if anything, should you do?

✦ 12 ✦

··

The Error of Our Ways

Managing Medical Error

Our feelings are with such errorists.

Blackwood's Edinburgh Magazine, 1849[1]

I. Medical Error

Errors and harm caused by healthcare are medicine's worst-kept secrets[2]. Little talked about in the past, they have been brought into the light of the public eye for over 20 years. "Life is short, the art is long, opportunity fleeting, experiment perilous, judgment uncertain," so wrote Hippocrates or one of his followers over 2000 years ago. Medicine is still a perilous and difficult profession. All clinicians can have bad days, and even the best make mistakes.

Case 12.1   "I'm Just So Tired!"

··

You are a busy family practitioner in independent practice. You are seeing Ms L, a 45-year-old corporate lawyer with two children, who complains of fatigue of several months' duration. She reports working very long hours preparing for a case and has been additionally stressed as her assistant is on maternity leave. She admits she is not eating properly nor getting enough sleep. She often works late into the night. You both agree she should strive for more balance in her life. Just to rule out other causes of fatigue, you send her that day for some basic blood tests, telling her your assistant will call her only if the results are abnormal. Otherwise, Ms L should come back to see you in three months.

When she returns for her three-month follow-up visit, you look over her chart just before entering the examining room. To your horror, you see that her bloodwork at that time indicated a significant reduction in her platelet, red, and white blood cell counts, most compatible with aplastic anemia. You have absolutely no recollection of ever having looked at the report.

"Doctor, I'm still feeling really exhausted even though I'm getting more sleep and worrying less about work," Ms L says as you sit down.

What should you say or do?

Errors and mistakes

Medical errors are considered preventable events, processes or outcomes which may or may not harm a patient, and which occurred in a medical setting as a result of a human or system fault [3]. They are common and are generally unexpected, unwanted, and unintended. Errors do not always cause physical harm but they can wound psychologically and undermine confidence. They can also be an impetus for learning and system change.

We will use the term "mistakes" interchangeably with "errors." Calling an action, process, or outcome an error (or errant) does imply some sense of responsibility in that it presumes you could have acted better or differently in the circumstances. If you reasonably could not or would not have acted any differently—in other words if the incident was not preventable—then there was no error by a practitioner, only an unfortunate incident. Systems can fail and err, too. As these can harm patients, the new approach to error involves examining the system's issues allowing error to occur, rather than seeing the system's adverse incidents as inevitable and under no one's control.

Adverse events and negligence

Adverse events are incidents caused by medical interventions that set back the interests of patients, causing them harm or threatening to do so. Studies suggest close to half of adverse events are considered preventable and so can be designated as errors. An unpreventable adverse event would be an unforeseen complication, such as a rash following the administration of penicillin in a patient with no prior history of drug sensitivity. It would be considered an error, however, if a rash occurred as a result of penicillin being prescribed again for the same patient due to, due to the physician forgetting the previous reaction, not checking the chart, or neglecting to ask the patient about their drug history [3].

Negligence, one of the main causes of malpractice actions against healthcare professionals, is something quite different. It is a legal determination, a finding by a court of law.

"Negligent events" refer to that smaller class of events that cause tangible harm, are preventable, and would not have been made by a reasonable and prudent clinician in similar circumstances[4]. Perfection is not the standard of care; "reasonableness" is—providing the "standard of care" has been followed.

Box 12.1

For an event to be considered negligent, it requires

- a duty of care by the doctor,
- a breach of the standard of care by the doctor, and
- an injury to the patient.

Importantly, the injury must have been caused by the breach.

Thus, re-prescribing penicillin in a patient with a known history of penicillin allergy might be found negligent depending on the circumstances and the seriousness of the harms caused to the patient.

Not all errors or adverse events are blameworthy. For example, a practitioner may make an error in diagnosis, such as mistaking heart failure for pneumonia. If they took a proper history, did a thorough exam, and took into account appropriate tests, as a similarly qualified clinician would have done, then the mistake may not be deemed negligent in a court of law.

Box 12.2

"The standard of care which the law requires is not insurance against accidental slips. It is such a degree of care as a normally skillful member of the profession may reasonably be expected to exercise in the actual circumstances of the case in question. It is not every slip or mistake which imports negligence."

Mahone v Osborne, 1939[5]

Size of the problem

The scope of the problem of medical error and adverse outcomes is huge. Studies done in Canada, Australia, the United Kingdom, and the United States reveal very similar adverse event and error rates[6]. Overall, preventable adverse events are connected with the deaths of about one in 200 patients admitted to hospitals. The mistakes in care cannot be said to have been directly causative but were implicated in the deaths of those patients, some of whom were very ill to begin with. Although this astonishing number has been disputed, the studies are very consistent.

Adverse events in medicine are universally acknowledged to be a common and serious quality-of-care issue for healthcare. They were the subject of influential reports released in 1999 and 2001e[7,8]. Research since then has shown remarkable improvements in some areas—for example, sepsis caused by central lines and wrong-side surgical error[9]—but there remains a long way to go as regards patient safety.

Discussion of Case 12.1

You cannot beat around the bush with this one. Ms L should be told without delay about the missed lab report from three months ago. You should tell her what you know about pancytopenia, its causes and management. Even if she fails to ask, you should tell her of the missed report.

A lawsuit might result but, quite frankly, this should be the furthest thing from your mind. You should be thinking, "How can I ensure this patient gets the best care possible without further delay?" Ms L needs to understand that part of the urgency stems from the missed lab report. It is doubly wrong to compound the original mistake by attempting to conceal it. The patient may also wish to hear what you will do differently going forward to ensure this will not happen to anyone else.

You should take a deep breath and begin to explain what happened with the lab report from three months ago. ("There is no easy way to tell you this, but . . .")

Cause and accountability

The etiologies of error and adverse events in healthcare are manifold and well-explored elsewhere in many books and journals[10]. Suffice it to say that systemic or human factors (or both) are typically involved in every case of significant error. An example of a human error is a nurse inadvertently, through fatigue or inattention, causing harm by giving IV KCl (potassium chloride, cardio-toxic), instead of IV MgSO4 (magnesium sulphate, used to prevent seizures). An example of a systemic error is a hospital stocking look-alike medications in a way that makes it easy to mistake one for the other. The systems error is an adverse situation waiting to fail: it facilitates or allows the nurse to make the error; the error could happen to anyone. Systems issues make it easy for health providers to fail—especially in the complex life-and-death situations in which they find themselves, under pressure and with uncertain goals[11].

We are human. No matter how good we are as clinicians, we will make mistakes—sometimes with grievous consequences. We need safer systems that plan for human fallibility and that allow for and encourage learning[12].

For example, as in Case 12.1, a common type of error is the missed or overlooked result. Sometimes clinicians say such mistakes—resulting in omissions of appropriate timely diagnosis and treatment—occur because they are "too busy" to follow up on all the tests they order. If so, they should try to get less busy[13].

The "Don't call us, we'll call you" system on which some clinicians rely is an outmoded one. It assumes perfect systems of return. However, no one is going to recall every test done on every patient. Electronic medical records may help with minimizing such errors, but even computer systems are fallible. It should help that motivated patients are increasingly allowed by hospitals to access and review their own records. But this, too, can be flawed: computerized records may be incomplete or not returned in a timely way; patients may not know what tests were ordered or what the implications of any abnormalities might be.

Legal expectations

There are few laws *per se* requiring healthcare professionals to be honest with patients (see Chapter 6). But even if the law isn't changing, professional practice is. The cases of medical harm particularly prompting patient and public ire are typically those where no one has assumed responsibility—especially if patients have been similarly harmed in the past. A perception of a "cover-up" by the professionals and institutions involved is a frequent addendum to the concerns about an unwanted outcome of care.

The failure of professionals to be thoroughly honest about such harms or hazardous situations is a violation of professionalism, considered to be deserving of sanction. A particularly egregious example is the 1999 British Columbia case of *Shobridge v Thomas* in which a surgeon accidentally left an abdominal roll in a patient's abdomen[14]. After recurrent infections and admissions to the hospital over the subsequent two months, the patient underwent another operation, at which time the abdominal roll was discovered and removed. The surgeon did not disclose this finding to the patient for over two more months and actively tried to cover up the error by telling the nurses not to record it on the operative record.

The judge found the nurses should have filled out an incident report but concluded the negligence causing Ms Shobridge harm was due to Dr Thomas's actions alone. The court described the surgeon's delay in informing his patient and his deliberate attempts to hide his mistake as demonstrating "bad faith and unprofessional behaviour deserving of punishment." In addition to "general damages" of $190,000, the surgeon was held liable for "aggravated damages" in the amount of $25,000 for the exceptional harm caused by the withholding of the information and an additional $20,000 in "punitive damages" for his deliberate deception of the plaintiff.

In modern healthcare, multiple specialties and professions are always involved in looking after a patient with serious illness [15], so deliberate camouflaging of error or poor outcomes is difficult to achieve. The failure to provide coordinated and transparent leadership can have serious repercussions, however. It is easy for care to fall through the cracks and for no one to feel responsible. The English psychiatrist, Balint, called this the "collusion of anonymity" [16]. Here is one such case.

Case 12.2   A Lapse in Care [17]

Dr V, a hospital-based obstetrician-gynecologist, did a Pap smear on Ms B in May 1992. The patient was not informed that pre-cancerous cells were found. Eleven months later, she was diagnosed with an advanced form of cervical cancer. Only then did she receive treatment. Despite this treatment, Ms B died of the disease a year and a half later. Her estate sued Dr V for negligence. Evidence was presented at trial that Dr V had left the country for an extended period shortly after doing the Pap smear. The hospital closed the clinic in which he worked without making any arrangements to handle his reports. As a result, Ms B's Pap smear report remained unseen by a clinician until almost a year later.

What is the central issue at stake here?

Discussion of Case 12.2

The central issue in this case was the lapse in routine clinical vigilance that might have prevented this error. Although the mistake was not deliberate, no one would defend missing an abnormal Pap smear for a year as an acceptable error, one that a reasonably careful physician would make. In this case, however, the lapse in care was not the doctor's alone. The Appeals Court ruled there is "a duty upon the physician to see to it that there is a reasonably effective follow-up system in place" as well as "a responsibility on hospitals to see to it that adequate procedures are in place to 'ensure' (but not guarantee) patient safety."

The Court, therefore, found liability for Ms B's outcome to be shared equally by Dr V and the hospital. This seems just about right.

> **Box 12.3**
>
> ....
>
> "Where a patient in a hospital is treated by more than one specialty, the hospital owes a duty to ensure that proper coordination occurs and that the treatment program it offers operates as a unified and cohesive whole."
>
> ....
>
> *Braun v Vaughan Manitoba Court of Appeal, 2000* [17]

Unexpected findings and cooperation

The responsibility for patient welfare does not end if one claims to be only indirectly involved in the care of a patient. If ancillary professionals have some information bearing on the patient's well-being, there is an evolving duty to ensure this information is received and acted upon. For example, when significantly new and unexpected findings are seen on an X-ray, issuing a timely and accurate report may be insufficient: in some jurisdictions, liability may accrue for radiologists who do not ensure that the findings are acted upon. Physicians ought to be familiar with the regulations as regards this matter in their hospital.

> **Box 12.4**
>
> ....
>
> "Where there is an unexpected finding which may affect patient management or where the severity of the condition is greater than expected, it is the responsibility of the radiologist to communicate this information to the clinical team either by direct discussion or other means." [18]

The requirement to report unexpected and possibly serious findings is an ongoing issue for medicine (see Chapter 18 for its impact on research). The interdisciplinary requirements regarding healthcare, insofar as different professions are essential to the comprehensive care of patients, are growing. To meet these needs, the following sensible and hardly onerous recommendations could apply to any healthcare professional:

- They must coordinate their efforts with those of other healthcare professionals involved in the care of the patient.
- They must have a system in place whereby unusual, hazardous findings can be communicated to the patient and/or the treating team.
- They may have a duty to communicate directly with the patient if they are unable to contact the most responsible clinician in a timely way [19].

The shared responsibility of healthcare professionals lessens the tremendous weight of responsibility faced by physicians, makes teamwork part of shared decision-making, and is definitely the way of twenty-first-century medicine.

Response to error

The automatic human response, when a mistake is made, is often to be defensive and embarrassed. Professionals involved in medical mishaps must learn to tame such automatic responses and try to be open and honest about such events. To be sure, this is hard to do. Admitting error may be like trying to, as someone once said, swallow a watermelon whole. The psychological harm—the shame, the embarrassment[20]—experienced by the erring practitioner should not be underestimated.

Disclosure can be difficult

Transparency as regards mistakes can be frightening for some clinicians—they can feel defenceless and alone. Case reports by clinicians remind us of the tremendous psychological strain healers undergo when they have harmed—or think they have harmed—the patients they serve[21]. But secrecy about error can be counter-productive: it can leave clinicians who participated in the incident with a never-ending emotional burden of guilt and shame.

Box 12.5

....

"Shame is so devastating because it goes right to the core of a person's identity, making them feel exposed, inferior, degraded; it leads to avoidance, to silence."[22]

Disclosure can be therapeutic

Disclosure of the event can be therapeutic for clinicians and prevent the corrosive effects of duplicity on their self-esteem as a healthcare professional. Admitting a mistake advances understanding of such incidents and promotes prevention efforts. Disclosing errors can also promote maturity and personal growth on the part of the clinician. Being open about our mistakes makes us humbler but wiser.

Unfortunately, it appears not all clinicians agree: one-third of US doctors surveyed in a 2012 study[23] did not completely agree with disclosing serious medical errors to patients. More reassuring is another 2012 study, this time of medical trainees[24], showing that interns are now, as compared with 10 years ago, more open about their errors and appreciate that honesty is the best path for dealing with errors. Thus, the habits of professionalism may be a generational issue: the new cohort of healthcare practitioners, perhaps as a result of the ongoing revolution in healthcare curricula, may be inclined to act in more morally appropriate ways.

II. Error and Being Responsive to Patients

Certain "facilitative" communication styles [25] by health professionals can guard against making errors and against complaints, regardless of patient outcomes. ("Do my recommendations make sense to you?" "Do you have any other concerns we haven't addressed today?" "Has anything about your illness or the treatment to date been a surprise for you?") Being "present" with the patient [26]—letting them know you care and are there for them, no matter what the outcome—cements the therapeutic relationship.

Patients and families who pursue legal action are often motivated by a need for explanation and accountability and a concern for the standards of care. Thus, it can be helpful to provide patients and/or their families with a full explanation of "unexpected events," even if minor. Informing patients and families promptly and honestly about harmful incidents fosters a healthier and more realistic understanding of medical care and may prevent anger [27]. Major events—such as the unexpected death of a person in a medical setting (see Chapter 10)—deserve close attention by physicians.

While disclosure and being responsive to patient concerns are not guarantees against lawsuits and complaints, timely transparency and attentiveness can reduce the punitive sting that sometimes accompanies complaints against clinicians. Kraman and colleagues [28] reported on the experience in an American Veterans Administration hospital that routinely informs patients and their families of any harmful incident and then offers them help in filing legal claims for compensation. This "proactive" policy of disclosure did lead to an increase in the number of claims made against the hospital but many were local, out-of-court settlements. As a result, this hospital had the eighth lowest total monetary payouts out of comparable VA hospitals. Similarly, the University of Michigan Health System [29] combined disclosure with an offer of compensation without increasing its total claims and liability costs.

Because of universal healthcare (which tends to make for a less litigious system), physicians and hospitals in Canada have been spared many of the worst excesses of the US malpractice system. However, compensation to patients and families harmed by error may still be an important consideration for some in Canada because universal healthcare does not cover all health-related expenditures—nor does it cover the devastating psychological impact some medically related injuries can have upon patients and families.

When to disclose

Do all medical errors need to be disclosed? In theory yes, but it depends on the circumstances and the patient. Minor errors that do not affect the patient, such as ordering an antibiotic four times daily instead of the three times daily, may not warrant disclosure, especially if no harm was caused. In general, disclosure is a proportionate duty that should take into account the preferences of patients and families, the clinical circumstances of the patient, and the nature and gravity of the incident:

- The greater the impact or harm an adverse event has or may have upon a patient, the greater the obligation to disclose the event to the patient and/or the family.
- By corollary, "non-significant events" do not require disclosure. However, just what "significant" means may depend on individual or subjective factors that need to be taken into account by clinicians when deciding whether they ought to disclose an unanticipated outcome to the patient.
- When in doubt, it is better for clinicians and institutions to err on the side of disclosure than non-disclosure.

The bottom line: honesty is the best policy. Clinicians should assume that patients and their families want to know what happened. They should routinely acknowledge and discuss an unexpected serious event with the patient (if they are alive and well enough, of course, to be able to participate) and the patient's network of support or their family (if the patient agrees). This should take place as soon as possible after the incident has been identified and may require more than one meeting, especially if the event is complex (as they often are).

The question, then, is not whether or not to disclose but how to do so.

III. How to Disclose Error

When a serious adverse event occurs, such as missing a critical test result leading to a delay or failed treatment, it is unwanted and may have been unexpected by the clinician and the patient and their family. If unexpected, it likely will not have been covered in the consent to treatment discussion that took place before the harmful incident occurred. Seriously harmful outcomes—such as the death of a previously well person in the ER or OR—require time and effort on the clinician's part to discuss. Whether or not medical care caused the demise, the family may see the healthcare professionals as responsible. Transparency, not silence, is critical to assuaging families affected by loss as well as to maintaining the trust in medicine. Clinicians should also avoid blaming others or assuming all the blame themselves. These events are complex and have multiple causes; they are not due to the actions or inactions of a single individual.

> **Box 12.6**
>
> ....
>
> The following are some suggestions for managing the disclosure of error:
>
> - Establish rapport with the patient and/or the patient's significant others. Express sympathy: "I am sorry to see that you are still feeling so tired/unwell/not right."
> - Don't prevaricate and don't wait for the patient to ask why they still feel so unwell. Instead say, for example, "I have something difficult to tell you: the abnormalities were also there the last time we did blood-work on you."
> - Provide information regarding the error and the missed result. Offer, "Would it be helpful for me to explain what I think happened?"
> - Provide an objective, narrative account.
> - Don't speculate: if you don't know what happened, find out. "Here's what I know now . . ."
> - Apologize for the event.
> - Avoid being defensive.
> - Try to empathize with/normalize the patient's feelings. Use reflective listening: "I know this must be hard for you . . ."

IV. Apologies

Apologizing for poor or unwanted outcomes should not be seen as an admission of liability or an admission that something wrong or substandard was done. Apologies are primarily empathic statements of regret and an attempt to identify with the emotional loss that families or patients may have. Seen in this way, they can prevent legal or regulatory proceedings that can follow from a perception that the professional does not truly understand or care about what the grieving families and patients may experience. Sincere apologies can cross emotional crevasses, reduce the burden of guilt, and help heal broken relationships [30].

Honest and sincerely offered apologies may be protective against lawsuits, and it is helpful to know many jurisdictions have passed "Apology Acts" that do not make the offering of an apology an admission of liability. In Canada, *the Uniform Apology Act* is recommended legislation and not required federal law. It excludes, as an admission of liability, a healthcare practitioner's admission of "*fault or responsibility*" for an untoward outcome [31, 32]. Not all jurisdictions in Canada have signed on to this recommended language in their legislation (Quebec and the NWT are two places that do not have exculpatory laws). Many, but again not all, American states do have such legislation. (See "Sorry Works!" website for a list of the states that do and the work to promote disclosure in healthcare [33].) However, the shadow of this law may loom large even in jurisdictions without formal apology laws as the standard for disclosure advances.

Box 12.7

Excerpt from Ontario's *Uniform Apology Act*:
"An apology made by or on behalf of a person in connection with any matter,

   a)   does not, in law, constitute an express or implied admission of fault or liability by the person in connection with that matter;

   b)   does not, despite any wording to the contrary in any contract of insurance or indemnity and despite any other Act or law, void, impair or otherwise affect any insurance or indemnity coverage;

   c)   . . . shall not be taken into account in any determination of fault or liability in connection with that matter." [34]

V. Large-Scale Adverse Events

Those medical errors affecting whole classes of patients can be particularly trying for healthcare professionals and their institutions. "Large-scale adverse events" are a series of related incidents or processes that increase the risk of injuring multiple patients. Well-known examples have included faulty cleaning of investigative technologies, such as endoscopes or EEG leads, or the dispensing of contaminated drugs [35]. Typically, in these large-scale events, the increased risk was unanticipated by healthcare professionals and was not recognized at the time of the occurrence of the incident. Thus, even with best management at the time, the event may or may not have been preventable [36]. The level of risk to the population potentially affected is typically not known prior to the review, but usually more people are *not* affected physically than are affected by the incident.

Case 12.3   The Newfoundland Breast Hormone Assay Inquiry

In 2005 in Newfoundland, a patient with advanced metastatic breast cancer not responsive to conventional treatment, whose hormone receptor test was initially negative, was re-tested and found to be positive. This represented an

continued

important finding, as the results of receptor hormone assays determine further treatment of breast cancer. It was subsequently demonstrated that the lab procedures were deeply flawed, and up to one-third of women tested had received incorrect diagnoses about their hormone status. An external audit of the lab noted poor quality control, deficient procedures, and frequent turnover of staff[37].

The errors in the lab had a significant impact. A review confirmed that 108 patients who died had not received adequate treatment. Another 383 of 1013 women had not received the recommended treatment[38].

What and when should the women have been told?

Discussion of Case 12.3

There should have been no ethical dilemma in this case. The women and the public needed urgent disclosure of the incident and the events leading up to it. Given the magnitude of the error and the tremendous implications for patients, there could be no defence of non-disclosure. Spokespersons for the Regional Health Authority, however, initially attempted to keep the findings out of the public eye. Why? Perhaps shock, perhaps uncertainty over its scope, perhaps concern over causing public panic. Unfortunately, this delay in disclosure meant many of those affected found out initially through the public media.

The bottom line: even if ultimately not physically harmed, all recalled patients suffered some psychological distress. A more timely and transparent disclosure process could have mitigated the impact of this recall.

Class action suits have been filed against hospitals alleging psychological harm caused merely by the warnings of possible adverse events. These have not yet found much support in Canadian courts—even in out-of-hospital contexts. A Court of Appeal in one well-known nonmedical case[39] found non-compensable events to be those "unusual or extreme reactions to events caused by negligence [that] are imaginable but not reasonably foreseeable." Thus, for example, a medical class action suit, seeking compensation for undue anxiety and depression after a hospital warned patients of a remote risk of tuberculosis[40]—although none did eventually contract the disease—similarly failed. Even where an event might be the result of negligence (falling below the standard expected of a reasonably careful practitioner or institution), warning a person about such an event should not *itself* give rise to a compensable injury. It is inappropriate in the Court's view to compensate people for every insult or psychological distress caused by living in a society.

While it cannot be certain that every court action concerning the disclosure of possible adverse large-scale events will be dismissed, transparency and full disclosure, done in a sensitive and careful way, should be recognized as best practice for healthcare professionals and their institutions. Just how best to do so is the subject of ongoing discussion. Policies and guidelines have been proposed for physicians and healthcare organizations facing large-scale errors or adverse events. These policies focus on preparing an institution for such an event, having clear lines of authority for communication, and clarifying the nature of the event and just what needs to be disclosed. The debate is no longer whether adverse events need to be disclosed, but how to do so in a timely and effective way.

Box 12.8

Guidelines for institutions faced with a large-scale event:

1. Promptly initiate a look-back investigation to identify the root causes.
2. Obtain broad input as to precisely what information needs to be disclosed by whom and to whom.
3. Get accurate information about the event (its causes and risks),
   a. ensure all potentially impacted patients are informed personally,
   b. ensure empathic delivery of essential information,
   c. for low-risk, low-harm events, give written notification,
   d. for events involving greater risk, also give oral notification.
4. Provide clear procedures as well as trained and trusted personnel to
   a. disclose all large-scale adverse events to affected patients,
   b. manage the disclosure process,
   c. notify patients and the public in a timely manner,
   d. coordinate follow-up testing and treatment,
   e. respond to regulatory bodies,
   f. communicate openly with media, and
   g. provide follow-up testing and treatment for patients.
5. Apologize sincerely and clearly for the event and accept responsibility.
6. Provide reasonable compensation to persons truly harmed by the event. [41]

Conclusion

> ## Box 12.9
>
> "Though error bee blinde, she sometimes bringeth forth seeing daughters."
>
> John Hall, 1646 [42]

Healthcare professionals do not seek to harm patients, but when inadvertent harm does occur, the professional assumes responsibility and asks, "What can I learn from this incident?" So, while the error may be blind, the evaluation of it need not be. Professionalism as regards medical error encompasses a broad scope of duties, attitudes, and behaviours by healthcare practitioners. Honesty and humility about medicine's limits and harms will better advance medicine. Although honesty about mistakes is considered important and praiseworthy in any domain of social life, truthfulness is particularly important for healthcare. Without honesty, the trust we require of medicine and the healthcare professionals will be lost (see Chapter 6).

What justice has to do with honesty and trust in healthcare is the subject of the next chapter.

Cases for Discussion

Case 1: An Rx for Dizziness

You are a physician caring for Mr S, a 45-year-old diabetic man, who is being investigated in hospital for dizziness. You write an order to give him 10 units of short-acting insulin. Shortly after receiving the insulin, he becomes lethargic and confused and has a cardiac arrest. He is resuscitated and taken to the ICU. It appears the order you wrote was not clear and that Mr S received 100 units of insulin, instead of 10, leading to hypoglycemic shock.

Mr S spends 22 days in the ICU, complicated by pneumonia and sepsis, but eventually recovers.

Questions for Discussion
1. How should you explain to the family, and eventually the patient, what happened?

2. Because a nurse gave the wrong dose, does this mean it is a nursing error and they should deal with it?
3. Should patients be notified of minor errors (such as receiving 12 units of insulin instead of 10) with no sequelae?
4. Can you think of general guidelines for dealing with patients and family when addressing situations of "medical error"?

Case 2: Lost in Transit

You know Mr P, your next patient, well—he has been your family practice patient for years. A retired bus driver of 75, he has a nice sense of humour. He tells you he is tired today. He didn't sleep that well due to an annoying cough that has been attributed to his new blood pressure medication. As well he had been in the local ER with another bout of blood in his urine. When Mr P had the same problem a year ago, an ultrasound found kidney stones. He had lithotripsy done at another hospital and was fine until this current episode of hematuria. When you saw him for hypertension a few months ago, he reported no more renal pain or blood in the urine.

He wonders if you can tell him about the CAT scan they did last night in the ER. He tells you he's not sure why it was done and says, "So, Doc, when will I get my next stone-pulverizing appointment?"

Able to electronically access his hospital chart, you are shocked to read the report: "The mass in the right kidney seen on ultrasound *one year ago* is now much larger, filling in the whole renal pelvis." There was also evidence of tumour involving the lower lobes of his lungs. The news could not be much worse. Terror grips your heart; you search for last year's report.

Last year's ultrasound indeed indicated Mr P had multiple kidney stones at that time. As well, however, an "incidental note" was made of a small mass in the right kidney for which "follow-up is recommended." You are shocked. You wonder to yourself what you did wrong. You honestly don't recall ever seeing that report . . .

Mr P is waiting in the examining room for you. His urologist is away.

Questions for Discussion

1. Why do you think the report from last year was not acted on?
2. What would you say to Mr P?
3. What are your responsibilities as his family physician?

✦ 13 ✦

Beyond the Patient
Doing Justice to Justice

The future belongs to crowds.

Don DeLillo, 2004 [1]

I. Justice in Everyday Medicine

It's hard to deny there is a malaise within modern medicine today. The recent past seems to have been a time of optimism and unlimited potential, when any disease could be cured, and price was no object. Now, things seem more complicated—diseases are more challenging and care is more complex, more expensive, less readily available, and can *itself* be the cause of significant medical injury. The fair distribution of the benefits of medicine—the justice of healthcare arrangements—will be examined in this chapter.

Though often not consciously considered, questions of justice come into play every day in patient care. Should access to a clinician be first come, first served? Or by whoever can afford it? Or should it be prioritized by medical need? What exactly is medical need and who determines it?

Case 13.1   Time Well Spent?

You are the primary care provider for Ms E, a 92-year-old widow who visits you monthly in the clinic. Her main complaints are fatigue and sadness connected with her experience of aging. Although she has the usual depredations of old age—arthritic joints, fatigue—she is not acutely ill in any particular way. Your main reason for seeing her is simply to listen to her concerns and be supportive.

> But after a number of visits, you wonder whether the time spent with this patient is justified, given your many other patients who also need your time. Just yesterday you delayed seeing a patient with a seemingly more urgent physical problem rather than disheartening Ms E by postponing her appointment.
>
> *Should you de-prioritize seeing Ms E?*

Doing justice

Like a cut diamond, the idea of justice is multifaceted. Amongst its many meanings, we will focus on the ideas of distributive justice. Distributive justice involves the opportunity or the right to access, and to receive, certain goods according to ways that are "fair" and "proportionate"[2]. The context for this notion of the proper distribution of healthcare assets may be considered at an individual level, at a society or state level as a whole, between peoples, or even globally in terms of what duties or obligations we owe each other as tribes, regions, or nations. There must also be consideration of "the system"—the wider set of medical and social resources clinicians and patients must be able to access.

Discussion of Case 13.1

Having taken her on as a patient, you do have a duty of care to Ms E, but how far does it extend? The patient can expect you, her primary care clinician, to spend the time with her that is proportionate to her medical needs. These do not have to be physical—they could be Ms E's psychosocial needs as an aging person. To attend to these is to show her respect as a person and is a part of compassionate care.

If she benefits from these visits and your time is not so stretched that worries about priorities arise, then you should continue seeing her. While Ms E may consider your visits to be an opportunity to chat, you should also use her visits to assess the depth of her sadness, the reasons for it, and what might be done to help her.

Determining whose need is more urgent than Ms E's is a clinical issue; if she is seriously depressed or suicidal, her needs are no less important than those of another patient. And her claim on the healthcare system is hardly excessive. One could argue from a consequentialist perspective that a little deontological caring (caring for her as a person) shown by her doctor may help prevent more serious (and ultimately costly) illnesses.

The effectiveness of healthcare may be defined as the use of resources that make a tangible difference to patients. What is effective care seen from the patient's point of view?

Case 13.2 Misfortune Begetting Injustice

You are a practitioner who has recently joined a community health centre in a poor neighbourhood. One of the patients assigned to your multidisciplinary professional team is Ms D, a proud woman of Ukrainian descent in her late 50s. She has had a difficult life, singlehandedly raising her own three children and now caring for her two young grandchildren since her daughter was murdered a year ago.

Ms D lives on a small disability pension from the university where she had worked as a cleaner for 20 years. She has been unable to work for some time due to her multiple morbidities—disabling osteoarthritis, emphysema, adult-onset insulin-dependent diabetes, obesity, and congestive heart failure.

In discussing her functional status, she reveals she is now confined to the front of her small house because of her inability to manage steps. Because she cannot get to her pharmacy easily, she sometimes goes without insulin for days. Anyway, the money it costs for diabetes care is not money she can readily afford. Even with a walker, she can negotiate only short distances. She stopped taking the publicly funded "Wheel-Trans" bus service when she found the drivers downright rude at times.

Now dependent on her two surviving children for transportation, Ms D is reluctant to bother them. She avoided her last medical appointment, as she knew her numbers would be bad and she didn't want to feel like a failure again.

"Life," she sighs, "hasn't turned out the way I thought it would" [3].

What are the responsibilities of her primary care providers?

Discussion of Case 13.2

The primary ethical issue is that Ms D seems to be receiving less than her fair share of medical resources. Her poverty and social situation conspire against her receiving the aids—customized support services, an electric scooter—that would allow her greater freedom of action and improve her quality of life.

It's easy for patients with limited resources to fall through the cracks. "[P]eople with disabilities are particularly susceptible to receiving substandard care"[4], as are patients from lower socioeconomic strata—perhaps because of a blinkered vision or a lack of skills on the part of healthcare providers in connecting such patients to helpful resources, perhaps also because these patients do not know how, or are unable, to speak up on their own behalf. The burden of disability and disease carried by members of socially disadvantaged groups is closely linked to the deprivations they experience in society, creating a healthcare gradient "in striking conformity to a social gradient"[5].

This cycle of poverty, deprivation, ill health, and injustice has so far been difficult to break, but Ms D has something going for her: *you and your team*. As the new practitioner at the clinic, you can help her get what she needs and deserves by ensuring she has

- an advocate (you and your team as a start), especially when it comes to ensuring she gets the care and resources she needs and deserves (as do her grandchildren who are also at risk);
- continuity in healthcare providers—ideally, a devoted interdisciplinary team, with an MD, a nurse or nurse practitioner, a social worker, and a pharmacist; and
- regular comprehensive care (from your multidisciplinary unit, regular home visits) that addresses her physical, mental, and functional needs.

One moral question healthcare professionals must ask is how obliged they are to pursue an amelioration of situations such as Ms D's, beyond focusing on the medical issue at hand. This will, no doubt, depend on the healthcare practitioners. Do they have the right skill set? Does their clinic motivate clinicians to go the extra mile for patients like Ms D? Finally, how amenable to access and change are the social circumstances? If there are no avenues of social support open in a resource-limited society, there may not be much anyone can do. On the other hand, there may be hidden assets in a more resource-rich society that could be accessed by an imaginative healthcare team.

This would seem to be a proportionate duty. Just where to draw the line between obligatory professional duties of aid and rescue and optional and supererogatory, or exceptional/saintly duties will depend on many local factors[6]. Although recognizing what care a patient needs and wants may be quite different than having immediate access to it, it is a first step in achieving it.

The bottom line: once a person has become a clinician's patient, the less effort required and the more necessary the resource is to the patient's condition of well-being, the more obligatory from a professional perspective is the clinician's duty to help, to act as their advocate (see Chapter 9).

II. A System of Mutual Recognition

The problem of justice in healthcare goes beyond individualized decision-making: the healthcare system must be viewed as a whole. There needs to be a way to decide among competing priorities. It requires, as John Rawls has written, "a mutually recognized point of view from which citizens can adjudicate their claims . . . on their . . . institutions or against one another"[7]. Such a "mutually recognized" system does not appear to exist at the moment in healthcare. Healthcare has become too politicized—physicians, other healthcare providers, patients, and the public not always working towards the same goals. (As we cannot avoid debate as regards its purpose and ends, healthcare is always political.)

Box 13.1

Acceptable criteria for allocating scarce resources include

- likelihood of benefit to the patient,
- expected improvement in the patient's quality of life,
- expected duration of benefit,
- urgency of the patient's condition,
- amount of resources needed for successful treatment, and
- availability of alternative treatments. [9]

Discrimination

At a minimum, justice requires that all people are due access to beneficial treatment regardless of disability, pre-existing illness, age, gender, sexual orientation, faith, culture, race, socio-economic class, or citizenship.

Discrimination is an unjust distinction, whether intentional or not, that

- is based on grounds relating to personal characteristics of an individual or group, and
- imposes burdens, obligations, or disadvantages on such individuals or groups not imposed on others, or that withholds access to opportunities, benefits, and advantages available to other members of society[8].

All people deserve non-discriminatory care. Beyond that, in the way of positive benefits, people deserve necessary care, care without which they will come to avoidable harm. The standard by which treatment is judged as warranted or appropriate is the "best interests of the patient," that is, the care that a reasonable professional would, under the circumstances, provide to the patient. Patients should expect to receive access to care proportionate to their needs. Box 13.1 lists factors to consider when attempting to distribute scarce resources appropriately and fairly[9].

Unjust care

Unfair discrimination among and between patients was common in the past and still seen in medicine today. There are many examples of apparent discrimination in medical care.

1. Age and racial bias were evident when dialysis machines were first introduced in Seattle, Washington, in the late 1950s. Because the machines were expensive and in short supply, one of the earliest ethics committees—a "God squad"—was set up in 1962 to decide who should receive treatment and, so, in effect, who should live or who should die. This was described at the time as "the moral burden of a small committee"[10]. Precedent and reliable advice were lacking, and it is perhaps not surprising to find that those patients who were single, elderly, female, black, or poor were not offered dialysis. This "odious practice," as one observer deemed it, did not end until 1972 when the US Congress passed a bill, Public Law 92-603, authorizing Medicare to pay for dialysis for all patients with end-stage renal disease[11]. Improved funding thus allowed more dialysis units to be set up to meet the previously unmet needs of those with end-stage renal disease.
2. Age bias persisted in end-stage renal care in the United Kingdom until the mid-1990s with the acknowledgement by nephrologists and health officials that dialysis was a viable option in older patients[12].
3. Gender bias at first glance seems to be present in cardiac care. It has been claimed that "women with ischemic heart disease [receive] less than a fair deal"[13]. For example, women presenting to the ER with acute coronary syndromes are less likely than men to be hospitalized or undergo coronary revascularization[14]. "Women with ACS, despite undergoing a coronary angiogram, continue to be treated with coronary revascularization only about half of the time and considerably less frequently than men," a 2017 Canadian study concluded[15]. However, there may be physiological reasons for this difference in care, so the alleged "[un]fair deal" for women may be illusory.
2. Gender bias has been claimed to occur in other areas as well. In a Canadian study of men and women presenting to physicians with equally arthritic knees, men were twice as likely as women to have surgery recommended[16].

The authors speculated unconscious biases against women might have been to blame.

Again, these studies do not prove bias; they show only that groups of people are treated differently.

These cases are but a few examples of what Aristotle may have meant by injustice: likes treated as unlikes and the latter receiving less than what they are due [17]. Patients similar in relevant ways should be treated in a similar fashion. Thus, if patients have the same burden of illness—be it coronary heart disease, depression, renal failure, or arthritic knees—they should be treated in the same manner, irrespective of gender, race, age, and so on—assuming, of course, that these factors are irrelevant to the success of the treatment. For example, the same principles should guide the treatment of a child with meningococcal meningitis whether the child lives in Moscow, New Delhi, or Pikangikum in northern Ontario. Of course, the standard of care cannot be the same for a child residing in a major urban centre with a modern hospital and state-of-the-art facilities as opposed to a very sick child living in the far nether regions of a country. However, it would be unjust not to see as a problem the lack of ready access to medical care by reason of geography. Living far from a hospital may not be advisable if you have an unstable health condition, but the right to live with your family where you please is an important right in democratic jurisdictions. Still, underserviced or non-existent rural medicine and the unavailability of even basic medical care in impoverished circumstances is a worldwide problem.

Acceptable use of patient factors

The use of patient-specific factors is ethical and *not* discriminatory, however, when it reflects a *real* difference in patient populations. For example, it has been suggested that women with heart disease should be treated differently than men because their blood vessels are smaller and their symptoms therefore different [18]. It has also been suggested that women present with heart disease later in life than men, and so naturally they should be treated differently than men are [19].

This is not to say Aristotle was wrong, but that his view of injustice doesn't always apply.

Box 13.2

Treating similar patients differently is appropriate when they are different in ways relevant to the treatment in question.

Another factor is, of course, patient preference. Treating patients with similar conditions differently is *required* when it accords with the patient's own wishes and values. Thus, it would be acceptable to put limits on life-saving care such as dialysis for the elderly if the patients themselves choose to forego life-sustaining treatment. That said, advanced age, on its own, is *not* a predictive factor for a poor outcome in surgery[20]. Clinicians need to ensure older patients' refusals of potentially helpful care are in fact informed refusals (see Chapter 6).

When asked, the very old often do decline medical interventions, especially when accurately informed of the foreseeably less-than-positive outcomes of aggressive surgical options[21]. However, one study found that while less well-off elderly patients were prepared to forego their place in a queue for heart surgery for younger patients, the more affluent were less inclined to do so[22]. This suggests that more financially well-off patients may feel more entitled to care and less likely to be self-sacrificing.

Case 13.3   Should He Wait or Should He Go?

Dr Q, a physician, originally from a war-torn country whose name he does not care to remember, is doing a six-month medical locum in northern Manitoba. As the only health professional around for hundreds of miles, he finds his medical practice has its challenges. A typical day can involve reading ultrasounds, casting broken limbs, and even deftly removing a fish hook embedded in a patient's cheek. The locals have appreciated his dedication and interest.

Mr V is a 55-year-old lumberjack of Métis heritage whom Dr Q has been treating for hypertension. Today, there is a new problem: he has had a severe headache for two days unresponsive to the usual medications. On examination, Dr Q finds a concerning sign in his left eye: what looks like early papilloedema (a swollen retina that almost always means the pressure in the patient's skull is very high). If he's right, this is an ominous finding requiring prompt intervention.

However, having not done many fundoscopic examinations, Dr Q is unsure of his findings. He considers sending Mr V to the city, but because it is midwinter, the only way out is via a special rescue by plane: the runway is the frozen lake. Dr Q also recalls a missive from the Ministry of Health reminding doctors to "use society's resources wisely." In his home country, doctors would not dare to ignore such governmental edicts.

What should Dr Q do? Should he call for an (expensive) air evacuation for Mr V? Or should he send his patient home and wait and see how he is tomorrow?

Lessons from the field of battle

The issue of holding back potentially helpful care—rationing—is not new. In almost any area of society, some resources are scarce or expensive and rationing is common. Consequently, some people, when ill, are denied potentially helpful measures. This is most evident on the field of battle. When not everyone can be saved, triage decisions must be made. War requires soldiers to be able to fight. In order to prevail, the focus of command is less on the individual combatant and more on the welfare of the group of soldiers as a whole. Soldiers who can be easily treated and so return to battle are treated first, while soldiers who have more serious injuries may be left to die. Under these harsh, typically time-limited conditions, hard decisions must be made as to who should get priority for treatment. This is true rationing: potentially helpful care is denied to some injured soldiers— who, in less extreme situations, would receive that care—in order to preserve the unit's combat readiness [23].

It is sometimes suggested that healthcare is like modern warfare with the enemy being the country's debt or the "fiscal cliff." But the rate-limiting factor in healthcare is usually not time—rather it is the resources (the healthcare professionals, the operating room time, the bed spaces, the drugs) needed for proper care. In healthcare, treatment options are much more operator- and place-dependant. As a consequence, some patients get too much care, some get too little. Untested practices, financial incentives, patient or family demands, bed availability, and physician practice styles (such as the *furor therapeuticus*; see Chapter 9) may lead, for example, to aggressive care being inappropriately offered to patients at life's end [24]. Impoverishment, lack of family resources, and illiteracy can also lead to undertreatment, as patients do not know what to expect or what to request.

Doctors have traditionally held much discretionary decision-making power and have, at times, tended to overvalue their interventions [25]. Oncologists, for example, sometimes have found it hard to say no to dying patients who wanted "everything." So if insurance covers it or there are hospital beds available or if patients/families want it badly enough and a physician is agreeable, some patients will get almost any treatment available. Thus, sicker patients requiring more complex care may be prioritized despite their costs of care and even when evidence suggests treatment will be ineffective. There are often no clear stopping rules for many conditions, just as there no clear starting rules either. Precision medicine may be changing that by ratcheting up the genetic evidence for and against treatment, demonstrating some aggressive treatment strategies (such as chemotherapy for early-stage breast cancer) are not effective and may do more harm than good [26]. This is, surely, better than basing treatment decisions on "managed care," which is a bureaucratic solution to a clinical treatment issue and pits patients against doctors [27].

Discussion of Case 13.3

What should not be traded off—at least not by the clinician at the patient's side—is potentially beneficial care for a patient. Although Dr Q may glance at the Ministry's missive, he would be unwise to apply it to Mr V's situation. Rather, he should warn him of the potential seriousness of his condition and not waste any more time before bundling him up and shipping him out (with his consent, of course!).

Mr V did go out by medevac. He was found to have a large occipital tumour and had indeed been showing signs of increased intracranial pressure when Dr Q examined him. He underwent a life-saving craniotomy.

The upshot: when uncertain of your findings, better to err on the side of caution than worry about costs to the healthcare system—without over-reacting. Finding the right balance between ensuring the patient gets helpful care they need versus avoiding the drain on society's resources is not easy to achieve. The challenge for clinicians and patients is that the need for medical services always seems to exceed the available supply. What can be done about this is dependent on the medical system as a whole, but also on practitioners' and patients' interest in and facility with addressing the problems of the quality and timeliness of healthcare delivery.

III. Distributive Justice

Distributive justice aims to fairly distribute social goods such as healthcare. There are ends (goods or rewards) that people should receive in ways that are right and proportionate. Just what ought to be proportionately divided up is the subject of some debate. Fairness is central to this idea of justice. But justice is a hybrid concept and also involves elements of autonomy (the respect for persons includes the right to unbiased consideration) and beneficence (this includes the right to affordable healthcare—depending on the available resources and what goods others similarly ill are getting).

Awareness of the need to balance economic costs of care against the benefits of interventions is appropriate and should influence clinicians' obligations to their patients. A single-minded focus on one patient can lead to ignoring the larger implications of clinical decisions[28]. Compromises in care must be made—not everyone can get or needs the most expensive artificial hip; sometimes cheaper drugs are just as good as the latest and most expensive designer pills; and generic drugs can be as effective as brand-name equivalents.

Choosing wisely

Saving money in fiscally tough times, as the costs of care threaten to soar through the roof, is a big push in contemporary healthcare. Some research has revealed a significant proportion—more than 50 per cent—of medical care is not appropriate, may not improve a population's health and may even detract from it [29]. This astonishing statistic should force us—patients and providers alike—to take a sobering second look at the value of healthcare interventions, from little-ticket items like blood tests and X-rays to big-ticket items like MRIs [30]. It has been said there is an epidemic of overtreatment of patients [31]. This has led to a series of initiatives— such as the Choosing Wisely initiative [32]—in both medical schools and residency programs to instruct trainees how to make more cost-effective and truly helpful healthcare decisions.

How are we to design a system that can fairly allocate scarce healthcare resources? Avoiding futile, ineffective, or marginally effective and consequently wasteful care is a less morally troublesome way of coping with difficult trade-offs in care 33. Public resources can potentially be freed up if we rationally evaluate the need for medical interventions before ordering them. Box 13.3 lists questions that clinicians should consider before ordering a test.

Box 13.3

Five questions to ask before ordering any test:

1. Will the test result change my care?
2. Did the patient have this test before?
3. What are the chances and risks of a false-positive test?
4. Is the patient in any danger if the test is not done?
5. Am I ordering the test simply to reassure the patient?

Case 13.4 Terms of Entitlement

Mr and Ms K, a wealthy and "demanding" (in this case, "having a sense of entitlement") older couple, come to see you, their general practitioner. They have just been to the Mr K's new internist (his old one has retired) and tell you they are disappointed because she has not ordered an EKG, a urinalysis, or a blood test for the prostate. On questioning, you discover the 75-year-old husband has no new cardiac or prostate complaints. All the same, the couple has come to expect these tests to be done yearly and asks you to order them.

Should you order the tests Mr and Ms K have come to expect as the standard of care?

Questioning the value of medical procedures is not just a task for healthcare providers, however. Patients and their families, too, must be involved in decisions about the value of medical care. In deciding whether to accept a healthcare professional's recommendations, there are four questions to which patients and their families ought to seek answers [34].

Box 13.4

Four questions for patients to ask before a medical intervention:

1. Do I really need this test/treatment/procedure?
2. What are the downsides?
3. Are there simpler, safer procedures?
4. What is likely to happen if I do nothing?

By seeking answers to these critical questions in Boxes 13.3 and 13.4, healthcare professionals and patients can exert a profound effect upon unnecessary spending and the appropriate use of healthcare resources.

Discussion of Case 13.4

Battles over the usefulness of medical interventions are common in healthcare. As with any other intervention, screening tests—such as an annual EKG and a prostate blood test—should be done only if there is evidence they will be beneficial to medical care.

continued

Rather than simply comply with this couple's request (which is not in keeping with the standard of practice for primary care), it would be better to find out why they seem so demanding. The request should be examined. Is there a legitimate *patient-based* reason for the request? Can it be met in any other way? Is the wife overly anxious about her husband's health? Was there a failure of communication with the new internist?

Try to sympathize with their fears while not denying their requests head-on. If you have time and are a skilled communicator, you might get away with not doing the tests. Then again, the day is short and this couple may be uninterested in dialogue. If so (as in Case 1.1), you may choose to battle another day and, reluctantly, give in to their wishes. But saying no becomes harder the longer you put it off. And if you say yes today and provide ineffective care, remind yourself not to do so tomorrow. There is a war to be won even if you lose today's skirmish!

IV. Squeezing the Balloon

On a world scale, injustice and inequality have been long ingrained in human society and will not be readily eradicated[35]. Millions are without even the most basic kind of healthcare. Resources are not infinite, and individuals are often limited by what they can access within their country's border. How healthcare should be paid for is a huge issue. Should there be, for example, one central payer for "necessary medical services," or should healthcare be available to those with the financial means to afford it[36]? Canada has adopted the first option.

Box 13.5

"Access to health care based on need rather than ability to pay was the founding principle of the Canadian health-care system."[37]

The Canadian healthcare system has a number of features that allow for the preservation of a "just" or more equitable distribution of medical services[37]. It has problems, as its supporters point out, but they are capable of being solved[38]. Ability to pay for medical care has largely been eliminated as a driver of the provision of most, but not all, key healthcare services[37].

Box 13.6

....

The five principles of the *Canada Health Act* are as follows:

1. **Portability**: Insured residents keep their coverage when travelling or moving within Canada.
2. **Universality**: All insured individuals have access to the same level of healthcare, regardless of their ability to pay.
3. **Accessibility**: There are no financial barriers to access of healthcare—for example, no "user fees."
4. **Comprehensiveness:** All necessary health services, including hospitals, physicians and surgical dentists, must be insured.
5. **Public administration**: Single payer for covered services minimizes bureaucratic overhead.[39]

Whether or not citizens of Canada have timely access to *all* "necessary medical care" is an important question to ask. The *Canada Health Act*[40] requires provision of those "services medically necessary for the purposes of maintaining health, preventing disease or treating an injury, illness or disability." Such care is "any medically required services rendered by medical practitioners." This is a very loose definition, as it would cover whatever practitioners are willing to provide! Not all medically useful treatments are covered, however[41]. Many drugs, most dental services, most eye care, mental health services provided by non-physicians, and most out-of-hospital physiotherapy services, for example, are not subsidized under provincial medicare schemes. While timely access to emergency services and urgent medical care (for illnesses such as acute coronary events and cancer care) is not generally a problem in Canada, there are delays in accessing innovative or elective services. Wait times for some elective services such as hip and knee replacements have been considered inordinately long in comparison with other countries with universal healthcare[37]. The Wait Times Alliance Canada has targeted areas such as this, with some successes in reducing wait times[42].

Concern that Canada's publicly funded system, due to scarce resources, would prevent some patients from getting needed and timely care led to a constitutional challenge in Quebec. *Chaoulli v Quebec* challenged the prohibition against private health insurance for medically necessary services. The issue, which came before the Supreme Court of Canada, centred on whether this prohibition was necessary to preserve the quality of healthcare and equality of access to it [43]. The challenge was successful, with a narrow majority of justices (four to three) holding that allowing people to purchase medical services would not threaten the system's quality. The minority argued this would undermine the *principle* of free and equal access to car [44]. This judgment did not address the question as to which services are necessary and which are not. Although the door for private healthcare insurance has opened, there have been no seismic shifts in Canada's medicare system to date. However, there is always the possibility that future court cases and political opinion may move Canadian society away from universal access.

Scarcity

Given the scarcity of resources, individual patients may not receive what they need in as timely a way as they might prefer. Delays in care may then lead to further harm and suffering. In such cases, justice would require persons in equal need to have an equal *opportunity* to access that care. In creating a just healthcare system, it can be challenging to objectively evaluate need and harm, at least in ways upon which people can mutually agree.

In the optimistic view, difficult rationing decisions will be avoided by eliminating inefficiencies and useless treatments. In the pessimistic view, even if this is achieved, there will still be insufficient resources to satisfy everyone. Changing the healthcare system has been compared to a balloon: squeeze it in one place and it simply expands in another [45]. Are hard rationing decisions unavoidable? Probably. Will we always have to deny some patients the treatment they may want? No doubt we will. Not everyone can get the treatment they want. The question is: will people get what they need?

For example, the cost of drugs is a problem in every country's future. The exorbitant cost of new biologic agents poised to fight diseases such as rheumatoid arthritis and cancers of the breast and lung with personalized or precision medicine (see Chapter 17 for more on these developments) threatens recommendations for equity of access and comprehensive drug coverage in universal healthcare programs. As a society concerned about the fair and just distribution of healthcare, when it comes to essential medical services, we will need to carefully consider whether such drugs are fairly priced and worth the price.

NICE work

A fully moralized healthcare system, as we have emphasized throughout this book, would be a "*disadvantage-reducing*" system. It would ensure that opportunities to access healthcare resources are as balanced and equitable as possible. Some inequalities—of disease, of disability, of finances *within* countries—are more easily addressed. Others—such as geographic distance from a healthcare facility, genomic predisposition to diseases, situations of extreme deprivation—will require much more work to overcome[46].

A just society has an ill-defined obligation to ensure the healthcare needs of its citizens are fairly met. Some patients, on account of severity of illness or disability, will require more or different care than others. This patient-specific care compensates those with disability and disadvantage, resulting in some levelling of the social playing field. Medical care offers the opportunity to surpass the unfair disadvantages caused by poverty, place of birth, accident, or illness. If equality of access to effective care is not present, the deprivation and absence of choice that can accompany impoverishment, rural life, illness, and disability are often viewed as natural misfortunes, as if they were simply "bad luck," as in Case 13.2.

Many jurisdictions have institutions for objectively assessing the costs and benefits of new drugs and interventions before they are widely introduced into practice. One of the most impressive is the National Institute for Health and Care Excellence (NICE) in the UK[47]. It provides guidelines for the use of drugs and medical technologies, based on a rigorous evaluation of the evidence—evidence such as that provided by the Cochrane Collaboration[48]. However, any such system will never be able to make choices or to evaluate new drugs or procedures in an entirely neutral or value-free way.

Box 13.7

....

Improved evidence is important and will help prevent some poor choices in how we apportion out our healthcare spending, but choices, based on ethical values and debate, will be unavoidable.

V. Guidelines and Rationing

To help healthcare professionals better evaluate clinical practice and make more appropriate care decisions, there has been great interest in outcomes research and in the development of clinical practice guidelines[49]. These are systematically developed statements that assist practitioners' decisions about what is appropriate healthcare for specific clinical circumstances. Guidelines or practice policies are meant to distinguish between what works and what does not work, based on best evidence. Trustworthy guidelines are those that are constantly updated, open to external review and public input, rigorous in their review of the evidence, and free from conflicts of interest[50].

Box 13.8

Guidelines are most influential if they

- critically reflect the latest advances in medical research (but are not over-awed by the new),
- allow for clinical discretion and flexible interpretation,
- are easily implemented,
- are seen as aids to decision-making and not as regulations,
- incorporate specialists' and generalists' perspectives, and
- incorporate the patient's point of view.

Some scholars, such as John Wennberg, believe that once we tell our patients the true, often poor outcomes of most interventions, many will decline them. Indeed, some well-informed patients do decline interventions—such as drug treatment for hypercholesterolemia or early screening for prostate cancer—that tend to be overvalued by physicians, but are of lesser relevance to the patient. This will save the system the expense of marginally useful, possibly harmful, and unwanted interventions. If so, it would be a nice by-product of outcomes research, since refusals of treatment by patients ("patient-choice" rationing) are the most morally defensible ones [51]. Outcomes research would thus expand, not contract, the patient's autonomy and could also save the system money, as Wennberg has argued [52].

Adhering to guidelines will not always reduce costs, however, as larger numbers of patients may then end up meeting criteria for treatment they would not have previously been offered [53].

The worry about the legal implications of practice guidelines—that some patients will be denied helpful treatment—drives some doctors to practice defensively and order every test under the sun. However, guidelines are unlikely to increase the risk of litigation because they are used to define the applicable "standard of care." The real test for malpractice actions will be whether, in a particular circumstance, the defendant doctor's actions deviated from a widely accepted standard of practice—something guidelines themselves may help define (and so in this way guidelines are part of the evidence for what will be considered the standard of care) [53].

Criteria have been proposed to guide the process of making appropriate decisions as regards priorities for effective care. Such criteria, however, cannot depend on economic evidence alone. The best known are those of the American philosopher, Norman Daniels [54].

> **Box 13.9**
>
> Daniels' "accountability for reasonableness": the deliberations and rationale for rationing should
>
> - be transparent,
> - be based on reasons recognized as relevant by "fair-minded" people,
> - have a mechanism for appealing any decisions made, and
> - also have a mechanism for enforcing rationing decisions.

These criteria make allocation or distributive justice decisions under conditions of scarcity more amenable to rational public debate and discussion. Rather than unfolding in secret and being controlled by powerful interests, an open decision-making process must involve patients and practitioners[55]. Wennberg has written that a change in medical culture is also needed, "a change that reduces the influence of medical opinion and enhances the role of patient preferences"[56].

If guidelines do limit patient access to available and *better* care solely on the basis of cost and deny patients helpful care, patients should be explicitly told this. Economic evaluation of healthcare, such as cost-benefit analysis and cost-effectiveness comparisons, is best done at the level of social planning—at the level of society in general—where all the costs and benefits of an intervention can be seen[57].

> **Box 13.10**
>
> "One of the best avenues to improve accountability is to make decision-making less opaque and more transparent. Unfortunately, health care decisions have been and continue to be made behind closed doors."[46]

VI. Justice for All?

The decision-making processes followed by national and regional administrators and government officials for allocation decisions about healthcare often remain hidden. Using Rawls's words, what is missing is an open "system of cooperation between free and equal citizens" for making hard choices about medicine's present and future. This should not stop clinicians from trying to do better in their areas of work. There have been notable successes at constructing just or fair systems of allocation in several areas of medicine. Vaccination and transplantation are two such areas.

Vaccination

Vaccination against infectious diseases has been one of humanity's most successful medical advances [58]. Achieving universal vaccination has been an important principle of vaccine programs throughout the world. The permanent eradication of smallpox is the most impressive success of these programs. Dramatic reductions in the incidence of measles and diphtheria, for example, have been possible only on account of the widespread distribution of vaccines. (This is why the current trend among certain parents not to vaccinate against childhood diseases is so worrisome—as it threatens herd immunity—and needs urgent attention [59].)

But pandemic infectious illnesses still occur with an unpredictable frequency. Often viral in origin, their spread may be prevented or ameliorated by timely vaccination. Decisions regarding who is to be vaccinated first have to be made early on in the course of an outbreak. In cases of known disease, such as polio or a familiar respiratory viral illness, a substantial proportion of the population may already have been vaccinated, so the supply of vaccine is adequate for the needs of the population and no difficult questions of justice arise. In novel and rapidly spreading infectious outbreaks, however, even if an effective vaccine is found, there may be an insufficient supply. Various authorities have proposed principles for prioritizing access to new vaccinations. One report from the United States recommended prioritizing the following groups for vaccination in pandemic conditions:

1. First, healthcare professionals who are essential to the pandemic response and/or who provide care for persons who are ill;
2. Second, those who maintain essential community services;
3. Third, all children; and
4. Fourth, those workers at greater risk of infection due to their job [60].

Notice the combination of utilitarian and deontological principles for allocating essential pandemic vaccines—first, distribute the vaccine to those essential to the vaccine's effective delivery (fundamental to all vaccination programs), second, distribute the vaccine to those needed to maintain community safety (both utilitarian reasons), third, to children (respect for persons would seem to justify placing children on the priority list, since they've had less opportunity to experience their "fair innings" of life), and, fourth, to those at greater risk on account of their occupations (if we want professionals to work in dangerous and essential jobs, we have to protect them). Further principles of distribution would aim for universal coverage starting with those populations at particular risk (priority groups would include people under 65 years with chronic conditions, pregnant women, people in remote and isolated settings, household contacts and care providers of people at high risk who could not be immunized) [61]. For equally situated persons in each group, random allocation by lottery would best serve fairness (as opposed to first come, first served, which would preference the swiftest or those with the best connections).

Transplantation

Organ transplantation in North America is another area in which significant progress has been made in fairly distributing scarce medical resources. Impartial criteria have been established: these include the likely medical benefit, time spent on the waiting list, the urgency of need, and the likelihood of success [62]. Patients are ranked according to a complicated computerized point system taking into account factors such as how close the patient is to death, how quickly the donor organ can get to the recipient, and how likely it is the patient will survive the operation. This system purportedly does not allow for prejudice or favouritism.

Case 13.5   A Transplant Tourist

You are a nephrologist with an interest in end-stage renal disease. One of your patients is a 45-year-old well-connected businessman, Mr C. He has insulin-dependent diabetes and has been on the waiting list for a kidney transplant for three years. He has survived on home peritoneal dialysis, but has been finding it increasingly burdensome and uncomfortable. He has no idea when, if ever, a kidney will become available for him.

Mr C decides to look into buying a kidney from another country. He has been your patient for many years and asks for your opinion.

How would you respond?

Organ transplantation is unique in being a closely monitored and relatively limited system [63] within which there is a great deal of agreement about the purpose of treatment. But even here disagreement can arise: should a 70-year-old with renal failure be lower on the waiting list than a 30-year-old? Should a 30-year-old abstinent alcoholic patient with end-stage liver failure be given lower priority than a patient whose liver disease was not self-induced? Should we always give preference to those who might benefit the most, or is some consideration owed to those who are less likely to benefit [64]?

Asking the public what should be done is one way of addressing the issue of who should get the available organs. Interestingly, public opinion polls do not support the position that organs for transplant should always go to the most "in need" medically (a loaded term) or the most ill. Even those less likely to benefit should be given a chance to benefit [28]. This position might indicate that the average citizen cannot imagine saying no to anyone or that the availability of organs is overestimated. It might also mean that, at some level, there is a deontological barrier to allocating organs by utilitarian criteria, a belief that anyone in need deserves a "kick at the healthcare can," even if they are unlikely to be successful. This attempt to balance benefit against the "right to be considered" is interesting and may be the most ethically defensible path to take since it considers need, efficacy, and opportunity. It thus takes into account three of the principles of ethics (beneficence, justice, and autonomy, respectively). It may also compensate for the tendency of some patients to exhibit entitlement, while others are self-effacing and consider themselves unworthy when it comes to receiving an organ.

All this leaves aside the fundamental injustice of transplant medicine: while organ donation and transplantation can be fairly carried out within advanced countries, there is never enough supply, thereby encouraging patients to look outside their country's borders. The massive inequality in wealth worldwide results in the asymmetrical purchase of organs: the well-off buy from the destitute. Some argue that impoverished people in the underdeveloped world should have the opportunity to sell a kidney if this is the only way to save their family from grinding poverty [65]. Others have argued this commercial relationship has no place in modern medicine as it leaves the poor open to exploitation and sets a bad precedent. Would we in more "developed" countries tolerate an internal market in organs? What is the experience of those who sell a kidney? Does the money really free them from impoverishment and exploitation? Would allowing a free market in human organs threaten to undermine the dignity of persons? Are there not some undertakings, such as life-saving care and transplantation, that should be considered beyond the amoral language of commerce [36]?

Discussion of Case 13.5

As Mr C's nephrologist, you might have negative personal feelings about "transplant tourism"—seeing it, for example, as a relationship of exploitation, but you should keep these views to yourself. At this juncture, it would not be helpful to engage Mr C in a discussion of its morality. Only those who have been ill and kept waiting for years on a transplant list can appreciate how emotionally and physically draining this experience can be.

Your first response should be one of empathy—acknowledging how hard the wait has been for him and his family. You should not presume to understand how he feels; you should try to elicit his concerns and find out what life has been like for him. Next, you could discuss the worries he might entertain about the whole enterprise. Is it unsanitary as some have claimed or is it just as safe as healthcare elsewhere? Mr C might face dangers in going overseas for an operation but he might face similar dangers in his own country. Finally, you should consider a discussion as to why the wait is so long at home and what might be done to hurry it up. It might be helpful for Mr C to make a call to the program itself to see how far down the list he is. As his doctor, you could call one of the transplant doctors to get an idea as to when he might be seen.

Trying to game the system by using Mr C's connections of wealth to get him moved up the transplant ladder would not be appropriate. He has already benefitted by the international inequities in the distribution of wealth.

What if a relative made an offer of a directed donation, that is, to offer a kidney to Mr C alone? Would that be acceptable? It would be, so long as the donation was not coerced [66]. Web-based solicitation of organs for transplant has been taking place in the United States for more than a decade (see MatchingDonors.com) [67]. When transplantable organs are in short supply, this public solicitation of organs is not surprising [68]. This practice raises the question as to whether the established social rules of fairness are being bypassed [66]. There are tens of thousands of people on waiting lists and thousands dying while waiting for organs. Advances in medicine may ameliorate this problem by promoting the use of organs hitherto considered unsuitable for transplant (such as those from older patients and from hepatitis C–positive patients [69]) and by using organs for transplant designed for, rather than harvested from, humans [70].

As an altruistic, empathic practitioner of medicine, your mind might turn to the impoverished millions prepared to sell their organs to the highest bidder but who themselves would be unlikely to ever receive one. In some parts of the world, easily curable illnesses, such as respiratory viral infections and cholera, go untreated and patients die who could be readily saved. This seems profoundly unjust. Legally, we may owe citizens of other countries nothing, but morally we would seem to owe them *something*. Just what that might be is the subject of much debate [71]. Currently, it is up to governments and organizations such as the United Nations and the World Health Organization to offer assistance. Medical professionals may contribute to or join an NGO or work in impoverished or underserviced areas [72], but the problems exacerbated by wars and famines will not be resolved by individuals acting alone.

Conclusion

"Fair" provision of healthcare applies to everyone. The healthcare professional's role is to open doors for patients, not close them. But it is unclear how far one must go in fulfilling this advocacy role. There may be a higher duty of care expected of healthcare professionals looking after patients with special needs and unique circumstances—due to the historical and institutional inequities and discriminations faced over many years by, for example, those with disabilities, Indigenous persons, and transgender persons. In this chapter, we have focused on care at life's end. But what about care at the beginning of life? It, too, can be very expensive. It also raises other unique ethical issues to which we will now turn.

Cases for Discussion

Case 1: A Modern-Day Robin Hood?

You are a healthcare practitioner working in a poor and medically underserviced area. You work long hours and have large bills to pay—alimony, children in private school, overhead on the office, mortgage on the house . . . it all adds up. But you worry more about the population you serve. Among your patients is a large group of destitute and frequently homeless men and women. With poor nutrition, minimal protection from the elements, and poor hygiene, they are sitting ducks for TB and protein and vitamin deficiency syndromes.

You feel a great deal of empathy for *les misérables*, the unwanted and uncared for, of society. "Talk about the social determinants of disease," you think to yourself as you walk through your crowded waiting room. "Surely, one important way I can help is to improve their nutrition." You decide to use a regional food aid program to prescribe socially funded "special diets" for your destitute and weary patients. After all, you reason, you will be helping the poor; you alone are their social advocate.

Your receptionist greets you as you enter your office. "You're booked to see between 50 and 60 patients today, Doctor. Remember, it's important to fully bill for each and every patient."

Questions for Discussion

1. Is your program ethically (as opposed to legally) defensible? Discuss using ethical theories of justice.
2. How is this program any different from ones that advocate prescribing money for impoverished patients?

Case 2: The Customer's Choice?

You work as a primary care physician with a large cohort of older patients. Many are snowbirds who spend months in Florida, returning periodically to ensure their medicare coverage is continued and they get their free drugs. One of these is Mr V, an aging but active retiree. Your patient for some years, he has developed wet age-related macular degeneration (AMD), a common cause of blindness in the elderly. In the United States he was started on Avastin, a recognized, but off-label, treatment for AMD. This drug is given by intraocular injections every month or two at a cost of $100 USD per injection. Mr V's AMD has not progressed since he started Avastin.

But Mr V is unhappy: he wants to be referred to an ophthalmologist in Canada to get Lucentis, a newer treatment for AMD. He has heard about this drug due to direct-to-consumer (DTC) advertising of prescription drugs allowed in the United States and learned that it is considered by some doctors to be superior to Avastin. Both drugs are biologic agents that counter the over-growth of new blood vessels characteristic of AMD and are considered "biosimilars," not bioequivalents. The problem is expense: Lucentis, given in the same way as Avastin, costs twenty times as much, or about $2000 USD per injection. You know the evidence for Lucentis having increased effectiveness in treating AMD is equivocal. "It must be a better drug," Mr V says, "It costs so much more. Anyway, it's free, so why not?" You work in BC, a province that pays for both drugs.

Questions for Discussion

1.   Would you send Mr V to an ophthalmologist for a consultation?
2.   What are the pros and cons of doing so?

✦ 14 ✦

....

Labour Pains

Ethics and New Life

Among the most important moral issues faced by this generation are questions arising from technologically assisted reproduction—the artificial creation of human life.

Former Chief Justice McLachlin, 2010 [1]

I. Birthing and Reproductive Choice

Ethics and New Life

There is a great diversity of opinion and unavoidable disagreement in discussions concerning birthing and reproduction. This chapter will focus on abortion, assisted reproduction, stem cell use, and women's and fetal rights, where some standards for practice exist. Although medical professionals are often taught there are two patients in a singleton pregnancy, are those two patients morally equivalent or not? When it comes to deciding what to do about matters of reproduction, one thing is certain: we can no longer simply depend on what is "natural."

Case 14.1   A Trivial Matter?

....

A 23-year-old woman, Ms J, who seems happily pregnant, is screened at 16 weeks for fetal anomalies. When the ultrasound reveals her fetus has a cleft palate, she requests a pregnancy termination. Considering this a trivial reason for a therapeutic abortion, her clinician, Dr I, shares this view with her.

Is it acceptable for the clinician to voice her opinion in this way?
Should the clinician simply keep quiet and fill out the referral form for the abortion? How else might she respond?

Modern medicine has helped make pregnancy and its termination safe and secure, giving women, at least in some parts of the world, more reproductive choice.

Discussion of Case 14.1

Dr I is not wrong, per se, to express an opinion—insofar as it is a professional, as opposed to a purely personal, view. In general, patients' beliefs should be questioned or probed by their clinicians, especially if they appear inconsistent. Affirming the right of a patient to access a service, such as pregnancy termination, does not necessarily require agreement with the patient or acceptance of the patient's reasoning. Counselling should only be offered "if the woman requests it or there is a perceived need for it" [2].

It seems curious that Ms J should now want an abortion if she was, at the outset, "happily pregnant." Why should the presence of an easily correctable lesion such as a cleft palate make Ms J decide to end a hitherto wanted pregnancy? What does she know about cleft palates? Is she aware these can be surgically treated with likely success? Is she using this as an excuse to end a pregnancy she no longer wants for other reasons? Does Ms J have a partner who ought to be informed or involved? These questions are worth exploring, and, by being asked in a non-judgmental way, need not be experienced as intrusive by the patient and the partner. Instead, they should help the couple come to a decision that is right for them.

For most, if not all, healthcare choices, medical practitioners should not interfere with their competent patients' right to decide for themselves, especially when it comes to intimately personal choices such as having children and family planning. Clinicians are there to assist patients by providing information and explaining any reasonable options to them.

Case 14.2   A Right to Be Tested?

You are a primary care practitioner looking after a professional couple in their early thirties with two young girls at home. The woman is in the first trimester of her third pregnancy. At low risk for congenital anomalies and accurate for time of conception, she nevertheless requests an "ultrasound or amniocentesis." Her spouse admits they are primarily seeking to know the sex of the fetus. If it is a girl, they will seek termination and try to get pregnant again.

continued

You know it is the standard of care to offer an ultrasound between 11 and 14 weeks of pregnancy (late first trimester) when it is too early to determine sex[3]. Amniocentesis, which would give this answer, is not done until the second trimester, by which time it might be too late to easily obtain pregnancy termination.

There are alternatives to consider, however. All women, regardless of whether they are high or low risk, are offered prenatal genetic screening for "aneuploidy syndromes" (chromosomal irregularities, such as Down syndrome)—testing covered by provincial and territorial medicare. Less well known is NIPT (non-invasive prenatal testing)—a maternal blood test that can be done as early as 10 weeks and can, if the patient so chooses, report fetal sex with a very high degree of accuracy. However, it is not a covered entity under all provincial medicare programs.

You personally believe abortion on account of sex to be wrong.

Must you tell the couple about the limits of ultrasound and the availability of other ways (such as NIPT) of determining the sex of the fetus?

A brief history of abortion in Canada

Prior to 1969, abortion was illegal in Canada under criminal law. A woman who underwent the procedure could be sentenced to two years in jail while a physician or other healthcare provider who performed the procedure could be sentenced to life in prison. In 1969 the law was amended to permit abortions in accredited facilities, if approved by the whims of a three-physician (typically male) committee (a "Therapeutic Abortion Committee")[4]. A 1977 report found that these committees were inconsistent in their decision-making and women faced significantly increased risks from the procedure, due to delays in referral[5].

Throughout this period, Henry Morgentaler, a Montreal-based physician, performed abortions in unaccredited private clinics. Complex legal battles ensued in Quebec and Ontario and finally at the Supreme Court of Canada (SCC). In 1988 the SCC struck down the 1969 abortion law, ruling that it contravened the Canadian Charter of Rights and Freedoms.

Box 14.1

"Forcing a woman, by threat of criminal sanction, to carry a foetus to term unless she meets certain criteria unrelated to her own priorities and aspirations, is a profound interference with a woman's body and thus an infringement of security of the person."

R v Morgentaler, 1988[6]

Canada is one of the few countries in the world in which abortion has been decriminalized and where no specific laws or restrictions to access exist[7]. Abortion rates have remained stable over the past decade[8]. Medical abortion using a combination of drugs (Mifegymiso in Canada, Mifeprex in the US) can prevent implantation or disrupt implantation and can be used safely into the second trimester. The "morning after" pill and the copper IUD can also be used as "emergency contraception." These may gradually replace some surgical abortions. Although safely used for over 20 years throughout much of the world, it took until 2015 for Mifegymiso to be approved by Health Canada and then only for use up to seven weeks' gestation[9]. In North American jurisdictions where pregnancy termination is widely available, early and safe abortions are the norm[10]. In developing countries, where 97 per cent of the world's unsafe abortions take place, maternal mortality is high and a major public health problem[11].

Box 14.2

Absolute prohibitions on abortion do not eradicate the procedure but simply drive it underground and make it much riskier.

Status of a fetus

The right to choose whether or not to continue a pregnancy arises from the asymmetry in the moral status of the woman versus that of the fetus. In this view, the pregnant woman has full standing as a moral agent. By contrast, a fetus, until born, has only potential status.

Box 14.3

"The value to be placed on the foetus as a potential life is directly related to the stage of its development during gestation."

R v Morgentaler, 1988[12]

This leading Canadian legal view does not mean the fetus has no importance at all. As a pregnancy advances to term, there is an increasing reluctance to terminate it. (In Canada, most legalized abortions take place in the first trimester[8].) This may be due to a "gradualist" view of personhood, to be contrasted with the view that a fetus is fully human and has, from the moment of conception, equivalent moral status to an adult ("the right to life of the unborn"). For this "vitalist" view, to directly end the life of a fetus by performing an abortion for any reason is the moral equivalent of murder [13]. A gradualist view is compatible with making compromises about pregnancy termination, while the vitalist view is less likely to be.

That said, it is not surprising that women can have difficulty finding a doctor willing to perform an abortion for late second- and third-term abortions, with the exception of cases where the fetus has died or has major malformations, or where the mother's life is at risk. Late-term abortions can be psychologically and ethically unsettling, given that healthcare providers are expected to try to rescue neonates of 24 weeks who are born alive [14]. The moral and psychological complexity of this experience should encourage more dialogue between opposing views over abortion [15].

Discussion of Case 14.2

On the face of it, this would seem quite simple: the couple seeks a medical service—prenatal testing—that is readily available. Suppose you disagree with their rationale for pregnancy termination. Is that a sufficient reason to not tell them about all the options they have? If you are truly concerned, counselling them would be acceptable—but it should be sensitive to the different personal, ethnic, and cultural opinions in this area and ought not be overly directive. It would be reasonable to have a discussion with the woman without the husband in the room. Does she share the same views as her husband? Has there been any pressure from her family regarding the decision? As long as the woman is making an authentic choice and does not appear to be coerced by her spouse or her culture, her choice must, ultimately, be respected. And just because a test like NIPT may not be covered by medicare does not mean you have no obligation to disclose this option to the patient.

It may seem odd but, although abortions are allowed for any reason in Canada, certain requests for prenatal testing—such as those made *simply* to find out the sex of the fetus—are frowned upon. This value judgment about patient motivation may not be made on discriminatory grounds but to prevent sex-selection clinics from springing up and professionals from profiting from providing such services. Regulatory authorities have tried to limit access to such testing by developing guidelines suggesting that prenatal ultrasounds for sex determination are "inappropriate." However, developments in medicine have meant there is no way to deny couples early access to accurate methods of identifying fetal sex. The clinician must then discuss all the options with the patient.

The US philosopher Judith Jarvis Thomsen offered in 1971 a novel defence of the right to abortion. Imagine, she wrote, you were to wake up one day to find you had been tethered to the circulatory system of a world-famous violinist [16]. He will die if unhooked from you before nine months have passed. Are you obliged to maintain your non-voluntary nine-month association with the violinist? The answer would seem to be no. It is a question of consent: my right to another's person's blood or kidney depends on that person's consent. Similarly, the right of the fetus to its life depends on the pregnant woman's ongoing consent. Thus, even if one considers the fetus a person, this does not mean the fetus has a right to life that trumps the woman's right to choose.

Lee and George have argued that this view does not justify abortion [17]. They have a very dramatic view of abortion (defined by them as "the killing of a human child, the act of extracting the unborn human being from the womb—an extraction that usually rips him or her to pieces or does him or her violence in some other way"). They also parse the requests for asking for pregnancy termination. There may be "less or more serious reasons for seeking the termination of this condition," but "the burden of carrying the baby is significantly less than the harm the baby would suffer by being killed."

The language of Lee and George (the intentional "killing of a human child," "a grisly deed," "rip[ping]" the child "to pieces") suggests how emotional this issue is for some. But can two men speak convincingly as to how burdensome it is to be a pregnant woman? This is not an *ad hominem* argument, but a reflection on the state and substance of the debate. They admit pregnancy may involve "considerable burden to the woman" but only for nine months and there is always adoption, they say. These arguments would not withstand scrutiny—burdensomeness is a judgment to be made by the individual patient, not by the doctor or some "therapeutic abortion committee." This is not the place, however, to examine the longstanding and complex philosophical and religious debates over the morality of abortion. The fact is, in many parts of the world, abortion is a legitimate choice for women and cannot be prevented.

Thomsen's story is not a perfect analogy for pregnancy nor is it a definitive argument against the view that pregnancy entails responsibility. For many people, in the context of a wanted and consented-to pregnancy, the woman has a moral and social responsibility to take care to protect her fetus during the pregnancy. A similar situation would be one in which an individual who, having agreed to donate some tissue (or provide a gift) to another, behaves in ways to imperil the donation (or takes the gift back). We might find this, like breaking a promise, morally objectionable or at least difficult to fathom and ask, "Why would they do that?" These qualms should not, however, lead to legal sanctions such as refusing to respect or cooperate with the would-be donor, since the donation, like a mother's support for her fetus, is a voluntary matter. Rather, we need to make an effort to understand the donor's (like the promise breaker's or the pregnant woman's) change of heart. The pregnant woman deserves a chance to tell her story and be sympathetically heard.

II. Termination and Choice

In the United States, denying a woman's right to choose whether or not to continue a pregnancy was struck down as unconstitutional in 1973 in the well-known *Roe v Wade* Supreme Court decision [18]. The right to privacy was used to protect women from interference with their decision to terminate a pregnancy—at least up until the point of fetal viability—in other words, the right to be left alone [19]. Even though it ruled that state laws restricting a woman's right to abortion were unconstitutional, the Court still left the regulation of the practice up to the individual states [20]. This meant that many states could create legislation indirectly impeding a woman's reproductive rights [21]. For example, various American states have tried to prevent abortions by defunding clinics that provide such services or that even simply refer women to abortion providers [22]. So, although abortion is currently legal in all American states, access to it is quite variable. In California, with virtually no restrictions, abortion is offered in hundreds of clinics. In Mississippi, by contrast, the restrictions are legion, and abortions can be performed in a single clinic only on certain days of the week [23]. Anti-choice groups have used considerable ingenuity to create barriers and disincentives for many women, such as creating legislation requiring women seeking an abortion to view an ultrasound of their fetus or changing the design requirements for stand-alone abortion clinics, effectively running them into bankruptcy [24]. In 2018 the right of a woman in the US to choose whether or not to continue her pregnancy now survives by the slimmest of political margins. It may yet be criminalized again.

Canadian laws regarding pregnancy termination were struck down in 1988 on much broader and more secure grounds. As mentioned above, the Supreme Court in Canada ruled that state interference with a woman's choice contravened section 7 of the Canadian Charter of Rights and Freedoms, specifically, the right to security of the person [25].

A mother's right, a father's obligation

A woman from Quebec, who became pregnant while in a two-year common-law relationship, sought to terminate her pregnancy. The father of the fetus obtained a court injunction preventing her from having an abortion. Clarification of the rights of the father and of the fetus were obtained through appeal to the Supreme Court of Canada.

This case, *Tremblay v Daigle*, both solidified the right of a woman to decide independently regarding her pregnancy and clarified the rights of the father.

1. "The foetus cannot, in English law . . . have a right of its own at least until it is born and has a separate existence from its mother"[26].
2. "No court in Quebec or elsewhere has ever accepted the argument that a father's interest in a foetus which he helped create could support a right to veto a woman's decisions in respect of the foetus she is carrying"[27].

That a father has no legal say in a woman's decision whether or not to end her pregnancy does not mean he is free from obligations regarding the pregnancy. Would-be "hit-and-run" fathers must provide support if a pregnancy they helped engender is successfully taken to term.

Given the serious and intimate nature of pregnancy and abortion, there is no more legitimate and reliable person to make the decision to continue or terminate a pregnancy and to take the responsibility for living with the decision than the woman who is pregnant (see Box 14.4). Whether or not the fetus is considered a person (and many opinions regarding this exist), in Canada the fetus, while *en ventre de sa mère* ("in the belly of its mother"), has no legal protection;[27] its continued existence should depend on the woman's ongoing autonomous and uncoerced choice.

Box 14.4

"Parliament has failed to establish either a standard or a procedure whereby any [state] interests might prevail over those of the woman in a fair and non-arbitrary fashion."

R v Morgentaler, 1988 6

Conscientious objection

If a healthcare provider has a moral objection to abortion, what role, if any, must they play if a patient requests one? Healthcare providers opposed to abortion on the grounds of conscience certainly do not have a duty to participate[28]. However, in some jurisdictions, such as Ontario[29] and Australia[30], physicians have a duty to disclose their beliefs and also to refer patients to another physician without an objection to abortion. The harm to the objecting practitioner's conscience in facilitating a referral is felt to be outweighed by the magnitude of potential harm to a patient should she be unable to obtain a timely termination. Failing to refer can put a woman at increased risk of a delayed abortion and a bad outcome (the later the termination, the greater the physical and psychological risks for women)[31]; not referring could be construed as negligence or patient abandonment.

Access to abortion services, however, remains problematic in many parts of North America. Finding someone to perform a timely abortion is generally not difficult in the larger cities in Canada but can be a challenge in many smaller communities, some provinces, and many American states where abortion providers have been assaulted and murdered. Hospitals in Canada are not required to provide abortion services, which makes equitable access a serious problem[32]. There is no good rationale for this in a publicly funded system which must respond to the legitimate health needs of the population.

III. The New Age of Reproduction

A woman can choose if, when, and even *how* she gives birth—albeit with substantial restrictions, depending upon where she lives, her finances, and her age[33]. In the past, infertility was usually less of a problem than the puerperal-related death of mother and child. As with so many other things in the past half-century, giving birth is now not nearly as straightforward as it used to be.

Some people go to extraordinary lengths to become parents. Sperm can be provided and joined with an ovum in a petri dish (an *in vitro* embryo); sperm can be injected directly into an ovum (ICSI, intracytoplasmic sperm injection); embryos can be transferred into the mother's womb (*in vitro* fertilization, IVF); the uterus may be that of a surrogate; gametes may be collected and stored prior to chemotherapy, bone marrow radiation, or surgery, or harvested after death; pathogenic maternal mitochondria can be identified and replaced. Reproduction has now been "globalized," often outsourced to countries where surrogate parentage is accepted, although in the US surrogacy contracts can be stratospherically expensive. Previously a popular destination for foreigners, India now allows "altruistic surrogacy" only for Indian citizens[34].

Assisted reproductive technology (ART) includes all the varied techniques of harvesting, preserving, manipulating, transferring, and conjoining gametes as well as the technology for analyzing, storing, sharing, and using the genetic material of gametes and embryos. Options now include preimplantation genetic screening (PGS) and preimplantation genetic diagnosis (PGD). PGS is now PGT-A (preimplantation genetic testing for "aneuploidy"—ensuring the correct number of chromosomes are present) and PGD is now PGT-M (preimplantation genetic testing for monogenic diseases—screening for known genetic diseases such as Tay Sacks, cystic fibrosis, sickle cell anemia.) Both involve taking five to ten cells from the embryo at the blastocyst stage. The results of these tests can be used to select unaffected desirable embryos to transfer to a woman's womb. Mitochondrial replacement therapy (MRT) can replace specifically the pathogenic mitochondria

DNA (mtDNA) from the intended mother with non-pathogenic mtDNA from an oocyte provider; however, this procedure is currently illegal in Canada[35].

ART has allowed millions of infertile or childless couples, individuals, and families a chance to have children of their own. It has also enabled those worried about heritable conditions to be reassured they will not pass on a serious illness. ART comes with the expense of creating tens of thousands of excess embryos, however[36]. It thus creates dilemmas, not only for parents but also for practitioners. What should be done with the excess embryos? Who are the parents for an embryo? What is its legal status? Are the products of ART conceptions—unborn but not implanted embryos—persons with rights and interests of their own? Or are they chattel, mere property, to be manipulated, bought, or sold? If the ordering parents die and leave an estate, does the estate now belong to the unborn embryo or is the embryo inherited along with the estate?

This is ground more safely and commonly trod by lawyers and regulators than by doctors. There is a burgeoning legal canon of which clinicians should be aware and wary.

The *Assisted Human Reproductive Act*

Following a long period of study begun in the 1990s, Canada passed the *Assisted Human Reproductive Act* (hereafter, the *Reproductive Act* or the Act) in 2004 in an effort to keep up with the challenges associated with advances in reproductive medicine (see Box 14.5)[37].

Box 14.5

The *Canadian Reproductive Act* is guided by five principles:

1. a respect for human individuality, dignity, and integrity;
2. a "precautionary" approach to protect and promote health;
3. non-commodification and non-commercialization;
4. informed choice; and
5. accountability and transparency.

The Canadian legislation criminalizes (and tries to prevent) certain activities that "threaten the security of donors, recipients, and persons conceived by assisted reproduction"[38]. It is meant to prevent the commercialization of surrogate arrangements and the "anything-goes" atmosphere that permeates ART in some parts of the world—as if it was merely a personal service to be bought and sold like any other[39].

Prohibited acts include the following:

- human cloning,
- commercialization of human reproductive material and the reproductive functions of women and men, and
- use of *in vitro* embryos without consent.

Permitted activities, so long as they are carried out in accordance with regulations made under the Act, are deemed "controlled activities" and include the following:

- manipulation of human reproductive material or *in vitro* embryos,
- transgenic engineering, and
- reimbursement of the expenditures of donors and surrogate mothers (although, as yet, there are no regulations for this).

(Note that the Act governs only the use of embryos and gametes. Once transferred into a woman, the Act's provisions do not govern the fetus's treatment and use.)

As in the United States, and unlike the United Kingdom, Canada does not have a single agency to oversee assisted reproduction. The Act addresses concerns that unregulated use of ART could undermine the fundamental principle of dignity and respect for persons embodied in the practice of medicine. This principle of respect attempts to exclude monetary gain as the primary motivation for healthcare professionals working in this field. For example, to prevent commercialization of the process and exploitation of persons involved, the following would not be permitted:

- Sex selection via embryo testing, except for medical reasons, for example, to prevent sex-specific disease such as Duchenne's muscular dystrophy. However, as there is no enforcement of this law, this still occurs in Canada and the United States[40].
- Payments to would-be gamete (egg or sperm) donors, except for "reasonable expenses." Many US states are more liberal as regards payment to gamete donors for their time, pain, and suffering; one worry is that the higher the payment, the more likely gamete donors will downplay the risks of being donors and be subject to exploitation[41].
- Payments to surrogate mothers. In Canada, unlike some American states, surrogates can be reimbursed only for "reasonable costs" and losses associated with pregnancy. The intention is to remove any financial windfalls to surrogates and prevent a market-driven traffic in babies for purchase and wombs for hire. People do attempt to get around the

prohibition against payment by making generous gifts to surrogates and donors. While such gifting is illegal in Canada, it does occur. Persons who mediate such "gifting" are subject to significant fines and even imprisonment[42].

Box 14.6

Under Canada's *Human Reproduction Act*, you cannot buy (or advertise to buy) sperm or eggs from a donor or a person acting on behalf of a donor. You also cannot buy (or advertise to buy) the services of a surrogate. You can reimburse a donor or surrogate for actual expenses related to the donation or pregnancy.

Sara Cohen, a lawyer working in this area, has written that the attempt to block commercialization of ART has not prevented private clinics, doctors, lawyers, psychotherapists, and others from making very handsome fees from these efforts. The palpable desire and desperation to have children (and, if possible, with one's own DNA) make people vulnerable to exploitation by commercial firms ready to cash in on their despair and anxiety. The cost for an attempt at pregnancy using ART in Canada is at least $8,000 to $10,000, with the total cost of a successful pregnancy being around $80,000. This is still a bargain compared with the United States where the estimated costs for a gestational pregnancy, including IVF, run from $100,000 to $175,000 USD[43]. Private firms offer services worldwide to ostensibly ease the surrogacy process[44]. Ironically or sadly, surrogates and gamete donors are left out of this market[45]. Where the market dominates in medicine, as in other nonmedical products or services, one can only say caveat emptor.

The right to know one's past

Another important area continues to be unresolved due to the Act remaining in limbo: while adopted children have a right to seek access to information on file about their biological parents, do offspring from ART (where gametes meet *in vitro*) and from donor insemination (where gametes meet *in vivo*) have similar access to their parental genetic information and other health risks? It appears not—at least not yet in Canada. The *Food and Drug Act*'s regulations (which govern trade in gametes) recommend, but do not mandate, for example, that non-identifying information on the sperm donor be kept on file[46].

The Act proposed a new federal agency that would hold a confidential registry for information on gamete donors. With the donor's consent, access to this information would be granted to a donor's offspring. Lacking implementation of this legislation, however, no federal registry has been established and so there are no effective routes for the offspring of donor insemination or ART to ascertain their genetic history.

This is unlike the United Kingdom where, under the auspices of the Human Fertilisation and Embryology Authority [47], a central registry of all gamete donors and all births as a result of assisted conceptions in licensed UK facilities has been kept since 1991. Although no unique identifying information will be provided, donor-conceived individuals 16 years of age and older can discover the donor's age, ethnicity, other children (if any), physical characteristics, health status and any other information the donor may have wished to have passed on.

In 2011 the BC Supreme Court found British Columbia, in failing to provide ART and donor offspring the same rights and protections as adoptees (among them the right to have access to donor information), to be in breach of article 15 of the Canadian Charter, the right to equal protection under the law [48]. While this went some way in recognizing the right of donor offspring not to be deprived of access, it did not take the further step of affirming a positive state duty to provide paternal genetic information [49]. Thus, while offspring may need and want to know their lineage, in Canada they currently have no right to this information [50].

Reproductive restrictions and access

Some studies suggest that US reproductive service providers allow their values to influence their clinical decisions [51].

Box 14.7

"[T]he majority of ART programs believe that they have the right and responsibility to screen candidates before providing them with ART to conceive a child. The key value that seems to guide programs' screening practices is ensuring a prospective child's safety and welfare and not risking the welfare of the prospective mother." [51]

This may be at times quite appropriate where the interest is in assessing the psychological suitability of a person to be a surrogate parent. However, it would be an offence to justice to exclude people in "non-traditional" relationships or gay or transgender individuals from accessing ART [52].

Box 14.8

Types of Surrogacy

1. **Traditional surrogacy**: the father's spermatozoa are introduced into the surrogate's uterus to be conjoined with the surrogate woman's ovum. The surrogate mother is genetically linked to the embryo.
2. **Gestational surrogacy**: IVF techniques are used to conjoin gametes from the parents-to-be (or donated gametes). The resultant viable embryo(s) is/are then placed in the surrogate's uterus. This severs any genetic link between the surrogate mother and the intended parent(s).

A **gestational contract** sets out the terms of the surrogacy relationship (1 or 2).

Denying choice?

In 1993, a BC physician directing an ART clinic, specializing in fertilizing the ova of women with sperm donated by unrelated men, decided to no longer allow lesbian couples access to the clinic's services. Several years earlier, he had testified in a child custody case involving a lesbian couple who had undergone successful insemination in his clinic. The resultant publicity had led to harassing phone calls criticizing him for inseminating lesbians; this eventually led, he said, to his decision to limit his practice[53].

Denied the clinic's service, a lesbian couple filed a complaint of discrimination on account of sexual orientation. The Supreme Court of British Columbia upheld this, finding the physician in violation of the *British Columbia Human Rights Act*[54]. This decision might have been controversial then, but is less so now. It is accepted in many, but not all, jurisdictions that ART services should be available to gay, lesbian, transgender, and/or unmarried persons[55].

Box 14.9

Physicians providing any medical services must ensure there is no discrimination in their provision.

Physicians can deny any medical service if there are legitimate safety concerns, such as serious threats to the welfare of patients or society. If the child-to-be is likely to be seriously harmed by the would-be parents, then the physician may be obliged not to help them [56]. Just what parental conditions would justify not offering ART? Drug abuse? Possibly—especially if the gestational mother-to-be is drug-addicted. Abject poverty? Not on its own, but impoverished would-be parents couldn't afford ART anyway. Advanced maternal age? Possibly. It would depend on the reason for requesting ART and the risks to the would-be mother. A history of child abuse and neglect? Almost certainly.

What the market will bear

In Canada, the prohibition of the sale of gametes is meant to prevent the commodification of ART (a good thing), but can create barriers and delays in accessing donor gametes and/or surrogacy (not a good thing). In the real world, the "right" of opportunity to access artificial reproductive services—or at least to join the queue to access ART—is a limited one, usually accessible only to those with significant financial means. There is no financial reimbursement for ART use by infertile couples or individuals in many countries.

The reluctance of governments to reimburse such services treats infertility differently from other medical conditions, arguably infringing on the infertile person's "equality rights." Should the "right" to become pregnant be on par with another patient's "right" to be free of limitations on lying flat because of Grade IV heart failure or another's "right" to be treated for an inability to mix socially on account of a pervasive social anxiety disorder? Infertility is not one thing: it may be congenital or due to disease or injury or due simply to older age. The desire for ART may run from the reasonable to the outlandish.

Illnesses are, in one broadly accepted view, deviations from the "normal" human range of functioning, which cause harm to patients or threaten to do so [57]. Such conditions are sometimes seen as unfair—blindness, deafness—so any helpful interventions tend to be compensated through social support programs. We do not generally reimburse patients for the merely unfortunate experiences of life, such as being born short or being unattractive. Many view infertility as an unfortunate occurrence, not an illness rendering persons so afflicted that they are any less able to participate in life.

The Supreme Court of Nova Scotia, for example, has held that not reimbursing ART is a legitimate policy decision, interpreting it as a "reasonable limit" on the provision of services "demonstrably justified" in a democratic society as permitted by the Canadian Charter of Rights and Freedoms. (See Chapter 13.) This judgment perhaps missed the nuances in the causes of infertility and the various rationales for seeking ART. The judge wrote:

Box 14.10

"It would be unrealistic for this Court to assume that there are unlimited funds to address the needs of all." [58]

This statement is true but why choose this group for discrimination? The reality is that very few provinces fund ART and then only in very limited circumstances. This has meant that some would-be parents—single, gay, transgender, some in non-traditional relationships—find the help they need, but most cannot. Many people perceive this arrangement as unjust [59]. The considerable expense of ART and lack of coverage by most provincial medicare plans, as well as a lack of clarity about regulations, have led some desperate people to pursue unsafe alternatives (such as going abroad to purchase less costly gametes that may not have been subjected to the same rigorous quality control found in Canada) [60].

There has been a very slow process of acceptance of ART throughout the world. For example, MRT (mitochondrial replacement therapy) that would produce offspring with *three* genetic parents is not legalized in most parts of the world—despite the fact that mitochondrial diseases can be devastating and lack effective treatment options [61]. Many jurisdictions also lack any legislation that would allow and regulate surrogate parentage.

At Quebec's urging, the Supreme Court of Canada in 2010 found that certain provisions of the Act exceeded the federal legislative authority for healthcare [62]. As a result, many parts of this Act were struck down and critical regulations, such as proper reimbursement to surrogates and to gamete donors or an agency to track gamete donors, are missing.

That the legal framework has not caught up to the rapid changes in reproductive technologies is not unique to North America. This is especially evident when it comes to members of the LGBTQ+ community seeking to become parents. When a single father returned to England in 2014 with his baby (born as a result of gestational surrogacy with his sperm and an ovum from an unrelated donor), a senior judge ruled that under the law he had no parental responsibility for his child (despite being both the genetic and intended parent of the child) and that the US gestational surrogate (who had no genetic or intended parental interests) was the sole person with parental responsibility for the child under UK law. However, in May 2016, a UK court ruled that English law violated the European Convention of Human Rights by preventing a single parent from securing parental rights to his child born via surrogacy. Changes in the law are pending in the United Kingdom [63].

The introduction of the *All Families Are Equal (AFAE) Act* in Ontario 2016 represents an attempt by the government of Ontario to address the changing nature of the family unit in Canada as it is being influenced by developments in ART. The Act is meant to ensure that all people who use assisted reproduction technologies, such as egg/sperm donation or surrogacy, to conceive children will be legally recognized as parents without having to go through a lengthy legal process to adopt their own children[64].

Case 14.3   Whose Baby Is It Anyway?

A childless lesbian couple, Ms K and Ms M, arrange for the creation of an *in vitro* embryo from Ms K's egg and sperm donated anonymously. Neither Ms K nor Ms M is physically able to bear a child. The embryo is successfully implanted into a surrogate mother, Ms L, contracted by the couple to give birth to the child, Baby B, whom the couple intend to raise. The pregnancy is successfully carried to term; however, Ms K and Ms M split up acrimoniously shortly before the child's birth. The gamete provider, Ms K, now says she wants her former partner, Ms M, to have nothing to do with raising Baby B. Ms M objects and seeks legal remedy.

Who should be considered the parents of this child?
What if Ms L decides to simultaneously apply to be legally considered Baby B's mother?
Does the source of the gametes make a difference?

Surrogacy means implanting a fertilized egg (which may or may not originate from the surrogate mother) into a surrogate's womb (the "birth mother"). In traditional surrogacy, one uses the male partner's sperm to inseminate the surrogate mother, using the surrogate's own oocytes. In modern gestational surrogacy, the surrogate mother uses gametes from a female donor in order to sever any genetic link between the birthing mother (the "gestational carrier") and the child and to forestall any claim by the surrogate that she is the "real" mother.

In Canada this does not appear to be a significant issue, as studies suggest that surrogate women, in Canada at least, abide by the terms of their contract and see their involvement in the birth of the child as a service to others. Arguments as to whether commercial surrogacy arrangements exploit women continue[65].

Discussion of Case 14.2

What if the woman supplying the ovum, as in this case, wishes to prevent her legally contracted partner from a role in raising the child once born? The language of a surrogate contract would seem to suggest a ready answer: the "intended couple" would be considered to be Baby B's parents. If they split up there would have to be a court decision as to which parent would be the "best parent" and what role, if any, there would be for the other ordering parent. This appears to be less about whose baby it is than a decision about custody arrangements with shared parentage—and no different from the legal proceedings when parents of a naturally conceived child split up.

Does it matter who contributed the gametes? It might—or it might not. There have been conflicting views on this in the courts in Canada and elsewhere. When a dispute arises over "whose baby is it?" some courts, relying on the traditional doctrine of "birthing-means-motherhood" (an old doctrine, from long ago, before the invention of ART), have deemed the baby to belong to the gestational carrier. Others have awarded the baby to the intended parents on the grounds the baby would not have been born were it not for their efforts. Yet other courts have found, irrespective of gamete origin, against the gestational carrier, if it seems the newborn child would be better off with the intended parents.

In contemporary legal proceedings in Canada the trend is to look less to the origins of the gametes and to consider more what is in the newborn's best interests, but this is not a sure thing. Parenting matters are complicated and, to paraphrase Tolstoy[66], each family is complicated in its own way.

Kelly Jordan, a lawyer familiar with this area, has written, "in none of the reported cases . . . was the declaration of parentage opposed by the gestational carrier or the gamete donor. There is, as of yet, no reported Canadian decision involving a contested declaration of parenting in an assistive reproduction scenario"[67]. However, in 2018, there was a contested (and what may be a precedent-setting) case involving ART[68]. A couple bought two viable embryos produced by gametes genetically unrelated to the ordering couple at a US facility. In 2012, using one of the viable embryos, the wife gave birth. The couple then divorced and the question was: to whom did the other viable embryo belong? The Ontario judge awarded the embryo to the wife of the by-now estranged couple, according to the terms of a clinical consent form. The embryo was her property and the woman had to reimburse her former husband his half of the embryo's "value." This may turn out to be an isolated event—an unusual set of circumstances—or it may become a more common scenario as ART becomes used more widely. Hitherto, in Canada, there has not been a storm of such cases, perhaps because gamete donors and surrogate mothers in Canada tend to act more for altruistic than for monetary reasons. Physicians working with infertile couples need to have some familiarity with the local laws regarding surrogacy in their jurisdiction. Prudent clinicians should listen to their legal counsel who can tell them what arrangements are in place. Such cases, like many other areas of modern reproduction, are for family law lawyers, not physicians, to resolve.

IV. Desperately Seeking Stem Cells

The use of human stem cells to enhance human reproduction and health is also controversial. Stem cells are primal cells capable of renewing themselves through cell division. They also possess the potential to differentiate into more special-ized cells. Human stem cells exist in two main forms: embryonic stem cells and induced pluripotent stem cells [69]. Embryonic stem cells, which have the greatest capacity to differentiate, are derived from early-stage human embryos prior to implantation at the blastocyst stage when around four to five days old. Induced pluripotent stem cells, in contrast, are derived from normally differentiated adult tissues, such as skin. These are tissue-specific cells reprogrammed to behave like embryonic stem cells. The skin is the primary source of induced pluripotent stem cells, but there are other sources as well, such as bone marrow. (By contrast, there are virtually none in the heart or brain.)

Stem cells have legitimately been used for over 60 years to regenerate bone marrow and blood cells in patients with diseases such as leukemia. Stem cells offer the hope of definitive, that is, disease-modifying, treatment for other conditions such as heart failure, macular degeneration, Parkinson's disease, spinal cord injur-ies, and juvenile-onset diabetes—diseases affecting tissues or organs where stem cells are not apparent in adults. Infused stem cells could, in theory, replenish the loss of differentiated cells, such as the loss of dopamine-producing neurons in Par-kinson's. They also could potentially aid in regenerating certain tissues, such as cardiac tissue damaged by myocardial infarction [70].

Stem cells are often used before evidence of their safety and efficacy is known. We do not know, for example, what microscopic factors influence stem cells to become fully functional cells in situ. Despite this, a host of private clinics offering expensive stem cell therapies for diseases such as heart failure [71] have sprung up and, along with them, a nest of nasty adverse events [72]. The use of stem cells is not without its dangers. However, this may be a temporary aberration as there is a deep and legitimate interest in the promise of an era of precise and personalized "regenerative medicine" [73].

> ## Case 14.4 The Saviour Child
>
> ....
>
> Although currently in remission, a three-year-old girl, Becky L, has been gravely ill with leukemia. Curative treatment is possible but requires bone marrow stem cell donation from a suitable donor. Without it, the child will almost certainly die when the disease recurs, as it almost certainly will. No suitable match is found. The parents decide to conceive a new child in the hope this will result in a suitable donor, but they need ART because Becky's mother, now 38, experienced premature ovarian insufficiency at age 36. The mother's twin sister is prepared to donate her eggs.
>
> *Is this an acceptable use of ART?*
> *Is doing prenatal genetic testing (PGT) to find HLA compatibility acceptable?*

Research and treatment using embryonic-derived stem cells have generally been more controversial than using adult stem cells. Some oppose using embryonic-derived cells because they come with a moral tithe, for example, where a surplus of embryos is to be created with no plan for their management or if the embryo is sacrificed to derive stem cells. Creating an embryo for the purposes of destroying it, or neglecting it as excess tissue, contributes in some people's eyes to the devaluation of human life[74, 75]. It seems wrong—and is indeed illegal—to treat gametes or embryos as mere property to be bought or sold to the highest bidder. These actions and attitudes seem morally repugnant because they treat human life as a means to an end, rather than an end in itself. (This, as you can tell, is a deontological argument.)

Supporters of embryonic stem cell use in research, by contrast, point to the tremendous potential for improving the quality of human life. (This, by contrast, is a consequentialist argument.) Most countries do not prohibit, outright, work with embryonic human stem cells but choose rather to regulate it. Such work, it is argued, need not be done at the expense of a respectful view of human life, if we adhere to certain restrictions. For example, harvesting stem cells from the umbilical cord at birth would seem to be far less controversial and in keeping with Canadian law.

Where to draw the line as to when life begins is obviously a point of controversy. For centuries, it was commonly held that life began at "quickening," the point at which the woman could feel the child move in the uterus (16 to 20 weeks typically). Many countries try to get around religious concerns by limiting the use of embryos to the preimplantation stage or up to 14 days, usually for technical reasons having to do with the feasibility of maintaining embryos *in vitro* (outside a uterus) for longer than two weeks[76].

The Ethics Committee of the American Society for Reproductive Medicine has recommended that discarded or abandoned embryos be used for specific kinds of reproductive-related research but only with prior consent from the donors[77]. This would make the donation of stem cells akin to parents donating the organs of a child who dies suddenly; they can give their tragedy meaning by donating their offspring's organs or tissue for the benefit of others.

Discussion of Case 14.4

Kant argued that human beings should never be treated merely as a means to obtain some supposed "greater good" because this renders them mere "stepping-stones" to someone else's welfare or happiness. This suggests parents ought never to see one of their offspring as mere fulfillments for their own needs or the needs of others.

If so, this seems too demanding. After all, parents are allowed to have children for all kinds of emotional, economic, and cultural reasons. There is no moral litmus test prospective parents must pass—we do not question why people want a new child. So, why not, then, produce an offspring, a so-called "saviour child," to rescue the life of an imperilled one? There is no guarantee, of course, the newborn will be a match for their child although PGT can be used to discriminate among the embryos conceived *in vitro*.

Conclusion

We will now move on from life's beginning to life's end. In the next two chapters, we examine some of the most recurring and disturbing issues in modern ethics, the issues connected with the care of the dying, the lost, and the dead. If life's beginning is about possibility and promise, then life's end may be more about destiny and purpose.

Cases for Discussion

Case 1: Fetus at Risk

You are a nurse practitioner in a clinic in the Lower East Side of downtown Vancouver. One of your patients, Ms S, is a 29-year-old woman in her second pregnancy. Her first child suffers from fetal alcohol syndrome (FAS) and is in foster care. Ms S continues to drink heavily during this second pregnancy. Alerted to this by her common-law spouse, you are concerned for the well-being of the fetus as well as of the mother. Someone suggests you get tough with Ms S by making an urgent application for court-ordered protection for the fetus and seeking involuntary hospitalization away from skid row for the woman to ensure compliance (with a plan to treat her alcohol problem and control her alcohol intake).

Question for Discussion

1. Would you go along with this suggestion?

Case 2: Judgment of Solomon

A 23-year-old healthy female, Ms N, has decided to donate several of her oocytes to an upper middle-class couple seeking reproductive assistance. She will also act as a gestational mother for the couple. Currently unemployed, she will find the money from the oocyte harvesting ($5,000 per oocyte) paid to her by a private fertility clinic quite helpful. She's unattached at the time of the donation and has never been pregnant. Her oocytes are successfully conjoined *in vitro* with male gametes and two are implanted in case one fails. Both are successful in achieving viability and she will deliver twins. The intended parents are delighted. Ms N receives a handsome monthly retainer fee (under the table, of course) to offset the cost and inconvenience of pregnancy [78].

During her pregnancy, she reads a magazine article arguing against surrogacy. It posits that surrogacy, such as she has undertaken, exploits poor women and treats offspring as chattel to be bought and sold, like calves at an auction. As her pregnancy progresses, she develops an increasing attachment to her embryonic duo and begins to consider keeping the babies. She then meets a partner who is willing to help her raise the children but is not able to support her financially. Ms N feels some twinges of guilt towards the contracting couple. She and her partner decide to offer one of the children to them at birth and to keep the other.

Questions for Discussion

1. This scenario raises a number of legal and unethical issues. What are they?
2. Is dividing the twins between the two couples a fair compromise?
3. Should the law prevent such arrangements? Why or why not?

✦ 15 ✦

···

A Dark Wood

End-of-Life Decisions

We are born in a clear field and die in a dark wood.

Russian proverb, anon.

Towards the end of the play *Waiting for Godot*, one of the characters, Pozzo, summarizes with chilling hopelessness some of the darkest fears which we all as humans have: "*They give birth astride of a grave, the light gleams for an instant, then it is night once more.*¹" Along with the Russian proverb above, Pozzo's view reflects the pessimism with which, for much of human history, death has been viewed—as a dark and forlorn stop at the terminus of an all-too-brief life. Although Hobbes described life at times as "nasty, brutish, and short," in modern times it is death that is nasty and brutish, and, for many people, all too frequently anything but short. Despite advances in medicine, death has until recently remained a solitary experience surrounded in fear, over which people have had little control. In this and the next chapter we look at how precedents in law and ethics have changed the process of dying in modern medicine and given people more control over the final chapter of their lives.

I. Allowing Death: Refusals by Patients

The right of a competent patient to accept or refuse treatments has been a primary development informing medical care over the past century. This has been discussed in numerous places throughout this book (see Chapters 4, 5, 6). It should be no surprise, therefore, that the respect for autonomous decision-making should extend to end-of-life matters as well. This is consistent both with our ethical attitudes and legal precedents. In the 1993 case of Sue Rodriguez, discussed in more depth in Chapter 16, the Supreme Court of Canada summarized the issue succinctly:

> Canadian courts have recognized a common law right of patients to refuse consent to medical treatment, or to demand that treatment, once commenced, be withdrawn or discontinued. This right has been specifically recognized to exist, even if the withdrawal from or refusal of treatment may result in death[2].

One of the precedent-setting cases referred to in this statement was that of Nancy B.

Case 15.1   The Story of Nancy B

Nancy B, a 25-year-old woman from Quebec, was hospitalized in 1988 with an unusual and extremely severe form of Guillain-Barré syndrome (an auto-immune condition affecting the peripheral nervous system that can result in severe muscle weakness or paralysis, but which usually resolves spontaneously within a few weeks). In Ms B's case, the condition did not resolve, leaving her permanently paralyzed, bedridden, on tube feeds, and dependent on a venti-lator. She was considered incurable, but not "terminal" (she could potentially be kept alive in that state for many years). Although significantly physically incapacitated, her mind remained intact and she could talk.

Discussion of Case 15.1

After two and a half years in that condition, Nancy B expressed a desire to be removed from the ventilator and be allowed to die. However, her physicians were reluctant to discontinue her ventilatory support, for fear of being charged with assisted suicide or negligence in failing to provide the necessaries of life. Unwilling to accept her ongoing suffering, her family pursued the matter in the courts on her behalf. The case captured national media attention, generating a great deal of discussion across Canada. A judge even visited Ms B in the hospital where she told him, "I don't want to live on a machine, I don't want to live anymore"[3].

The Quebec Superior Court ruled that discontinuing the ventilator was her right and that, because she could not do so herself, it was not a crime for her physicians to do so on her behalf. They would simply be allowing the disease to take its natural course[4]. On February 13, 1992, her ventilatory support was discontinued and she died minutes later.

Withdrawal/withholding of potentially life-sustaining treatment

To begin, we need a word about terminology. It is not uncommon to hear or encounter the terms "withdrawal of care" or "withholding of care" when discussing end-of-life issues. Both are unfortunate phrases, as it is never the case that *care* is withdrawn or withheld. Care will always be provided. It will just be a different type of care—with different goals. When making end-of-life treatment decisions, patients and their families often express fear they or their family member will not be cared for as deeply and fully as if they were in the ICU on a ventilator, receiving medications, tube feeds, and the like. It is important to clarify at the outset that this is not the case. In many instances, the patient will be cared for more deeply and fully when the ventilator and tube feeds have been discontinued.

We therefore, along with most commentators, prefer the more accurate, albeit cumbersome, terms: "withdrawal of potentially life-sustaining treatment" and "withholding of potentially life-sustaining treatment."

Box 15.1

A patient's refusal of treatment takes one of two possible forms:

1. requesting the withdrawal of potentially life-sustaining treatment, or
2. requesting the withholding of potentially life-sustaining treatment.

End-of-life studies

Care that concedes the inevitability of death and focuses on quality (not quantity) of life is increasingly recognized as not only appropriate but also desirable. Any kind of treatment, whether it is the administration of antibiotics or ventilatory support, may be stopped or withheld if not contributing to the quality of a patient's life. Numerous studies have demonstrated that voluntary discontinuation of dialysis is one of the most common causes of death in North America and Europe for patients with end-stage renal disease (ESRD) [5–9]. Data from the United States indicates that withdrawal of dialysis consistently accounts for 20 to 25 per cent of deaths in patients with ESRD [10,11].

Other forms of life-sustaining treatment, including cardiopulmonary resuscitation, intravenous fluids, antibiotics, and artificial feeding, are frequently stopped for patients with irremediable multi-organ failure, terminal malignancies, advanced cognitive impairment, coma, and other end-stage conditions. Up to 85 per cent of all ICU deaths are preceded by a decision to forego life-support on the basis it is either incompatible with the patient's wishes or no longer helpful[12].

Due diligence in refusals of care

The refusal of life-sustaining treatment by a patient (or a family) should not always be accepted at face value as an autonomous choice. A prudent and caring professional must always consider other aspects of the patient's life—such as disabilities, addiction, and mental illness—that may undermine autonomous decision-making. Sometimes treatment refusals are precipitated by problems such as unhealthy family relationships, poor communication, or a perceived lack of empathy by healthcare providers. Patients who feel uncared for may seek out novel and sometimes self-destructive approaches in order to get *more* care or attention.

Other patient-related factors can negatively influence decisions to refuse care as well. For example, in a 2008 case from the United States, a father sought to discontinue life-sustaining treatment of his profoundly injured son in order to have the perpetrator of the violent crime charged with murder, not simply assault[13].

Health professionals are not immune to negative motivations when it comes to complying with refusals of care. If their experience with a patient is very unpleasant, they may project hostile emotions onto that patient—and ultimately regard them as not worth saving. These reactions become evident when clinicians (and sometimes even patients themselves) appear too ready to accept the death of patients with severe disabilities[14]. We can guard against this by ensuring certain criteria are met (see Box 15.2)[15,16].

Box 15.2

Conditions for the "proper" cessation of treatment include the following:

- the request is made by a competent informed patient;
- the request is consistent with the patient's beliefs, values and attitudes;
- the decision is freely made neither with coercion nor under circumstances such as severe depression, drug use, and the like;
- alternative forms of treatment and support have been explored and offer no further help to the patient; and
- the patient's condition or illness would be considered by a neutral observer to be reasonable grounds for the wish to stop treatment.

Case 15.2 No Crap, No CPR

Mr X, a 58-year-old homeless man with no known relatives, is admitted in respiratory distress with resistant tuberculosis. Emaciated and dishevelled, he looks 20 years older than his stated age. Uncooperative and resistant to care, he yells at staff, complains about the food, and repeatedly pulls out his tubes. Nonetheless, he undergoes various procedures including bronchoscopy and urinary catheterization.

A few days into his hospitalization, Mr X is approached about the issue of cardiopulmonary resuscitation (CPR). If his heart stops, he is asked, would he want them to try to restart it?

"What kind of crap is this?" he responds. "I don't want any more treatment!"

The staff takes this to mean he does not want CPR. They enter a "No CPR" order into his chart and do not return to discuss this with him.

A week later, Mr X suffers a cardiac arrest and dies. CPR was not performed.

Why might there be cause for concern in Mr X's care?

To CPR or not to CPR: That is the question

Until the 2000s, the approach by most physicians to end-of-life decision-making in acute care hospitals in Canada consisted of asking patients whether or not they wanted CPR should their heart stop beating. In most instances, CPR was a euphemism for "beating on a patient's chest, sticking a breathing tube down their throat, and taking them to the ICU," not a particularly subtle way of addressing end-of-life decision-making. It also made CPR sound as easy as re-starting a stalled car.

In the past several decades, however, the question of whether to perform CPR has largely been supplanted by the much more nuanced approach to end-of-life planning known as "goals of care." These changes notwithstanding, whether to perform CPR is still a relevant question in many situations.

Discussion of Case 15.2

Although Mr X certainly had the right to refuse potentially life-saving treatment, there is reason to be concerned that his care was not optimal.

Mr X had several "red flags" which may have contributed to less-than optimal-management—he was homeless, impoverished, and difficult medically and personally; he had resisted treatments and looked as if he was at the end of his life. Maybe he was, but his care providers could have been a little more diligent in assessing his wishes. The decision about CPR did not appear to have taken place as part of an overall treatment plan (that is, the goals of care). His refusal of "treatment" may have been more an expression of fear and frustration about his illness than a true refusal of care. This is not how end-of-life decisions should be made.

II. Competent Decisions, Living Wills, and Advance Directives

"Do not resuscitate" (DNR) and "No Cardiopulmonary Resuscitation" (No CPR) orders were early examples of advance directives. Another word about terminology: while the terms "living will" and "advance directive" are often used interchangeably, there is a subtle distinction. A living will expresses wishes dealing specifically with end-of-life medical decisions, in the event a person is not capable of making such decisions. It often specifies who can make decisions on their behalf—a substitute decision-maker (SDM)—and provides guidance in how they would like to be cared for at the end of life. In addition, it may include such matters as organ donation or gifting one's body to science.

An advance directive, by contrast, is broader in scope. It specifies not just end-of-life wishes, but also general healthcare preferences, such as where a person might live after an illness and what non-emergency and non-end-of-life treatments they would be willing to accept. Although the expression "living will" is still frequently used, it has generally been supplanted by the more contemporary and more comprehensive term "advance directive."

Box 15.3

Both living wills and advance directives can name a substitute decision-maker and/or specify wishes regarding care.

- A living will specifically directs end-of-life care
- An advance directive governs general healthcare preferences

All provinces and territories (with the exception of Nunavut) have legislation specifying the requirements for a valid advance directive [17]. Unfortunately, the terminology associated with such legislation frequently differs from one jurisdiction to another. For example, in some provinces, the terms "personal directive," "healthcare directive," "representation agreement," and "power of attorney for personal care" are used in lieu or alongside of the term "advance directive." The terms "proxy decision-maker," "attorney," "agent," and "surrogate" are used instead of "substitute decision-maker." It is therefore important for healthcare professionals to become familiar with local terminology.

Case 15.3 Don't Leave Home Without It!

Ms H, a 56-year-old otherwise completely healthy woman, is admitted to hospital with acute cholecystitis. Just as she is being wheeled into the OR for gallbladder surgery, she informs the surgeon, anaesthetist, and nurse: "Oh, I forgot to mention to you before, but I have an advance directive. If something should happen to me in the OR, I don't want to be resuscitated."

How should the team respond?
Should her comments guide her care in the OR?

As mentioned above, an advance directive is a legal document outlining how an individual would like to be cared for at some future time in the event they are not capable of making healthcare decisions for themselves. Scenarios where advance directives might apply can vary significantly. For example, an advance directive might come into effect when a person involved in a serious motor vehicle accident is unconscious and ventilated in the ICU, with a decision needing to be made as to whether they should have a tracheostomy to help wean them from the ventilator. An advance directive might apply when a person with moderate vascular-related dementia no longer possesses the insight to make decisions about their own healthcare, and a decision needs to be made whether to carry out extensive investigations for weight loss. In both situations, an SDM is designated to make healthcare decisions on behalf of the incapacitated person.

Advance directives are frequently assumed to specify in great detail how a person wishes to be treated in the event of illness with loss of capacity to make treatment decisions. However, the types and characteristics of medical issues facing patients and families are often unpredictable and far too complex and variable to be accounted for in this way [18]. For these reasons, advance directives tend to deal in general hypotheticals and provide broad directions for SDMs [19]. They may include a few specific requests, such as a wish never to be administered blood or resuscitated in the event of a cardiac arrest. But in most circumstances an advance directive functions primarily as a compass for an SDM. While this guides them in a general direction towards how the author of the directive would like to be treated, it also allows the SDM latitude and discretion when making decisions consistent with the values and beliefs of the individual. That said, a well-crafted directive can certainly help an SDM align treatment decisions with the patient's preferences [20]. At times common sense must be exercised by healthcare professionals when faced with advance directives (see Chapters 9 and 10).

One often-overlooked detail of advance directives is the need to discuss the contents with family and loved ones, especially with the designated SDM. No matter how well the SDM knows the person or how detailed an advance directive is, an open and honest discussion is an invaluable guide for an SDM when making decisions of the gravest nature and ensuring that the author's wishes are respected (see Case 8.3 and the discussion preceding it). It is important to also emphasize that such communication should consist of not just one isolated discussion, but rather an ongoing dialogue.

Discussion of Case 15.3

This case illustrates a common misconception about advance directives by both the lay public and many healthcare providers. Advance directives are generally designed to provide guidance in extended medical situations, in the event of loss of capacity to make healthcare decisions. Its role is primarily in the setting of long-term medical care, not in one-time, acute situations such as an intraoperative emergency during a routine procedure.

In a circumstance such as this, most patients do not really mean that in the event of a serious intraoperative event they do not want to be resuscitated. It would be tragic, for example, if Ms H suffered an acute allergic reaction and nothing was done to resuscitate her. She almost certainly intends that should she suffer a catastrophic complication and find herself on extended life-support (usually, in the ICU), she would not want extensive heroic measures to keep her alive.

Even though she has raised this issue somewhat cavalierly at an inopportune moment, it is important to address her concerns. Does she really *not* want resuscitation in the event of an intraoperative event? Does she understand the difference between a potentially easily remedied intraoperative emergency and prolonged life-support in the ICU? An appropriate response in this situation

continued

would be to clarify her understanding of these issues and reassure her of your commitment to respect her wishes. If after this brief discussion she still feels strongly about no resuscitation in the OR, then it may be worth delaying surgery in order to confer in more depth with her, her family, and an anaesthetist.

In this case, Ms H really meant that she did not want to be kept alive on life-support in a vegetative state. She agreed to intraoperative resuscitation and underwent an uneventful procedure.

III. Decisions to Withhold or Withdraw Life-Sustaining Treatment

It is a testimony to the increasing acceptance of the concept of "death" in our society that decisions to withhold or withdraw life-sustaining treatments are in actuality only rarely contested. In the vast majority of cases, patients, families, and healthcare professionals do arrive at a consensus around end-of-life treatment decisions. When further aggressive interventions offer no hope of relief or recovery, there is usually little disagreement [12]. But this is not always the case. Occasionally it is the patient who wants to persevere with futile or ineffectual treatment, but, in many instances, it is family members who resist discontinuation of life-sustaining treatments. These situations pose unique ethical and legal dilemmas.

Case 15.4 "She's Not Dying!"

Ms L, a 70-year-old widowed mother of six children, has been treated for multiple myeloma for the past three years. Over the past month, there has been a dramatic deterioration in her health. Her body is shutting down. Along with kidney and liver failure, Ms L has developed respiratory failure from pneumonia, requiring ventilation in the ICU. She has been unconscious for several days after suffering a major stroke. The circulation to her lower limbs has been very compromised and now both legs are showing signs of impending gangrene.

Ms L does not have an advance directive. Her oldest daughter, Anita, has been designated her guardian and substitute decision-maker. The ICU team meets with the family to explain that further aggressive treatment offers no hope of recovery and will only serve to prolong her suffering. They advise discontinuing the ventilator and reassure the family Ms L will receive supportive treatment to keep her comfortable until she dies.

Anita and the rest of the family, however, will not agree to this treatment plan. Not only do they dispute that Ms L is dying, they also question the diagnosis of multiple myeloma in the first place. They also make it clear they harbour deep suspicions about the hospital system and what they see as the trend to save money by not caring for people like their mother. They request a transfer to a centre where doctors will try to save their mother, not kill her.

How should the ICU *physicians and team respond?*

Discussion of Case 15.4

Intractable disagreements with families deserve careful thought and ethical analysis before going the legal route. While this case is not yet "intractable," it could become so if improperly handled. More information is needed before a decision can be made. Are there particular issues Ms L's family have with her care? Are the family's requests based on their mother's previously expressed capable wishes and/or her best interests? Or, do they arise out of family issues, for example, not being able to let go, unresolved guilt, or something as venal as financial considerations? In such difficult situations with families, healthcare professionals must demonstrate great tact and compassion [21]. Here lies the value of narrative medicine: to find the stories that help elucidate patient or family "resistance." Exploring how the patient/family is feeling and learning about the family dynamics rather than getting into an adversarial relationship is important. Unfortunately, this may not always be successful in resolving such conflicts.

For many healthcare providers who deal with life-and-death matters on a daily basis, it is easy to forget how bewildering and alienating a big hospital and ICU can be. It is also simple to overlook the fact that significant portions of the population harbour deep-rooted suspicions about "Western medicine" and the motives of physicians and other healthcare workers. That Ms L's family questions her central diagnosis indicates there has likely been less-than-optimal communication with them in the past.

Taking time to answer the family's questions, avoiding confrontation, and trying to get a sense of their values and beliefs may go a long way toward resolving this dilemma. Most physicians would also appeal to the family's sense of what Ms L would want under the circumstances. Offering to bring in other

continued

physicians to provide a second, third, or even fourth opinion may also help the family accept the inevitable. Most families, when treated in an honest, open, and respectful fashion, will eventually come around and make the right choice for their loved one.

With time and effort, Ms L's family eventually agrees after several meetings with the ICU team that keeping her alive is prolonging her suffering. They agree to discontinue the ventilation. Ms L dies shortly thereafter.

Box 15.4

Take the following steps when working with families:

- Assess understanding: "What have you been told about your [relative's] condition?"
- Acknowledge feelings: "It must be very hard to see your [relative] like this."
- Assess cultural factors: What are their fundamental beliefs? What are their views about suffering? The nature of death? The role of technology?
- Assess for guilt or fears: listen for statements such as, "I can't live without [relative]."
- Allow time to share and process information: "You may have more questions later. Write them down and we'll discuss them." State a definite time and be there.
- Avoid using jargon and value-laden terms such as "vegetative" (demeaning); "doing everything" (not possible); "brain dead" (harsh).
- Avoid loaded questions like, "Do you want to keep [relative] alive?" Ask instead: "How would [relative] want to be cared for in these circumstances?"
- Avoid asking the family to shoulder too much of the burden of decision-making. Part of being an expert and professional is shepherding families through difficult decisions. For example: "As experts in this area and having cared for many people in similar circumstances, we believe strongly that the most caring and humane approach to [relative] is . . . ."[22]

Not all such dilemmas are so readily resolved; some dilemmas lead to significant discord and conflict between healthcare providers and family. We will discuss two such cases (Jin and Rasouli) in the coming sections of this chapter.

IV. Persistent Vegetative States and Prognostic Error

In most cases when life-sustaining treatment is withheld, there is little ambiguity about the prognosis of the patient. Patients with advanced cancer and multiple organ failure, who end up mechanically ventilated in the ICU, simply do not survive for very long. (The issue of brain death and family disputes will be discussed in Chapter 17.)

However, one area where controversies arise is that of patients who appear to have significant brain injury and remain unconscious. Not dead yet, such comatose patients are often described as being in a persistent vegetative state (PVS). They may breathe on their own, move their limbs in non-purposive ways, and at times even open their eyes, but remain, for all intents and purposes, unconscious and unaware of their surroundings. They survive usually because of the wonders of modern medical, nursing, and other care.

One of the most well-known cases of such patients, Karen Ann Quinlan in New Jersey, United States, established the precedent to withdraw potentially life-sustaining treatment for patients in a PVS. Quinlan was 21 years old in 1975 when found unresponsive after overdosing on recreational drugs. Despite resuscitation, she never regained consciousness but was kept alive by means of ventilatory support and feedings through a nasogastric tube. Her parents requested her ventilator be discontinued and she be allowed to die peacefully. However, the physicians and hospital refused to comply for fear of being prosecuted for homicide. The New Jersey Supreme Court ultimately resolved the matter by ruling ventilatory support could be discontinued. To everyone's surprise, Quinlan continued to breathe unaided for another nine years. Nonetheless, the Quinlan ruling established a precedent permitting the withdrawal of potentially life-sustaining treatments from patients in a PVS[23].

The Quinlan case notwithstanding, there is some debate about the degree of awareness and potential for recovery of patients in a PVS. We will not go into great depth regarding the research and work done on PVS but, as the following cases of Zongwu Jin in Alberta and Juan Torres in Ontario illustrate, prognosticating in such circumstances can be fraught with error.

Cases of Recovery: Zongwu Jin and Juan Torres

Zongwu Jin, a previously healthy 66-year-old man, fell late one night in September 2007, sustaining a traumatic brain injury. Brought to a large tertiary care hospital in Calgary, Alberta, his condition steadily worsened over the course of the next 10 days. Eventually lapsing into unconsciousness, he was transferred to the ICU, where he was placed on a ventilator[24].

After five days in the ICU without improvement, he was considered by the attending physicians to have little chance for recovery. If he did survive, they told the family, at best he would be in a persistent vegetative state. Initially his physicians recommended he be designated care status Level Three, meaning no further ICU care. Later they revised their prognosis, deciding Level Two care most appropriate. This meant Mr Jin would continue to be cared for in the ICU and provided with ventilatory support. In the event of a cardiac arrest, however, no aggressive resuscitative measures, such as CPR, would be undertaken.

Mr Jin's family, believing his situation not to be as dire as the physicians maintained, wanted CPR to be offered. In addition, although his son was making arrangements to travel to Calgary from overseas, he would likely not show up for three or four more days. The family wanted the physicians to do whatever possible to keep Mr Jin alive until he arrived.

When the ICU physicians insisted on maintaining the DNR order, the family engaged legal counsel and petitioned the court to grant an injunction and lift the DNR order. The matter was heard urgently one evening by Justice Sheilah Martin of the Alberta Court of Queen's Bench. Acknowledging the complex issues at play, she granted a temporary injunction to lift the DNR order until a full legal determination could be made. The Calgary Health Region announced its intention to appeal this decision.

However, neither the full legal determination nor the appeal was ever made. A few days after Justice Martin's decision, Mr Jin began a dramatic recovery. Within a few weeks he was talking, reading, and starting to walk again. He left the hospital under his own power a month later, leaving behind a large piece of humble pie.

The case of Juan Torres also emphasizes the perils of predicting outcome in patients in a PVS. Mr Torres, age 21, was found unconscious one morning by his mother, apparently having choked on vomit during the night. He was resuscitated and stabilized at a local hospital, and initially kept alive through ventilatory and nutritional support.

Eventually, the ventilator was discontinued as Mr Torres began breathing on his own, but the physicians caring for him felt he would remain in a PVS for the rest of his life as a result of anoxic brain injury. He was also assessed by an independent expert research team from the University of Western Ontario conducting research on PVS. Their findings concurred with the diagnosis of the treating physicians.

Three months after his initial injury, Mr Torres began making purposive movements. A short time later he began speaking and communicating rationally. He was able to tell his family and physicians about actual events he recalled during his so-called "vegetative" state. His recovery has continued. Although he has not regained the same level of function as his pre-injury state, Mr Torres lives at home, studies at a college, and plays music[25].

Both of these cases are not typical of patients in a PVS state. Most do poorly neurologically although they may be kept alive for years. However, in the end, there are two important messages from the Jin and Torres cases. First, medical prognostication is fallible. Adopting a humble attitude is always appropriate. And second, good communication, an open mind, and a non-confrontational approach are indispensable when dealing with such cases.

V. Unilateral Decisions Regarding Life-Sustaining Treatment

An important question is whether healthcare professionals have the authority to unilaterally withdraw or withhold life-sustaining treatments in severe cases, such as those of Mr Torres and Mr Jin. The answer is both complicated and controversial. There have been numerous legal decisions supporting both views. It is not an understatement to say that the matter remains unresolved.

Box 15.5

"The law makes clear that consent is a sufficient condition for the withdrawal or withholding of treatment. But is consent also a necessary condition? Whether a physician or hospital can legally withhold or withdraw potentially life-sustaining treatment without the consent of either the patient or the patient's substituted decision-maker, is currently under much debate."

Carter v Canada, 2012 [26]

At the heart of the issue is a fundamental conflict between medical personnel who believe continuing treatment is not just futile but actually degrading and harmful to the patient and the right of families and SDMs to make decisions they believe are most consistent with the values and beliefs of a loved one. The case of Hassan Rasouli exemplifies this dilemma well.

The case of Hassan Rasouli

After undergoing surgery for a benign brain tumour in 2010 in Toronto, Mr Hassan Rasouli, a 59-year-old engineer from Iran, developed meningitis and lapsed into a coma. Subsequent CAT scans and MRIs demonstrated significant injury to his brain. Initially felt to be in a PVS, he was subsequently diagnosed as being in a minimally conscious state. Regardless of the specific term for his impairment, since that time he has not demonstrated awareness, appeared conscious, made purposive movements, or communicated verbally—at least not to the healthcare professionals caring for him. At the writing of this book, he remains on a ventilator.

His physicians informed the family there was no hope of meaningful recovery after exhausting all appropriate treatments and recommended that withdrawing life-sustaining measures, such as the ventilator, and providing palliative care would be the most humane way to care for him. Mr Rasouli's wife, Dr Salasel, his SDM (who had been a pediatrician in Iran), refused to consent to the withdrawal of any life-sustaining measures, arguing this was not consistent with their religious beliefs and would not be what her husband would want.

After the medical team indicated that consent was not required for cessation of non-therapeutic measures, Dr Salasel applied for and received a court order to prevent the withdrawal of life-support for her husband without her consent. The issue was subsequently appealed through the Ontario Court system and eventually to the Supreme Court of Canada, which made its ruling three years after Mr Rasouli's tragic complication.

The issues in dispute in the case of Mr Rasouli at the Supreme Court were in large part specific to Ontario, which has its own consent legislation (*Health Care Consent Act 1996*) and its own quasi-judicial mechanism for resolving such issues, the Consent and Capacity Board (CCB). But some of the conclusions from *Rasouli* have implications for all jurisdictions. The questions before the Supreme Court were twofold:

1. Is a treatment that serves no therapeutic benefit really a "treatment"?
2. Does common law permit the discontinuation of life-sustaining treatment without consent from the patient or the SDM?[27]

Regarding the first question, the medical team made a somewhat technical argument that, under Ontario's *Health Care Consent Act (HCCA)*, treatment not serving any therapeutic benefit is not really treatment and therefore withdrawal or withholding of such treatment does not require consent from an SDM. The Supreme Court rejected this, pointing out that withdrawing treatment always involves some degree of therapeutic intervention. It serves a "health-related purpose" and so, even if it is just providing sedation when removing a patient from a ventilator, requires consent from the patient or their substitute decision-maker[28]. As the family would not consent to this or to palliative care, the provision of life-supporting care could not be stopped.

Regarding the second issue, the Supreme Court indicated that while the question of whether consent is required for the withdrawal of life-sustaining treatment remains unresolved, in the Rasouli case, there is already a statutory mechanism for resolving such issues: namely, by way of application to Ontario's Consent and Capacity Board (CCB). In this case, since the CCB had already ruled that Dr Salasel's consent was necessary, the issue was already resolved.

The net result in *Rasouli* is that consent from the SDM is required in Ontario to withdraw life-sustaining treatments, even if the providers believe their continued use is of no benefit to the patient. This is because consent must be sought for any treatment provided for a "health-related purpose" [29]. In jurisdictions where there is neither a Health Care Consent Act nor a CCB, the Supreme Court left this matter unresolved; future cases will have to be adjudicated by the courts [30]. It is possible there will never be an overarching common law resolution of this matter, as the unique details of each case must be considered when making a judgment.

By way of follow-up, Mr Rasouli was subsequently transferred from the ICU in late 2013 to another non-acute healthcare facility where he continues to reside [31].

Box 15.6

"The SCC found that life support was still 'treatment' under [Ontario's] HCCA even if it served no medical benefit as it had a 'health-related purpose' and that the patient [or their SDM] should have the right to determine when it should be withdrawn." [29]

Indecision in common law

We have already noted the courts have been split on the issue of whether physicians can unilaterally decide to withdraw life-sustaining treatments or whether consent from family or the SDM is necessary. Some rulings favour "consent required," some favour "no consent required," and others openly acknowledge that the "law is not settled."

The lack of clarity on the part of the legal system leaves healthcare providers not only in legal limbo, but in an ethical one as well. Healthcare providers may find themselves providing care they consider deeply harmful and unethical, but unavoidable because of legal uncertainty. The impact of this is not to be underestimated. In *Golubchuk*, the chief physician caring for Mr Golubchuk, an elderly Jewish man on indefinite life-support in an ICU, resigned his post in protest because he felt it was deeply immoral to continue the care the patient was receiving. In his letter of resignation, he wrote: "To inflict this kind of assault on him [Mr Golubchuk] without reasonable hope of benefit is an abomination . . . I can't do it" [39].

Box 15.7

The following outlines rulings on major cases in Canada. These lists are not exhaustive.

Rulings favouring "consent required":

1. *Rasouli v Sunnybrook Health Sciences Centre* (2013)
2. *Barbulov v Cirone* (2009)

Rulings favouring "no consent required":

1. *Child and Family Services of Central Manitoba v Lavellee et al* (1997)
2. *I.H. v (Re)* (2008)
3. *Children's Aid Society of Ottawa-Carleton v M.C.* (2008)

Injunctions/rulings indicating "law is not settled":

1. *Jin (next friend of) v Calgary Health Region* (2007)
2. *Golubchuk v Salvation Army Grace General Hospital* (2008)
3. *Sawatzky v Riverview Health Centre Inc.* (1998) [28,32–38]

Fortunately, there are very few end-of-life situations where common ground cannot be found between healthcare providers and the families of patients. When conflicts do arise, however, there are ways to address and resolve them without involving the courts. These are outlined in Box 15.8.

VI. Palliative Sedation

Any discussion about ethical issues at the end of life should also include recognition and discussion of the therapy known as palliative or terminal sedation. Continuous palliative sedation therapy (CPST), as it is now officially known, refers to a form of deep sedation, administered intentionally to a person during the final week or two of their life, with the goal of relieving refractory symptoms and intolerable suffering [40]. While CPST does not cause death, it always ends in death. It is to be distinguished from any form of assisted dying by the fact that the goal of treatment is to relieve symptoms, not cause death.

There is considerable debate and controversy as to whether CPST actually shortens the life of a patient or simply controls symptoms while the disease runs its course. It is hard to deny that, in some circumstances, it may potentially shorten a patient's life. From an ethical point of view, however, this does not seem

---

Box 15.8

Five ways to prevent and resolve conflicts over end-of-life care:

1. Communicate honestly and frequently with family; be frank but avoid abruptness and paternalism.
2. Involve support services, including pastoral care, social work, ethics review, and counselling services.
3. If religious views play a role in the conflict, attempt to understand the perspective and consider discussion with religious authorities.
4. Make the medical record available to the family and encourage them to obtain a second opinion.
5. Offer to have the chart reviewed independently by physicians un-involved in the patient's care. [30]

---

terribly problematic. Given that the primary intention is to try to control intoler-able suffering, even if this does on occasion result in shortening of life, one might simply regard this as a risk of the intervention. In this regard, it is analogous to other interventions in medicine with known associated risks. For example, for some types of open-heart surgery, the risk of death might be three to five percent. Most patients accept this risk, as the alternative option (that is, living with debili-tating heart disease) may be intolerable or much riskier.

In the case of CPST, although the risk of shortening life may be significant, given the degree of suffering, it is a risk some people are willing to accept. Sup-porting this view is the acknowledgement by the Supreme Court in *Carter* that "[s]ince *Rodriguez*, it has been clear that potentially life-shortening symptom relief is permissible where the physician's intention is to ease pain." This is commonly known as the doctrine of "double effect" [41].

Box 15.9

"The administration of drugs designed for pain control in dosages which the physician knows will hasten death constitutes active contribution to death by any standard. However, the distinction drawn here is one based upon intention—in the case of palliative care the intention is to ease pain, which has the effect of hastening death, while in the case of assisted suicide, the intention is undeniably to cause death."

Rodriguez v British Columbia, 1993 [2]

Conclusion

In many areas of medicine, such as reproductive and genetic technologies, it is primarily advances in technology that give rise to bioethical dilemmas and help shape our attitudes and beliefs. In the case of ethical issues at the end of life, while technology clearly plays a role in keeping people alive for longer and longer, the issues of refusing, withholding, or withdrawing life-sustaining treatments appear more timeless. Regardless of the technologies we employ, decisions about end-of-life care will always remain central to issues of autonomy and self-determination. Nowhere in medicine is this more relevant than in the domain of medically assisted dying, which represents in many ways the centrality of autonomy in bioethics and patient care. Societal attitudes towards assisted dying have undergone significant changes in the past quarter century. We address this timely topic in the next chapter.

Cases for Discussion

Case 1: A Slow Recovery

Mr Z, a 75-year-old widowed and retired lawyer, has planned meticulously for his care at the end of life. He has recently undergone open-heart surgery to repair his mitral valve. He has been in the Cardiovascular ICU for one week, on mechanical ventilation, making a very slow, but steady recovery. His advance directive specifies his oldest son as his substitute decision-maker. Of the many wishes he specifies in this document is one indicating he would not want to continue aggressive care if dependent on a ventilator for more than a week. His son asks the physicians, given Mr Z's advance directive, to discontinue mechanical ventilation and see how he does. He says his father would not want to continue living like this.

Questions for Discussion
1. What should his doctors do?
2. Should they honour the explicit request in his advance directive?

Case 2: A Painful Decision

Ms W, a tiny but feisty 91-year-old, comes to hospital with a history of severe back pain and difficulty breathing of a week's duration. Initially the team thinks she may have pneumonia, but it turns out to be right-sided heart failure. Treatment options are limited— she needs a longer course of hospitalization than initially expected. She has a large family and many friends who come to visit. Bright as a pin, her social interactions are "well-preserved." On admission to the ward, Ms W agrees to a level of care that would not include CPR or aggressive resuscitative interventions, but has otherwise not completed an advance directive. Her back pain was a red herring—it had nothing to do with her heart failure. Ms W has very severe degenerative spinal arthritis for which she is prescribed a low dose narcotic.

Two days after admission, Ms W is accidentally given a much larger dose of the prescribed narcotic. She lapses into a comatose state with very shallow breathing and is in danger of acute respiratory failure and cardiac arrest.

Questions for Discussion

1. Should CPR be performed on this patient despite the No CPR order? Should any resuscitative efforts be attempted?
2. Should age be a factor in deciding to perform CPR?

Medical Assistance in Dying

The Triumph of Autonomy

A country like Canada could not, without violating its social traditions and history, tolerate and give a legal veneer to a policy of active euthanasia, not even voluntary euthanasia.

Report of Law Reform Commission of Canada on Euthanasia,
Aiding Suicide and Cessation of Treatment, 1983[1]

If I cannot give consent to my own death, whose body is this? Who owns my life?

Sue Rodriguez[2]

Over the past 50 years, public opinion in favour of legal medically assisted dying has been steadily increasing in Canada, the United States, and Europe[3]. Recent surveys on public attitudes in Canada have shown that more than two-thirds of the population support the right for individuals to choose an assisted death[4-6]. There are likely several factors that have influenced this shift, including the impact of an aging population, the ongoing secularization of society, advances in medicine which have led to prolonged lingering at the end of life, and an increasingly strong commitment to individual autonomy and self-determination[7]. There are still many vociferous and articulate critics of legalized assisted dying. Their arguments tend to be based on the risks of slippery slopes and the inviolability of human life within the rule of law[8-10]. In the final analysis, however, it appears the general public's desire, at least in a Canadian context, has triumphed. The questions now being addressed are no longer whether physician-assisted dying should be permitted, but rather under what circumstances it should be allowed and how appropriate safeguards can be put in place to protect vulnerable persons.

Case 16.1   An End Foretold

Born and bred in Newfoundland and possessing a wry sense of humour, Ms C is the picture of health when she is diagnosed at age 65 with widely metastatic gallbladder cancer. This uncommon cancer rarely responds to chemotherapy and is often fatal within six to 12 months. After some ineffective chemo that makes her miserable, Ms C accepts her fate with grace.

Told of her prognosis, she quips, "Well, I want to enjoy what time I have left on this earth. But when I have to go, make it quick! No point in hanging on."

What Ms C does not anticipate, however, is how this cancer takes control of her life. A few months after the surgery and chemo, she develops numerous openings in her abdominal wall, which start draining feces. No matter how much the nurses attempt to control the drainage, they cannot contain the leaking stool, nor the foul odour of rotting flesh. Ms C's life becomes intolerable.

Increasingly despondent, she finally begs her palliative care physician, Dr E, "Surely to God, you can do something about this, Doc. Enough is enough. I mean, come on, what are we waiting for?"

How should Dr E respond to Ms C?
What options are available to Dr E—and to Ms C?

Discussion of Case 16.1

This request represents an opportunity for Dr E to discuss with Ms C various options to help control her symptoms. Medications to decrease intestinal secretions, in conjunction with nurses who have greater expertise in managing complex abdominal drainage, might be able to mitigate the symptoms related to her abdominal wall. Aggressive attempts to control her pain, including the option of "palliative sedation" (see Chapter 15), could also be explored.

In this situation, it would also be appropriate for Dr E to broach the topic of a medically assisted death. While this may not be something Ms C would want, it is now a legal option in Canada and she has a right to be informed

continued

about it. All provinces have their own protocols for medically assisted death and provide comprehensive resources (online and elsewhere) to educate and inform patients and families exploring this topic. Even though a significant number of people who inquire about assisted dying do not ultimately opt for it, the process of exploring this option can be instructive and therapeutic for many patients and their families. Many patients express the sentiment that just knowing they have control provides comfort [11–13].

I. Assisted Death: Terminology and Other Jurisdictions

In the past, medically assisted death has been referred to by many terms: "assisted suicide," "physician-assisted dying," "physician-accelerated death," "aid in dying," and "voluntary euthanasia." However, Canadian federal legislation passed in 2016, Bill C-14 [14], has subsumed all these terms into one designation: medical assistance in dying (MAID). We will use the term MAID to discuss any form of legal assistance to accelerate death in Canada.

Box 16.1

MAID refers to one of two scenarios:

1. With the consent of a competent patient, a physician or nurse practitioner administers one or more substances to the patient, causing the patient's death.
2. With the consent of a competent patient, a physician or nurse practitioner provides a prescription for substances or provides such substances, which a patient can self-administer to cause their own death.

A note about the term "euthanasia"

The term "euthanasia" derives from Greek, meaning a "good death," traditionally construed as the intentional killing of a person (or animal) to end their suffering—so-called "mercy killing." When used in the setting of medically assisted dying it is sometimes sub-defined as voluntary, involuntary, or non-voluntary. Voluntary euthanasia refers to a competent individual voluntarily consenting to ending their life, as in the case of MAID. Involuntary and non-voluntary euthanasia refer to situations where a person's life is ended either against their wishes or without their knowledge, respectively[15]. These latter two scenarios are illegal in Canada and the United States, and considered a form of homicide, although this is not the case in some European countries.

In the United States, the terms "euthanasia" and "physician-assisted suicide" are frequently used to describe different scenarios. "Euthanasia" refers to a physician administering the lethal drugs (MAID scenario 1 above). "Physician-assisted suicide" refers to a patient self-administering the lethal drugs (MAID scenario 2 above). This distinction is based in part on legal precedents derived from the actions of Dr Jack Kevorkian, a well-known and controversial American crusader for assisted dying who aided over 130 people in committing suicide in the 1990s. He was charged and tried numerous times over this period, but was never convicted of a crime until 1999, after a recording showing him actively administering lethal substances to a patient aired on the American television program, *60 Minutes*. This resulted in a conviction for second-degree murder and a significant penal sentence. In 2007, suffering from hepatitis C, he was paroled, and died in 2011.

Kevorkian's crusade on behalf of the right for assisted dying had a great many short-comings, not the least of which were the absence of appropriate safeguards, oversight, and quality control. There is evidence several of those whose suicide he assisted did not suffer from lethal diseases or even serious medical conditions[16]. However, his actions did generate discussion about the right to control how we die and likely influenced the legalization of assisted suicide in some states.

In all US jurisdictions where assisted dying is presently permitted, it is legal only if lethal drugs are self-administered by the patient (that is, physician-assisted suicide). It continues to be considered homicide if a physician administers the medications. In states where assisted suicide is permitted, no Kevorkian-like "suicide device" is involved. Instead, after physicians have ensured that eligibility criteria and safeguards have been met, they write a prescription for lethal doses of specific medications (usually secobarbital) with the express purpose of causing death, and which can be self-administered only by the patient (that is, not family) at a time of the patient's choosing[17].

Assisted dying in various jurisdictions

The first country to permit assisted dying was Switzerland, which decriminalized it in 1942. Other European countries, such as Belgium, the Netherlands, and Luxembourg followed suit in the 1990s and 2000s. In the United States, there is no federal law permitting assisted dying, but several states (Oregon, Washington, California, Montana, Colorado, Vermont, and the District of Columbia) have legalized it in some form over the past 20 years. Most recently, Colombia (2015) and Canada (2016) have created legislation to permit assisted dying[18, 19].

There is considerable variation in approaches to assisted dying in different jurisdictions. In Switzerland, for example, it is legal only if the patient self-administers the medications (similar to the United States). In Belgium, the Netherlands, and Luxembourg, it may be either self- or physician-administered. Belgium and the Netherlands permit assisted death of infants with terminal diseases (so-called non-voluntary euthanasia), but only under very strict controls.

The eligibility criteria and safeguards also differ considerably from country to country. For example, in Belgium, there is no minimal age criterion, whereas in most other countries, a patient must be at least 18 years old. Most jurisdictions require a person undergoing an assisted death to be a resident of that jurisdiction. Switzerland is an exception, allowing persons travelling from elsewhere to undergo an assisted death, as long as they meet the Swiss eligibility criteria. There are a great many other variations in the way different jurisdictions deal with assisted dying[3].

II. Medically Assisted Death in Canada: A Brief History

The forerunner of MAID in Canada: Sue Rodriguez

In 1991, at the age of 42, Sue Rodriguez was diagnosed with amyotrophic lateral sclerosis (ALS), a motor neuron disease causing progressive muscular paralysis and respiratory failure. As she approached the later stages of her disease and became increasingly incapacitated, she found herself no longer able to fully care for herself. She sought help to be able to end her life with the assistance of a qualified physician—at a future time when she no longer wanted to continue living. Although suicide had been decriminalized in 1972, assisting or counselling (that is, aiding and abetting) someone to commit suicide was still a crime as per section 241(b) of the Criminal Code. Rodriguez, through a series of court challenges, pursued the issue all the way to the Supreme Court of Canada, where she argued that the prohibition against assisted dying contravened her rights under sections 7, 12, and 15 of the Canadian Charter of Rights and Freedoms.

The Court ruled against her by a slim majority of judges (five to four), maintaining section 241(b) did not contravene her Charter rights. While many of the justices were sympathetic to Rodriguez's argument, the majority also expressed concern there was no way to safeguard vulnerable persons in matters of assisted death[20].

Despite the Court's decision, four months later, Rodriguez, with the aid of an anonymous physician, ended her life by ingesting lethal amounts of sedatives. Although an investigation was carried out, no charges were ever laid[21].

Quebec: *An Act Respecting End-of-life Care*

In response to increasing interest and concern about assisted death, the province of Quebec in 2009 went its own way and set up a select committee to study the topic of "dying with dignity." The commission's 2012 report outlined a series of recommendations for improving end-of-life care in Quebec and a process whereby an individual can obtain a medically assisted death [22]. In response to the report, Bill 52, *An Act Respecting End of Life Care*, was put before the Quebec National Assembly and passed in June 2014 [23]. This bill provided a comprehensive and integrated approach to end-of-life care in that province, including the right of patients to receive high-quality palliative care and, if desired, medical assistance in dying.

The march towards MAID: Gloria Taylor and Kay Carter

At the same time Quebec was studying the topic of assisted dying, the cases of Kay Carter and Gloria Taylor were disrupting the status quo in the rest of Canada. Carter, an 89-year-old woman living in a nursing home in Vancouver, British Columbia, suffered from degenerative spinal stenosis. As she became increasingly incapacitated, unable to walk, eat, or care for herself, and in unrelenting pain, she expressed to her seven children a desire to be able to end her life. Because this was illegal at the time in Canada, Carter and some of her family travelled to the Dignitas Clinic, in Zurich, Switzerland, where, in January 2010, she self-administered a lethal amount of barbiturates, dying a short time later. The procedure was legal and carefully regulated by Swiss law. The entire process, including mandatory Swiss medical examinations, fees, paper work, cremation, and travel for both Carter and several members of her family, cost approximately $35,000 CAD [24].

After her death, Carter's children, with the assistance of the British Columbia Civil Liberties Association (BCCLA), filed a lawsuit in British Columbia, challenging the prohibition of assisted dying in Canada on the same grounds as Sue Rodriguez twenty-two years earlier.

Shortly thereafter, they were joined in the lawsuit by Gloria Taylor, a 63-year-old woman also from British Columbia, who had been diagnosed with ALS in 2009 at the age of 61. Taylor had always believed an individual should be able to control how they die. As her disease progressed, she joined the BCCLA lawsuit challenging the ban on assisted dying, becoming the lead plaintiff.

The arguments for this case were heard by the British Columbia Supreme Court in late 2011. Six months later, in June 2012, Justice Lynn Smith released a comprehensive 398-page decision, in which she ruled that the Criminal Code prohibition of assisted dying (section 241[b]) *did* contravene the rights of citizens under sections 7 and 15 of the Charter. As well, she declared the section invalid and unconstitutional. However, she suspended her judgment for a year, in order to permit the federal government time to remedy the matter. She also granted Gloria

Taylor a constitutional exemption from the law, making her the first person in Canada to win the right to die with the assistance of a physician[25]. Taylor never needed to exercise this right, as she died suddenly in the fall of 2012, about three months after the ruling, from complications of a perforated bowel[26].

Carter v Canada

The decision by Justice Smith was subsequently overturned by the British Columbia Court of Appeal on the grounds of *stare decisis*—the lower court did not have the authority to overturn the precedent set by the Supreme Court of Canada in the Rodriguez decision. The BCCLA subsequently filed leave to appeal to the Supreme Court of Canada. In 2014 the Court agreed to hear the case.

A year later, the Supreme Court ruled unanimously that the prohibition of assisted dying in section 241(b) of the Criminal Code violated section 7 of the Charter. Similar to the British Columbia ruling, the Supreme Court gave the federal government just over a year to remedy the Criminal Code before the unconstitutionality of section 241(b) would come into effect and the law no longer apply.

Box 16.2

"It is a crime in Canada to assist another person in ending her own life. As a result, people who are grievously and irremediably ill cannot seek a physician's assistance in dying and may be condemned to a life of severe and intolerable suffering. A person facing this prospect has two options: she can take her own life prematurely, often by violent or dangerous means, or she can suffer until she dies from natural causes. The choice is cruel."

Carter v Canada, 2015[27]

III. Legislating Medical Assistance in Dying: Bill C-14

In response to the *Carter* decision, the federal government introduced Bill-C14[14], which amended the Criminal Code and other Acts to permit Medical Assistance in Dying (MAID).

Bill C-14 permits both physicians and nurse practitioners to carry out MAID. In addition, while the legislation does not disaffirm the prohibition for aiding and abetting suicide in Canada, it acknowledges that numerous individuals, including family, friends, psychologists, social workers, nurses, and pharmacists may play a role in both the decision and provision of MAID. These people are protected from prosecution.

The bill established general inclusion criteria and safeguards for MAID. However, because the provision of healthcare is primarily a provincial matter in Canada, it left the detailed mechanisms by which MAID would be implemented and performed to the provinces.

Box 16.3

Federal eligibility requirements for MAID require an individual to

- be eligible for publicly funded health services in Canada;
- be 18 years of age and capable of making decisions about their health;
- have a grievous and irremediable medical condition;
- make a voluntary request for MAID that was not made as a result of external pressure; and
- provide informed consent for MAID after having been informed of various means available to relieve their suffering, including palliative care. [14]

The legislation also stipulates the criteria for a person suffering from a "grievous and irremediable medical condition":

- they have a serious and incurable illness, disease or disability;
- they are in an advanced state of irreversible decline in capability;
- that illness, disease or disability or that state of decline causes them enduring physical or psychological suffering that is intolerable to them and that cannot be relieved under conditions that they consider acceptable; and
- their natural death has become reasonably foreseeable, taking into account all of their medical circumstances, without a prognosis necessarily having been made as to the specific length of time that they have remaining. [14]

Recognizing that there will always be some ambiguity in the interpretation of such terms as "reasonably foreseeable" and "enduring physical or psychological suffering," the legislation provides a framework for permitting individuals to seek assistance in dying under fairly strict conditions. In addition to specifying inclusion criteria for MAID, the legislation also specifies a number of procedural safeguards to protect vulnerable persons and prevent abuse of the procedure.

Box 16.4

MAID safeguards require a physician or nurse practitioner to

- be of the opinion that the person meets all inclusion criteria;
- ensure the request is made in writing and is signed and dated by the person after they have been informed of their grievous and irremediable medical condition;
- ensure the request is witnessed by two independent witnesses;
- ensure an independent second physician or nurse practitioner confirms the eligibility of the request;
- ensure there is a 10-day waiting period between the signed request and the day MAID is actually provided (unless death or loss of capacity is imminent and the patient may not be able to tolerate the wait);
- ensure the person is given an opportunity to withdraw their request and also reconfirm their express consent immediately before providing MAID; and
- ensure that all necessary measures are taken to assist persons who have difficulty understanding the information or communicating their decision. [14]

Finally, Bill C-14 also includes a number of monitoring and review stipulations, ensuring that there is ongoing oversight on a national level. For example, provinces must establish mechanisms for keeping detailed statistics about MAID and monitor its provision on a regular basis. There is also a requirement for a formal parliamentary review of the provisions of the Act five years after its enactment.

IV. MAID: Minors, Advance Requests, and Mental Illness

Canadian legislators also acknowledged three exceptional situations under which MAID is considered particularly controversial, and which would require further study before they could be considered in future iterations of the legislation: requests by mature minors, advance requests, and requests by those with mental illness as the sole underlying medical condition. Although these reviews were still ongoing at the time of writing this section, they warrant a brief discussion here.

Requests by mature minors for MAID

Case 16.2 A Minor Problem

William was 12 years old when he was first diagnosed with osteosarcoma of his right thigh. He underwent state-of-the-art chemotherapy and surgery with good effect. Unfortunately, a year after he completed his treatment, the cancer recurred in his lungs, brain, and spine. Despite experimental chemotherapy, the cancer progressed and led to partial paralysis below his waist. Having exhausted all curative treatments, his oncology team suggested he pursue a palliative approach at that point.

Now, after three tumultuous years, William and his parents have come to accept he is going to die from the cancer. Although his symptoms are reasonably well-controlled at present, he tells his physicians and his parents that when he is no longer able to tolerate the pain, he would like to be put out of his misery. William is a thoughtful, self-possessed, and articulate 15-year-old. He not only meets the criteria to be designated a mature minor, but shows more wisdom, insight, and maturity than many adults. Although grateful for everything that has been done for him, he would like assurance he can have some control over the timing of his death.

Should William have access to MAID?

The "mature minor" doctrine acknowledges that some persons under the age of majority (that is, 18 years of age in most jurisdictions) may possess the capacity and maturity to understand and appreciate the nature, risks, benefits, and foreseeable consequences of a proposed medical intervention. In such situations, their autonomy should be respected and they are permitted, in most jurisdictions, to make appropriate decisions about medical care[28]. When this involves MAID, however, the question is whether a decision to end one's life is ever "appropriate" for a mature minor to make.

The issues facing mature minors and MAID are very similar to those facing mature minors and refusal of life-sustaining care. The courts have given mixed messages with regard to the latter: sometimes siding with the right of the minor to refuse such care and sometimes superseding this right (see Chapter 8).

In a 2016 survey conducted by the Canadian Paediatrics Society, 11 per cent of the 1050 respondent pediatricians reported having had MAID-related discussions with parents and/or patients over the previous year. Just over 4 per cent of all participants recalled parents making an explicit request for MAID; among these, two-thirds actually dealt with children under the age of one year. In another Canadian Paediatrics Society survey, of the 29 per cent of pediatricians who responded, 46 per cent favoured permitting MAID for mature minors experiencing progressive or terminal illness or intractable pain, while 33 per cent indicated this should not be available to mature minors under any circumstances.

Currently, the Netherlands and Belgium are the only two countries in the world permitting MAID for minors. In the Netherlands, minor children aged 12 to 15 may request and receive MAID, but only if their parents agree. Children aged 16 to 17, on the other hand, may receive MAID without parental consent, but their parents must be consulted and participate in the decision-making process. Needless to say, in order to be accepted, any such request must also meet the Dutch eligibility criteria for MAID [29]. Belgium introduced its assisted dying law in 2002, allowing children 16 years of age or older to seek an assisted death, as long as they demonstrated appropriate maturity. In 2014, the law was amended to permit any child, regardless of age, to make a request for assisted death, as long as it meets certain strict requirements: it must be made in writing and include an assessment from psychologists or psychiatrists as well as parental consent [30]. Since this change in the law, a nine-year-old child with a brain tumour and an 11-year-old child with cystic fibrosis have undergone assisted deaths in Belgium [31, 32].

As we saw in the discussion of mature minors and refusal of life-sustaining treatments (see Chapter 15), the issues are multifaceted and complex. Ultimately, the decision as to whether to allow mature minors access to MAID will be determined by the opinions of society as a whole, as well as by the views of affected minors, their parents, bereaved parents of children who have already died, and healthcare professionals who care for such children. If the trend towards recognizing the autonomy and self-determination of youth in Canada is any indication, it is very likely that access to MAID by mature minors will be permitted in future amendments to the legislation.

Discussion of Case 16.2

As of the writing of this book, providing William with an assisted death is not yet legal in Canada. Certainly, there is a great deal that palliative care can do to help him, if and when his symptoms worsen. But sometimes symptoms just cannot be adequately palliated.

If this were simply a matter of William refusing life-sustaining care, there would likely not be much opposition, given his maturity and insight. Indeed, there might also not be much resistance if he requested palliative sedation to relieve his symptoms. But for many, an assisted death is a different matter. Undoubtedly, there will be vigorous debate as to why a mature 15-year-old cannot choose MAID, while an immature 18-year-old can. Assuming appropriate safeguards are created, it is our opinion a mature minor like William should be permitted to choose an assisted death.

Future challenges of MAID for persons under age 18 will likely go beyond requests by only mature minors. As we deepen the discussion around assisted dying, questions will undoubtedly arise as to whether those who will never achieve competency should be considered for assisted death. This might include neonates, infants, or older incapable children with terminal or profound disabilities who appear to be suffering extraordinarily. As difficult and controversial as these matters are, they are real and cannot be ignored.

Advance requests for MAID

Case 16.3   Advance Notice

Dr D is a physically healthy 65-year-old retired spinal surgeon who lives with his spouse in Toronto. In the past few years, both he and his wife have noted issues with his memory. He not infrequently forgets people they have met recently, discussions they have had, and movies they have seen together. After seeing some specialists in cognitive assessment, he is diagnosed with early dementia of the Alzheimer's type. Although he still functions very well, enjoys life, and continues to manage his own finances and healthcare issues, Dr D has strong recollections of how his mother with advanced dementia lived her final years. He can picture her still, just sitting around all day in the nursing home, incontinent, blankly watching television, and unable to recognize even her family.

This is not how Dr D wants to spend the last years of his life. After much thought and consideration, he and his wife draft a meticulously worded advance directive expressing his wish to have a medically assisted death, if his dementia reaches the point where he no longer recognizes his children.

Can his request be honoured?

The prospect of being able to make an advance request for MAID would seem commonsensical, given the other precedents that exist already for stipulating how a person wishes to be cared for when they no longer have capacity (for example, *Malette v Shulman* in Chapter 4 and *Fleming v Reid and Gallagher* in Chapter 8) [33, 34]. Nowadays it is commonplace for patients to have advance directives specifying how they wish to be cared for in the event of a catastrophic illness with little chance for meaningful recovery.

However, because informed consent must be reconfirmed just prior to the provision of MAID, Canadian legislation is not compatible with advance care directives requesting MAID, at least not if the person is suffering from a form of cognitive decline such as dementia. This state of affairs, however, was not an oversight. In contrast to advance requests for refusing future care, advance requests for MAID pose numerous challenges.

Given the gravity of the decision, it is appropriate for legislators to require informed consent as part of the MAID process. As with any treatment decision, a patient must be informed about risks, benefits, and alternatives, including other means to relieve suffering, such as palliative care. Since most advance directives are generated by lawyers, this sort of healthcare information is not generally part of the process. Even if a healthcare expert were to be present during the drafting of an advance directive, it would be impossible to provide meaningful information about alternatives for relieving a patient's suffering, without knowing the specifics of their condition. The possibilities of future illnesses are often far too complex and protean to be determined in advance. Advance directives address broad "hypotheticals" of future illness, and can only provide general "wishes that must be interpreted and incorporated into the decision-making process by substitute decision-makers" [35] (see Chapter 15).

When it comes specifically to advance directives for MAID in dementia, the challenges are even greater. Dementia exists on a spectrum. Cognitive impairment may also wax and wane, depending on circumstances, time of day, medications, and general health issues. Determining precisely when dementia has reached the critical point to initiate MAID is not a simple matter. Would the threshold be reached when they can no longer manage their own finances? When they can no longer carry out basic activities of daily living? When they no longer recognize their spouse or family? What if they recognize some family members, but not others? Or only sometimes? It might be relatively easy to make these decisions for someone in a persistent vegetative state, but if someone's dementia is gradually worsening, it can be very difficult to know when the line has been crossed.

Other questions arise when considering MAID for dementia. Breslin argues that many patients with dementia still have a reasonable quality of life and can derive significant pleasure from their activities. He asks: "[s]hould their wish to die be acted upon out of respect for their former capable wishes or should their current best interests take priority?" [35]. That they may appear perfectly content in their existence and not display any obvious physical or psychological suffering implies they would not meet the MAID criteria for intolerable suffering. Finally, Breslin also points out that up until 2010, even in the one jurisdiction where advance requests for MAID are permitted (the Netherlands), there has never been a reported case of assisted death exclusively for advanced dementia[36]. Nevertheless, somewhere along the inexorable decline, relatives may say the person with dementia has lived far longer than they would have wanted to—their personhood and capability for personhood are extinguished. But who can say with certainty when that point is reached?

It has been suggested that clinicians and patients should focus on nutrition as an indicator for when dementia has reached its final stages. Loss of interest in food is a hallmark of advanced dementia and may serve as an appropriate time to limit nutritional intake in concordance with a patient's prior wish not to be kept alive when their cognitive impairment has reached a critical state[37].

Although these obstacles to advance requests for MAID are not necessarily insurmountable, they illustrate just how complex and challenging the issue is. Nonetheless, it warrants serious consideration—otherwise some patients may opt to prematurely end their lives for fear they might not be competent to make a decision about MAID at a later date. Although some have argued that requests for assisted death in advance directives will never be feasible[38], work is currently being done in Canada and other jurisdictions to come up with acceptable legal and ethical frameworks for this[39]. Because of the finality of MAID and the need to protect vulnerable persons, there will always be practical and ethical challenges to getting the balance right.

Discussion of Case 16.3

Dr D's request for MAID when no longer competent cannot be honoured under Canadian law at this time. The law very clearly specifies a person making such a request must not only be capable of providing informed consent when making the request, but must also be capable of confirming this decision just prior to the provision of MAID. In this regard, MAID differs significantly from advance requests refusing future treatments.

As his cognitive symptoms worsen in the following months, seeing no other alternative, Dr D obtains a prescription for lethal amounts of sedatives. He opts to end his life before he loses the capacity to make this decision.

Box 16.5

"In some situations, such as AIDS and Huntington's disease, the courts have already accepted that the prospect of impending humiliation could qualify as unbearable and hopeless suffering."[40]

MAID for psychiatric illness

Case 16.4   A Depressing Condition

Mr S is a 45-year-old man, living alone, who has suffered from severe depression since the age of 15. He subsists on a disability pension, having been unable to work for more than a decade due to his unrelenting depression. He has several times attempted suicide but has always somehow survived. While he is not afraid of dying, he is afraid of the pain and violence involved in jumping out of a building or shooting himself. Despite consulting the best psychiatrists in the field and trying all forms of therapy, including innumerable types of antidepressant medications, psychotherapy, group therapy, ECT, and even experimental treatments, nothing has helped. His depression has become "treatment-resistant."

Mr S finds it impossible to interact with people, even his family. He cannot concentrate, read, or carry on discussions. He stays in bed most days and gets up only to eat. He feels hopeless and insignificant. His life is a constant torment. His sense of overwhelming hopelessness is so deep that the only thing providing any relief is the thought of being dead. His feelings in this regard have not changed for over five years. He desperately wants to die. In response to Bill C-14, he writes his psychiatrist, requesting help through a medically assisted death.

Should his psychiatrist arrange a consultation with a MAID team?

While the majority of Canadians support MAID for patients with grievous and irremediable physical conditions, such as advanced cancer and neurodegenerative disorders, most do not support it for patients suffering intolerably from psychiatric illness, such as treatment-resistant depression [41]. Although severe mental illness might be considered in many ways grievous and irremediable, and the associated suffering intolerable [41, 42], one important criterion of the Canadian legislation is not satisfied: namely that an individual's natural death must be reasonably foreseeable. Although the word "terminal" does not expressly appear in the MAID legislation, the requirement for the natural death of an individual to be reasonably foreseeable effectively limits MAID in Canada to terminal conditions—at least in a general sense. As we will see below in the case of *Lamb v Canada*, the requirement for a "reasonably foreseeable death" is already being challenged in the courts with regard to chronic physical illnesses. There is also little doubt it will eventually be challenged for chronic psychiatric illnesses.

In jurisdictions where assisted dying is permitted for psychiatric illness, such as the Netherlands and Belgium, it is nonetheless an infrequent indication for assisted dying, and its occurrence is strictly controlled and monitored for abuse. In Belgium, "unbearable mental suffering due to irreversible disease" (that is, psychiatric disease) was reported as the indication for an assisted death in 40 (3.5 per cent) of a total of all 1133 reported cases of assisted death in 2011 [43].

Advocates of MAID for patients with intractable and unrelenting psychiatric illness argue that prohibiting such patients from an assisted death condemns them to grievous and irremediable suffering without any recourse [44, 45]. It can be seen, in some ways, as discriminating against those with mental illness. Advocates also emphasize that while many persons with depression do achieve remission, almost 40 per cent have a chronic, relapsing course—and some patients never obtain any relief [44]. Vanderberghe and others have also argued that although the goal of treatment for much psychiatric disease is to help prevent patients from taking their own lives, there are some situations when suicide is a reasonable option—so-called "rational suicide" [45]. Ultimately, they point out, we can either opt to help such individuals end their lives humanely, or we can stand by while they frequently make violent and ineffectual attempts to kill themselves.

Miller and Appelbaum, on the other hand, make a number of compelling arguments against MAID for patients with exclusively psychiatric illness. Because of the distorted nature of their thinking, patients with psychiatric illness tend not to see their options objectively: "It is difficult, if not practically impossible, for clinicians to be reasonably certain that such a request is not related to the effects of the disorder" [46]. Moreover, they argue, it would undermine the physician–patient relationship, which assumes the inherent value of a patient's life. It would imply the physician agrees with the patient that their life is, indeed, hopeless and worthless.

It is also impossible for clinicians to be certain a psychiatric condition is truly irremediable. In cases of physical deterioration and suffering related to malignancies, it is relatively straightforward as to when we can conclude further curative treatment is futile. A body ravaged by cancer will not suddenly recover. With burgeoning research in psychiatric disease, however, it is very possible new developments could occur in the next few years, allowing patients to recover from their disease [46]. In addition, the majority of persons saved after a suicide attempt are ultimately grateful and never attempt suicide again [47]. Given that psychiatrists and other mental health professionals devote so much time and training to preventing suicide, sanctioning MAID for patients with mental illness does appear antithetical to much of their work. Along the same lines, MAID for psychiatric illness also appears to be inconsistent with the generally accepted public policy that physicians, police officers, and others are legally authorized to try to prevent people from committing suicide (see Case 9.5). That said, there is already a legal precedent from Alberta, in which an individual was permitted access to MAID on the basis of psychiatric illness alone [44, 48].

In summary, it does seem discordant to devote significant resources to suicide prevention for the mentally ill, while simultaneously sanctioning it through MAID. Advocates who argue vociferously to permit MAID for psychiatric illnesses, such as Vanderberghe, have pointed out that the safeguards in the Netherlands and Belgium are still deeply inadequate and they devote much of their arguments towards outlining safeguards to ensure that vulnerable psychiatric patients are not exploited or victimized[42]. But even if adequate safeguards are possible, is it worth the price? The debate will undoubtedly continue.

Discussion of Case 16.4

Mr S's story is sad and deeply disconcerting for most of us. While currently under review, at the present time assisted dying for psychiatric illness is not permitted under Canadian MAID legislation. Whether his psychiatrist should still refer him for a MAID consultation is a personal decision on the part of the psychiatrist. Mr S is not eligible, but going through the process may be partially therapeutic and reassure him as to why he is not eligible. It is very possible that at some point Mr S will succeed at taking his own life. Regardless of whether this occurs by his own hand or with the assistance of MAID in the future, it will be tragic.

Lamb v Canada: a reasonably foreseeable death

One of the more contentious aspects of the Canadian legislation permitting assisted death is the requirement that an individual's death be "reasonably foreseeable." It took only 10 days after passage of Bill C-14 for a challenge to this requirement to be mounted. The case of *Lamb v Canada*, like previous challenges dealing with assisted death, focuses on the constitutionality of the Criminal Code's restrictions under sections 7 and 15 of the Canadian Charter of Rights and Freedoms[49].

At the time the legal challenge was lodged in 2016, Julia Lamb was a 25-year-old woman with spinal muscular atrophy type II (SMA2). This rare genetically inherited neuromuscular disorder is characterized by progressive weakening and deterioration of voluntary muscles of the body. Julia Lamb has a severe form of the disease. In her Notice of Civil Claim, she explained she required the support of three aides to assist her with almost all her activities of daily living, even just turning over in bed.

With progression of her disease, she has developed severe pain from muscle and tendon contractures as well as severe osteoporosis. She is fearful she will eventually lose the ability to control her motorized wheelchair, use her computer, or even talk or express herself in any way—a situation which may go on for years and which she would deem intolerable. Yet, because this deterioration may occur very gradually and her death from natural causes may not be "reasonably fore-seeable," she is concerned she will not meet the eligibility requirement for MAID when she has reached a time of "enduring and intolerable suffering." For this reason, she has challenged the constitutionality of the "reasonably foreseeable death" requirement of this legislation [50]. Lamb and her legal counsel argue that many Canadians with chronic, progressive debilitating disorders, such as multiple sclerosis, spinal stenosis, locked-in syndrome, Parkinson's disease, and Huntington's disease, will not meet the eligibility requirements of the MAID legislation and thus experience "enduring and intolerable suffering." Ethically, however, requests for MAID based on degenerative neurological illnesses seem less troubling than requests based on psychiatric disease or those made in advance for dementia.

Whether in practice the "reasonably foreseeable death" requirement truly infringes on the individual's access to MAID remains to be determined. The term is vague and non-specific enough that it may well permit enough discretion to include people with chronic, non-terminal illnesses, if they are truly grievous and irremediable. This appears to have been the case in 2018, when a Toronto couple in their 90s underwent MAID together, although neither had a "terminal" illness per se [51].

V. MAID and Issues of Conscience

In its ruling in *Carter*, the Supreme Court was careful to specify that nothing in its decision would "compel physicians to provide assistance in dying." Referring to similar issues raised during decisions on abortion, it recognized that "a physician's decision to participate in assisted dying is a matter of conscience and, in some cases, of religious belief" [27]. These acknowledgements notwithstanding, the issues involved in conscientious objection regarding MAID may not be as simple as these declarations by the Supreme Court suggest. Some of the reasons for this include the following:

- There are many allied healthcare professionals, such as nurses, pharmacists, psychologists, and social workers, affected by MAID. Their right to conscientious objection must be respected.
- If MAID is truly comparable to abortion, conscientious objectors then have a duty to "effectively refer" or facilitate patient requests for MAID, even though they personally oppose it.
- As publicly funded institutions, there would seem to be an obligation for all healthcare facilities and hospitals to provide MAID. This would apply

not only to facilities with religious affiliations, but also to facilities such as hospices, which may be opposed to assisted dying for various non-religious reasons.

The conscience of physicians

Case 16.5 A Conscientious Objection

Dr G is a palliative care physician who manages patients in a hospice. While she is not religious, she has found the recent developments with regard to assisted dying very disconcerting. She has made it clear this is not something she would be willing to perform or facilitate. She does occasionally administer palliative sedation to patients, but sees that as fundamentally different from MAID, given that her goal with palliative sedation is to relieve symptoms, not accelerate death. Many of the nurses at the hospice share her reservations about MAID, although a few do support it.

One day, Mr Z, a patient with pancreatic cancer who has been under her care at the hospice for almost two months, tells her he is ready to "go." Although he has a partial bowel obstruction, suffers from unrelenting pain, and has become increasingly weak and tired, his death is not imminent. He might live for another three or four weeks. He tells Dr G he'd like to explore the option of MAID.

Given her opposition to MAID, what should Dr G do?

Although surveys of public attitudes in Canada and the United States over the past decades have consistently shown strong support for assisted dying (66 to 75 per cent in favour) [3-5], physician support over the same period has typically lagged behind that of the public. A 2013 survey by the Canadian Medical Association, with 2125 physicians responding, revealed that only 34 per cent of physicians felt assisted dying should probably or definitely be legal in Canada. Only 20 per cent indicated they would be willing to participate if it were legal. Another 42 per cent of physicians said they would refuse to participate. The fact that physicians in many countries tend to have a more guarded attitude than the public towards assisted dying has been demonstrated by numerous studies [3]. Although there is a great deal of heterogeneity in the methodology of such surveys, it appears that, on average, between 40 to 55 per cent of physicians in various developed countries (such as the United States, Europe, Australia) support assisted dying laws. The exceptions to this are the two European countries with the most experience in this matter, Belgium and the Netherlands, where physician support for assisted dying is over 80 per cent.

It should not be a surprise that physicians' enthusiasm for assisted dying is lower than the public's. There are several likely reasons for this:

1. Support for assisted dying exists more on a theoretical level for the public than it does for physicians. Physicians are on the front line and aware of the day-to-day challenges of what assisted dying means.
2. The concept of assisted dying is foreign to the culture of "curing and caring" in medicine. Most physicians will tell you they went into medicine to cure disease and relieve suffering. Intentionally ending someone's life seems antithetical to the basic mission of medicine for many physicians [52].
3. Many physicians believe that other end-of-life therapies, such as withdrawal of life-sustaining measures, proper opioid use, and palliative sedation provide sufficient ways to care for patients' suffering at the end of life.
4. Many physicians feel that the ready provision of MAID will undermine initiatives to improve palliative care [6, 52].

These reasons notwithstanding, physician attitudes towards MAID in Canada do appear to be changing significantly and catching up to attitudes among the general public. A survey by the College of Family Physicians of Canada carried out shortly after the *Carter* decision in 2015 revealed that 58 per cent of Canadian family physicians supported the Supreme Court's decision and that 65 per cent would be willing to help a competent, consenting, dying patient to end their life [53].

A duty to refer or a duty to cooperate?

While there is likely little disagreement that physicians and other allied healthcare professionals have a right to conscientious objection when it comes to the provision of MAID, there is controversy as to whether conscientious objectors have a duty to facilitate or to refer patients when met with a request for MAID. Depending on the licensing authority, the approach to this question will likely differ somewhat across Canada.

The College of Physicians and Surgeons of Ontario (CPSO), for example, requires physicians to make an "effective" referral if they decline to provide MAID for reasons of conscience. An "effective" referral is defined to be one made "in good faith, to a non-objecting, available, and accessible physician, nurse practitioner or agency" [54]. Some physicians feel that this makes them complicit in the process of MAID and have legally challenged the CPSO policy [55].

Several other organizations, including the College of Family Physicians of Canada, the Centre for Effective Practice, and the Canadian Medical Association, have outlined approaches for physicians who oppose MAID on grounds of conscience or religion. All these organizations also stipulate clinicians should not abandon their patients but continue to provide ongoing care separate from MAID [53, 56].

Discussion of Case 16.5

Within the MAID legislation, there is only a cursory reference to freedom of conscience and religion on the part of healthcare workers. While Dr G has no obligation to provide MAID, most would agree she does have an obligation to ensure Mr Z accesses the appropriate information and sees a healthcare provider who can educate and aid him in this matter. Even if she has strong moral opposition to MAID, Dr G has an equally strong obligation to respect Mr Z's autonomy.

A key aspect moving forward will be ensuring there is a space and mechanism for physicians like Dr G to opt out of MAID, while guaranteeing patients can access this option if they wish. Any facility dealing with end-of-life issues, especially hospices, will need to address how they will respect requests for MAID, while also providing moral space for those who do not wish to be a party to it.

The Conscientious Facility

The ability of healthcare facilities and institutions to opt out of participation in MAID on conscientious or religious grounds poses a slightly more complex situation. While it may be easy to arrange for another physician to attend to a patient requesting MAID, it is considerably more challenging to transfer a weak and frail patient to a facility that will provide them with the care they wish. Transferring patients from facilities, such as hospices, where they may have resided for some time and where they may have developed close relationships with staff, may represent a significant hardship to patients and their families as they navigate the final days of life [6].

While one might argue that publicly funded institutions, like hospitals and hospices, should be compelled to provide MAID as part of their public mandate, enforcing such a position is often not popular or practical. In the case of pregnancy termination, for example, 84 per cent of hospitals in Canada do not provide abortion services on the basis of religious or ethical grounds [57]. For this reason, the vast majority of therapeutic abortions take place in separate stand-alone clinics [58]. There are no simple solutions to these challenges. However, a few general concepts may minimize strife in such environments:

- Establish a policy of respect for everyone's views.
- Create a space for ensuring everyone has an opportunity to speak their mind.
- Establish a policy for how such facilities will address requests for MAID and accommodate the wishes of both staff and patients.

Conclusion

Few areas in society demonstrate the speed of changing ethical mores than approaches to assisted dying. The quotation from the 1983 Law Reform Commission Report, in which the authors argued that legalizing any form of assisted dying would violate the social conditions and history of Canada, illustrates just how much Canadian society has changed.

Assisted dying is still in its early stages in Canada. Like abortion, it will always generate some degree of controversy, and, like abortion, it is likely here to stay. There will also undoubtedly be unique challenges, such as addressing the impact of MAID on those who provide the service [59]. These issues will inevitably be resolved as we work through the challenges of implementation and MAID becomes more integrated into the medical system.

Cases for Discussion

Case 1: Nothing Minor About This

A few months after the birth of their third child, Robert and Helen, a young Jewish couple, are informed the baby has Tay-Sachs Disease and will likely not survive past age four or five. Over the next few years, as he is cared for by his parents, Noah becomes deaf and blind, develops extensive skeletal spasticity, requires a feeding tube, and experiences regular seizures, despite high doses of anti-epileptic medications. At age four, he is unable to engage with his parents at all, but continues to live, mostly because of tube feeding and compassionate care.

His parents approach the palliative care team to ask for help. They do not want to prolong Noah's misery, but are reluctant to discontinue the feedings,

continued

concerned he will suffer as a result of being starved and dehydrated to death. They request their son be put to death compassionately to end his suffering.

Questions for Discussion
1. Should Noah's parents' request to end his life be allowed?
2. What are the ethical issues in this case? The legal issues?

Case 2: Night Terrors

For five years you have been the physician caring for Ms Y, a 94-year-old woman, who lives alone with occasional assistance from social agencies. Although she has multiple medical problems causing great suffering (such as severe arthritis, fecal and urinary incontinence, and poor eyesight and hearing), she has no obvious condition which will lead to her foreseeable death. She continues to deteriorate slowly. During each of your visits to her home, she reiterates the same thing.

"I wish I were dead," she states. "Can't you just prescribe me something to help me get a good night's sleep? I hear barbiturates are good for that," she says, winking at you.

Questions for Discussion
1. Would it be wrong to prescribe Ms Y some barbiturates?
2. What if she intentionally starved herself, until her death was foreseeable? Would she then be eligible for MAID?

....

Nature and Culture

Of Genes and Memes

Cultures differ from one another, sometimes radically. The nagging question remains: What, if anything, follows from the facts of cultural relativity?

Ruth Macklin, 1999 [1]

"Every patient tells a story" [2], practitioners of modern healthcare are told. That story is the unique product of a patient's biology—their genetics—and of their culture, their memes. In this chapter we first examine the rise of genomics in healthcare, the discipline that crosses all cultures, and then we consider what culturally sensitive care might look like.

I. All in the Genome?

It is trivial to say that genetic knowledge is transforming medicine. Since the completion of the Human Genome Project (the complete sequencing of the human genome) in 2003, work on genomes and genomics has expanded exponentially.

Case 17.1 A CRISPR View

....

Daniel and Laura L have an eight-month-old son, Ryan, who has seemed a little floppy since birth. His doctor, having noted this as well but unable to determine the cause, refers the child to a local university-affiliated children's hospital. There, Ryan is diagnosed with Canavan disease, a rare disorder causing irreversible neurological decline due to a single mutation in a gene that codes for an essential brain enzyme. Absence of this enzyme leads to breakdown

continued

---

in the myelin sheath protecting nerve cells and subsequent irreversible brain atrophy. There is no treatment for the disease.

Ryan's parents are devastated by this news. Faced with the terrible prognosis, they search for alternatives for Ryan. They read on the Internet about a clinical trial of CRISPR, a revolutionary new way of treating genetic illness through genetic manipulation.

Ryan's parents are eager but wonder about the safety of a gene trial. Are they right to be concerned?

Box 17.1

"Genomic studies do not raise wholly new ethical issues, but they cast these issues [of biomedical research] in a fresh light." [3]

"Genome" is an amalgam of the words "gene" and "chromosome." The genome, be it of a cell, an individual, a group, a population, or a species, refers to all of the hereditary material of the individual, including nuclear and mitochondrial DNA (mtDNA). Medical care customized to individual patients and their genomes—"precision medicine"—takes some of the guesswork out of medicine [4]. The US National Institutes of Health have identified precision medicine as "an emerging approach for disease treatment and prevention that takes into account individual variability in environment, lifestyle and genes for each person" [5]. Precision medicine is personalized medicine.

But the path of personalized medicine is neither simple nor inexpensive. For example, research on small-cell lung cancer and on malignant melanoma, two of the commonest causes of death from cancer, has led to the development of drugs acting on the genes responsible for these malignancies' ability to grow. [6] These drugs, however, are dizzyingly expensive ($10,000 USD per month) and only marginally effective, extending life only by months [7]. At that cost, who will be able to afford them? Will the poor and the rich have equal access (see Chapter 13)? The hope may be that, in the long run, genomics will allow for more effective and cheaper drugs, but that is not the reality now. And it may never be.

Proceed with caution: CRISPR tools

Since the 1980s, scientists have been looking to change human DNA using the processes of gene or genome editing. In 2012, a more accurate and powerful technology using CRISPR (Clustered Regularly Interspaced Short Palindromic Repeats) and CRISPR-associated (Cas9) genes was introduced. The new technology allowed a more precise identification and replacement of defective segments of DNA causing illness[8].

These tools have the potential to help treat diseases with a genomic basis, such as Tay-Sachs, cystic fibrosis, and Canavan disease, by "disrupting endogenous disease-causing genes, correcting disease-causing mutations or inserting new genes with protective functions"[9].

The way forward, however, has been blocked by technical difficulties and regulatory challenges. There are three kinds of issues that must be addressed in order for the safety of CRISPR technology to be established[10].

1. Gene manipulation may expand in unpredictable ways. CRISPR/Cas9 are akin to molecular scissors that can identify and cut defective genes. They may not be precise enough, however, and could potential cause unexpected mutations in other cells. Changing a gene locus in one cell may lead to an unanticipated cascade of alterations in other cells. Cas9 may also misidentify the target cells. It is not known whether and how other tissues or organisms will be affected—so-called "off-target" changes.

2. CRISPR technology may alter an individual's germline genome, leading to genetic changes in subsequent generations. It is one thing to change the genes of a person's somatic cells, but it is an altogether different matter to alter the germline cells posing unknown risks to future generations. There are clearly unknown hazards if changes in the human genome are passed on to other species[9].

3. Just as worrisome is that some people may wish to use CRISPR for non-therapeutic or enhancement purposes[11]. It is one thing to want to have healthy children, free of heritable illness, but the spectre of parents seeking designer babies worries many people. There is the added concern that these technologies will only be available to the well-off, exacerbating social inequities. This could in turn lead a new form of eugenics (see Chapter 9) where certain people are discriminated against on account of unwanted traits.

While there is a diversity of views on the use of gene-altering technologies, most researchers would concede that there are serious risks of unintended consequences when altering a human genome. Regulating the field is uniquely challenging, because it is changing so rapidly and the risks cannot be quantified. The impact of altering an individual's or a species's genome with CRISPR technology is reminiscent of Mickey Mouse in *The Sorcerer's Apprentice*. Taking up the sorcerer's magic wand, Mickey is unable to control the forces he unleashes and is quickly overwhelmed by hordes of the sorcerer's avatars.

Discussion of Case 17.1

Given the lack of viable treatment alternatives and the seriousness of his condition, Ryan's parents would be justified in pursuing various treatment options. CRISPR technology may offer some prospect of hope. But, as with other
"orphan illnesses," finding a genuine and respected experimental trial may be
difficult indeed. It is certainly reasonable to pursue this as a treatment option
(see Chapter 18), but the parents need to be aware of the treatment's novelty
and its dangers.

Return of results

A tremendous gain in information about individuals and populations is provided
by genomic research. It has been argued that "the incorporation of genetic risk
markers into prevention science has the power to enrich preventive interventions,
such that researchers and practitioners can more efficiently and effectively target
those at greatest risk for disorder development" [12].

But with more knowledge here, too, comes more moral complexity.

For example, genetic researchers, while having one set of genetic objectives
in mind, may incidentally make other discoveries. While much of this information might be "noise," important genetic information may come to light—such
as mistaken diagnoses, misattributed parentage, or unexpected inheritable disorders. This information may have implications for the patient or other family
members. Do the researchers have a duty, a professional requirement, or simply
an allowance legally, to return these "secondary" results to the patient and other,
potentially affected, family members? Or should they be prohibited from disclosing such information [13]? Some have suggested that if there is a duty to disclose incidental findings, there is also a duty to search for them [12]—although,
as one researcher has sagely pointed out, if so, the findings would no longer be
incidental [14]! The American College of Genetics and Genomics has released a list
of 25 conditions for which it recommends testing be done when Whole Genome
Sequencing is being carried out for other clinical reasons. The focus is "on secondary findings related to monogenic disorders for which there is evidence of
clinical utility" [15].

There is a developing consensus that "valid, clinically significant, and actionable information"—"medical actionability" [16]—ought to be shared with a patient,
unless the patient has expressed a wish *not* to be informed [12].

> **Box 17.2**
>
> "Discovering an incidental finding can be lifesaving, but it also can lead to uncertainty and distress without any corresponding improvement in health or well-being."
>
> President's Commission on Bioethics, 2013 [17]

The standard utilitarian rationale for disclosure is this: inform patients if it might make a difference to their health. Of course, some patients will want to know about their condition even if they cannot do anything with that information. "Just so that I know," some patients will say (see Chapter 6). It is their health information and they have a "right to know." (This is the deontological view.) Others, however, will want to know only if something can be done in the way of disease treatment and amelioration.

But one concern in returning genetic testing results to a patient is that the researcher might be engendering a physician–patient relationship. This is similar to a radiologist unexpectedly discovering an X-ray finding with grave implications for a patient. Even if there is no prior personal physician–patient relationship, a radiologist may still have a duty of care to the patient. It may not be enough to write a report. Radiologists are expected in some locales to ensure that the ordering physician is made aware of any significant unexpected findings. They may, in some jurisdictions, even have a responsibility to directly communicate with patients themselves [18].

And then there is the issue of third parties, such as other family members, whose well-being may be affected by information released to the patient. One of the unique aspects of genetic testing is its potential impact on others who share a related genome. When carrying out genetic tests, you are never just testing one individual. Genetic testing may have ramifications for siblings, parents, and progeny, as the following case illustrates.

> **Case 17.2** All in the Family? [19]
>
> You are a primary care provider looking after a 24-year-old man, Mr M, who develops ataxia and paranoid ideation. Noticing unusual copper-tinged rings in his pupils, you make a diagnosis of Wilson's disease, a disease affecting
>
> *continued*

copper metabolism with protean manifestations that has genetic markers and is amenable to treatment [20]. After the diagnosis is confirmed through further biochemical and genetic testing, the patient is started on standard treatment.

Mr M has two siblings also in your practice. You advise him to disclose his diagnosis to his siblings, recognizing they each have a one-in-four risk of also having the disease. Mr M refuses to do this, saying he has never gotten along with his siblings and they can "rot in hell" as far as he's concerned.

Does the duty to prevent harm to others outweigh the duty to protect the confidences of Mr M?

Discussion of Case 17.2

The tension in this case exists because of conflicting duties: respect for confidentiality owed Mr M and beneficence owed to his siblings. Although the patient's wishes are clear, the possibility of serious harm to his siblings, if not informed of the risks, is also evident. In general, in a conflict between prevention of serious harm to others and preservation of privacy, beneficence should prevail. It would be unconscionable for a medical professional to allow serious, preventable harm to another person to occur simply on the basis of a blanket principle to protect another's right to privacy (see Chapter 7). Genetics raises the question: whose responsibility is it to warn the potentially affected family members?

A careful clinician—genetics advisor, nurse, social worker, or doctor— would spend time with Mr M in an attempt to understand the reasons for his decision. This is an unusual circumstance as most people notified about genetic risks are keen to warn relatives who may also be at risk. Is Mr M's desire to allow potential harm to befall his siblings a manifestation of a paranoid illness? Is it an extension of a resentment he has harboured for years? Are there deeper cultural differences at stake? Or is he just a nasty guy?

Whatever the reason for Mr M's attitude, the right thing to do is to warn his siblings. Clearly, the best outcome would be if he were to tell them himself. However, if you are also their healthcare provider, it would certainly be within your professional responsibilities to bring them in for an examination to look for evidence of Wilson's disease. Although it would be better to be upfront with them, you may wish to approach the matter a little circuitously in order not to explicitly breach your duty of confidentiality to Mr M. It might also be wise to seek legal counsel and advice from colleagues.

> ### Box 17.3
>
> "Persons who undergo genetic testing must be provided full information on the procedure and that they freely give their informed consent. Patients also have the right to be informed of the results or, if they so desire, the right not to be informed of them."
>
> *From the International Declaration on Human Genetic Data (October, 2003) and the Universal Declaration on Bioethics and Human Rights (2005)* [21]

Preventative ethics

The ethical dilemma in Case 17.2 might have been avoided if the informed consent requested prior to genetic testing had been more carefully obtained. The patient could have been warned in advance that if testing revealed a serious inheritable disease, others potentially affected must be informed. This is especially important for conditions like inherited breast cancer or familial colorectal cancers, where early detection may literally save the life of a patient.

Where practitioners are uncertain about what advice to give to an individual regarding their relatives, help should be sought from more experienced consultants. Although the information is derived from one individual, it has been suggested that this information should not be seen as theirs alone. Rather, it should be seen as part of a familial "joint account" that ought to be shared [22]. This seems reasonable enough as long as there are protections from scrutiny by those outside the family's circle such as employers or insurance companies.

In the era of genomic medicine, large "anonymized" genomic data banks and direct-to-consumer genomic testing can be used to identify specific individuals if they have a distinct genetic aberration or variant [23]. This may be done for some very good reasons: identifying at risk individuals or catching criminals [24]—or for bad reasons: limiting insurance coverage or job opportunities. Hence, non-traceability may be a relic of the past. As well, whole groups of people or communities may be identifiable by linkages established through genetic predispositions and genomic associations. One must be sensitive to local mores and local jurisprudence in this area. In many parts of the world there are few, if any, laws protecting privacy of genetic data. This does not give researchers free rein over such data [25].

Indigenous objection

In 2010, a settlement of $700,000 USD was levied against an American university for having allowed its researchers to study blood samples from an Indigenous community in Arizona for genetic purposes to which they had not consented[26]. Assuming their samples were being used for the study of diabetes, research subjects did not realize these were also being examined to study schizophrenia and the effects of "inbreeding."

This case is a reminder that some populations with an increased prevalence of certain diseases may have a unique interest in research due to the increased medical and social burdens such diseases (for example, diabetes and addiction) can place on their communities. They may also be motivated by a desire not to be further stigmatized by the disease and may see such research as potentially helpful or as burdensome. Unfortunately, Indigenous communities have long been used (and abused) by researchers; they are now looking to benefit more directly from the results of research in which they might be asked to participate.

It is not surprising now to find Indigenous peoples creating guidelines for ethical research involving their communities, advising researchers they are owed a role in "shaping the conduct of research that affects [them]"[27]. It is no longer acceptable for researchers to drop into a community, conduct whatever research interests them, and then promptly leave. Such behaviour is now considered exploitation of Indigenous people and a legacy of colonialism. "Aboriginal ownership, control, access, and possession of research process and products" guidelines, developed by Indigenous scholars, promote the interests of local populations and allows them to help set the agenda and reap some of the benefits of research[28].

To avoid such disputes, it is important to clarify at the outset to what the research participants are agreeing. Some participants and communities will have particular needs to control information concerning them. However, too strict controls by donors over genomic information gathered from thousands of individuals might seriously hamper accurate population-wide research and thereby unduly slow down medical progress[29]. Too lax consent, on the other hand, provides donors with little or no control over how their genetic material is used and by whom. Many individuals will not object to the scientific use of their genetic specimens if they are confident that researchers will only use them for the benign purpose of treating and understanding disease; but they might object if their genetic data is collected for eugenics or for purely commercial uses.

While genetic knowledge can be beneficial to patients, clinicians, and researchers alike, it also creates new professional responsibilities not only to protect that information, but also to ensure it is used appropriately. Genetically based risk assessments are complex and fraught with uncertainty. Conducting a greater number of genome-wide association studies on larger populations is one way to resolve such uncertainties[25]. This involves rapidly scanning markers across the genomes of many people to find genetic variations associated with a particular disease.

There is now a much clearer, if still only partial, sense of the potential impact of genetics and genomics on humankind and medicine. Does medicine have a similar understanding of the impact of culture and cultural change on humankind and medicine? The brief answer is that we do not, although we do know how important culture can be.

II. Cultural Connections

"Culture matters. The question is: how does culture matter?" [30]. Culture matters as ideas matter and cultures are distinguished by their distinctive ideas about the world. Peter Landstreet, a Canadian sociologist, lucidly explains the idea of culture this way:

> In the most general terms, culture serves as a contrast word for nature. Some examples: An edible root is a fact of nature, but the same root, ground and cooked into a porridge according to a people's customary ideas about how it should be prepared for eating, becomes part of that people's culture. The human sex drive is a fact of nature, but "sex magazines" are cultural. Human vocal organs are a fact of nature, but the Spanish language is cultural. Virtually all conceptions of culture, however, have one thing in common: shared ideas. [31]

Members of one culture rarely adopt one consistent set of beliefs. Within one and the same culture, some may consider a family and the individual's place within it as all-important; for other members, a person's own autonomy and independence ("to live as they please") is pre-eminent. A culture can tolerate, indeed, thrive on, diversity. A modern culture can include gun lovers and gun haters, flag wavers and flag burners. What unites them is a belief in some higher order: the Nation, the Constitution, the Greater Good, God.

Under pressure from within and without, cultures are always changing. An appreciation of the changing nature of cultures and respect for the ideas behind cultures are indispensable to the practice of modern medicine. One issue is whether healthcare professionals and trainees receive the kind of education they need in order to be sensitive to the values and beliefs of their patients. Will they be equipped to understand and appreciate the cultural mores and conduct of others?

Case 17.3 A Cultural Gap

Dr R, a primary care physician early in his training and working in a family medicine setting in downtown Halifax, is carrying out a complete physical examination on an anxious young man. Mr W is a 24-year-old patient who recently

continued

immigrated to Canada from rural Nigeria and as yet lacks health benefits. Dr R has only done a complete examination on a few patients as a medical student and never on someone from Africa. He wonders what issues he should raise with Mr W. In particular, he cannot help but notice deep scars on his face and back: Are they perhaps ceremonial ritual scars or has he been tortured? He wonders if he should ask about these scars or not. Should he ask about Mr W's background? Dr R feels uncertain about what he should do and wishes he had someone else present for the examination.

Does Dr R need someone to supervise this encounter?
What other steps might he take to become more culturally sensitive to this patient?

Box 17.4

Culturally sensitive healthcare has been described as care that reflects "the ability to be appropriately responsive to the attitudes, feelings, or circumstances of groups of people that share a common and distinctive racial, national, religious, linguistic, or cultural heritage." [32]

To be culturally sensitive is thought to be a good thing, even when we encounter aspects of a culture that seem unacceptable to us. Cultures vary tremendously, yet they also overlap and are enmeshed with each other. A person can simultaneously be part of a consumerist culture, a scientific culture, an African culture, and a transgender culture. In terms of basic beliefs or commitments, different cultures overlap like Venn diagrams, sharing some attitudes and rejecting others. People and cultures are "diversely different" [30], despite their shared genomes.

Nursing education is particularly notable for its attention to improving the cultural competence of its practitioners [33], likely on account of the greater time nurses typically spend with patients and the more intimate and familiar nature of the care they provide [34]. Sensitivity to the cultural characteristics of various groups of patients is now recognized as increasingly important for physicians [35]. Guidelines have been provided for those caring for members of the LGBTQ community [36-38], adherents of various religious faiths [39], Indigenous peoples [40], members of ethnic minorities [41], and victims of torture [42]. The deficiencies in practice due to misogyny, racism, homophobic attitudes, and other prejudices are gradually being recognized and rectified in mainstream medicine.

Box 17.5 lists some of the understandings and attitudes "culturally competent" trainees and practitioners require.

Box 17.5

To be "culturally competent" means having the knowledge, attitudes, and skills to be able to

- accommodate patient/family "culture-dependent" views;
- ask about patient/family experience of illness and what matters to them, without imposing your own values on others;
- avoid bias towards and stereotyping of patients;
- avoid presumption of a patient's allegiance to their identified group;
- recognize the patient may "belong to" more than one culture;
- appreciate the diversity within the relevant groups;
- recognize that cultures are rarely self-sufficient or self-enclosed;
- appreciate the need to negotiate resolutions;
- realize that cultures can overlap and share values; and
- understand that not all conflicts of value need to be resolved in order to address ethical issues/problems.

Adapted from Epner and Baile, 2012 [34]

To be culturally sensitive can seem a huge task. Although a healthcare practitioner would rarely fulfill or address all these considerations in a single interview with one patient, they do represent some of the prerequisites permitting and facilitating the process of communication between patients and professionals. There is no suggestion that in becoming aware of another's culture one has to uncritically accept its basic beliefs, attitudes, or practices. There is more room for negotiation and compromise, however, if one knows and appreciates where the other person is "coming from." We have seen already how cultural norms can affect conceptions of autonomy (Case 4.1), privacy (Case 7.2), truthtelling (Case 6.2), and consent (Case 5.3). Not all of these situations were resolved to everyone's satisfaction, but reasonable compromises were made. When it comes to ethical dilemmas, a successful resolution may require accepting less than perfect results.

Cultural biases are present when it comes to gender in almost all aspects of our interactions with patients. For example, physicians rarely involve chaperones (someone to supervise an encounter—usually a nurse) when they examine patients of the same sex. Physicians and other healthcare professionals will tell you there are two main reasons for using chaperones when examining patients. The first is for the benefit of the patient: it can be reassuring to have a third party present, someone whose attendance can prevent any untoward interaction between patient and clinician. The second reason is for the benefit of the physician: having a third party observing the proceedings can protect the physician from any subsequent false accusations.

There are, however, many other reasons for having a chaperone present. At times the physician needs assistance during the exam. And sometimes patients are uncomfortable or in pain and need a hand to hold. But for some patients—the victims of torture, for example—it can be intimidating to have an unknown third party in the room. Wendell Block, a family physician who has worked with refugees for many years, has commented on the potential downside of mandatory chaperoning[43]. The interview can become a "two-on-one" situation involving a third party who could be making silent judgments or could break confidences. But if the chaperone is someone known to and trusted by the patient— a family member or a friend—this could encourage the trust necessary for a good medical encounter. On the other hand, having someone known to the patient present may inhibit the patient from responding frankly.

The presence of a third party can lend a degree of professionalism to the encounter. As healthcare trainees may lack the maturity and experience required for a comprehensive examination of certain patients, having a cultural chaperone or mentor present may help reduce anxiety and fears for patients as well as trainees. This depends on the cultures of the doctor and the patient.

Discussion of Case 17.3

In this case, Dr R probably could benefit by having a chaperone (if he can find one) to help, not so much with the physical examination of sensitive areas, as to help address delicate aspects of Mr W's history. If one is not available, he'll have to learn as he goes and make do with less information, much as he would if there was a language barrier.

It is clearly important, in this case, for Dr R to distinguish ritual scarification from the effects of torture[44]. Novices may find this subject embarrassing and difficult to address. Having another person such as a nurse known to the patient in the room may help him raise the issue in an appropriate way. Dr R could prepare himself for Mr W's next visit by familiarizing himself with the patient's culture and becoming comfortable enough to simply take the time to converse with the patient about his background.

III. Worlds apart?

Anne Fadiman's *The Spirit Catches You and You Fall Down: A Hmong Child, Her American Doctors, and the Collision of Cultures* is a stark and powerful book about the influence of culture on medical practice[45]. The book concerns a Hmong Laotian refugee family arriving in California in the 1980s. Speaking little English and having next to no understanding of American medicine, they do have very strong beliefs about why illness strikes some people and not others; in their culture, illness is felt to result from the spirit separating from the body.

When the young daughter, Lia, develops a complex and increasingly serious seizure disorder, her healthcare professionals never come to understand her illness from the perspective of her parents. Language is a problem and the parents' ideas about their child's illness are never adequately translated; neither side finds a bridge to the other. The result is a tremendous informational and emotional downward spiral as Lia and her parents go from one clinician to another, seeking treatment and answers.

Due to the unscaled barriers in language and understanding, Lia appears not to have received proper and timely treatment from anyone's perspective. The conventional Western treatment she did receive may have, in fact, contributed to her decline. But Lia's parents are blamed and suffer legal consequences for failing to provide her with what was thought to be necessary care. The misunderstandings deepen, the confrontations escalate, the child's illness worsens, and, ultimately, as the doctors have the power over the parents, she is removed from them and put in foster care.

Reading this story is like watching a train wreck in slow motion. You see the inexorable terrible conclusion coming straight at you. In the end the child will die—or so everyone expects. After a prolonged anoxic seizure from which recovery is not expected, Lia is taken off life-support and allowed to go home with her parents. The book ends with a Hmong healing ritual.

This tragic tale is characterized by a series of seemingly avoidable misunderstandings, of failures to communicate across a cultural divide, and a total breakdown in trust. As it turns out (and this is not in the book), Lia did *not* die but fell into a persistent vegetative state. Meticulously cared for by her loving parents, she remained in that twilight existence for 26 years, dying in 2012[46].

The lesson of *The Spirit Catches You and You Fall Down* seems simple, perhaps deceptively so. The world is populated by different interpretations of illness, each with dissimilar approaches that can verge on the incommensurable. There is an idyllic quality to the memories Lia's parents have of their old country before it was destroyed by war; this contrasts with the rigid, cold world of Western medicine. Regarding children with illnesses as severe as Lia's, who is to say which approach is better and which is worse? We can only avoid this kind of tragedy by trying to see the world from the point of view of the "other." By being open and sympathetic to a patient and their culture, treatment options, both modern and ancient, are more likely to be acceptable to each side[47].

The following questions, based on the work of the well-known medical anthropologist, Arthur Kleinman, can help healthcare professionals better appreciate the "explanatory model" which a patient or family can bring from a different culture[48].

Box 17.6

....

Questions for Patients/Families to Help Bridge a Cultural Gap
As regards their troubles/sickness, ask them their thoughts on the following questions:

- What is the illness?
- What caused it?
- Why did it start when it did?
- What other problems/difficulties has it caused?
- How severe is it?
- What are their greatest worries/fears?
- Is it treatable and by what?
- How will they know if treatment is working?
- Who else should be involved in the healing process?[48]

These kinds of questions encourage effective cross-cultural communication and can reveal whole new worlds for clinicians. For any particular case, some questions in Box 17.6 will be more pertinent and so more easily answered than others. It depends on how different a patient's culture is from one's own. Many of the questions, quite frankly, should be asked of *every* patient and/or family in order to get a sense of a patient's/family's experience, priorities, and beliefs concerning the problem or illness.

During the 1980s, when Lia's story took place, there were apparently no courses on cross-cultural communication for medical trainees in their region of the United States. The message from Fadiman's book is not that we cannot communicate across cultures and language—we can and must do so. But it is challenging where empathy is lacking, communication skills are poor, respect for others is missing, and cultural biases predominate.

IV. Culture and Defying Death

Certain cultural convictions can at times seem to be at odds with dignified care. One such circumstance is around death: Is it culturally sensitive to allow a family to dictate the terms of life and death in an ICU? Or should the clinicians play the leading role? There is no one right answer but, where the stakes are high, principled and respectful negotiation should be sought. Ultimately though, while many aspects of ICU care are sensitive to the values and wishes of the patient and/ or the family, death is not one of them.

Case 17.4 A Dispute Over Death

Mr. N, a 44-year-old man with a large extended family, is admitted to an ICU with raised intracranial pressure from an untreatable cerebral malignancy. Despite various measures, he has continued to decline and is now on a ventilator. It is obvious to the ICU staff that the patient's brain is too compressed to respond to any treatment. On no sedatives, he has been in a deep coma for several days, completely unresponsive to any stimulation. His score on the Glasgow Coma Scale (GCS), poor from the outset, has been declining for several days. It is now 3—as low as you can get—and there is complete absence of any brainstem reflex activity on two assessments.

Mr N is in every neurological sense dead, "brain dead," as that term is used. As is usual practice, confirmatory clinical testing by way of an apnea test is arranged. This entails temporarily removing the patient's attachment to the ventilator. In response to rising carbon dioxide levels in the body, a brain-dead patient will fail to initiate respiration as would normally occur [49]. The lack of cortical responsiveness, the absence of brainstem reflexes, the lack of movements or breathing, a flat electroencephalogram, are all consistent with death, whatever the state of the patient's circulation might be [50].

Mr N's loved ones disagree strongly with the diagnosis of death—they are a religious family and feel everything possible must be done to extend his life, arguing: "If God wanted him to die, He wouldn't have allowed mankind to invent ventilators. He's not dead until his heart stops beating."

As the ICU resident and attending neurologist are about to perform the test on Mr N, a family member exclaims, "Don't touch him! If you remove him from the breathing machine, we'll sue you!" According to the family's (and the patient's) religion, where there is a heartbeat, there is life, and one may not disconnect a breathing apparatus.

What should the response of the ICU staff be?

"Reasonable accommodation"

The idea that death may be defined or defied by modern medicine seems a widely held view and may be one source of cross-cultural conflict in the ICU. In most jurisdictions, however, religious objections to brain death are not acceptable. Even where they are accepted, such as in the states of New Jersey and New York, it is expected only that clinicians offer families "reasonable accommodation" [51, 52]. A "brain-dead" person is dead, full stop, and only remains in an ICU for exceptional reasons (for a coroner's/medical examiner's inquiry or while awaiting organ retrieval). Out of respect for a family's wishes, one may delay removing a ventilator (sometimes called "removing life support," but this is a poor choice of words as it suggests the person is still alive) to allow time for grieving and/or any religious rites to be performed. How long this period of accommodation should last cannot be fixed in advance: as with many other medical and moral conditions, the right answer is, *it all depends on the circumstances* [53].

The inevitability of complete somatic collapse following entire brain death (within seven days even with cardiovascular support [54]) used to limit how long a body could be kept perfused after death [55]. In some cases, with maximal ICU support, this limit can now be extended much longer—not forever, perhaps, but for weeks or months [56]. This means increasingly one cannot wait for "nature to take its course" and assume time will solve all ethical problems. Clinicians need to play a more active role in directing the resolution of such cases—especially as such care is so expensive (see Chapter 13 for a discussion of this thorny issue). How the healthcare team manages the grieving family requires extreme patience.

Discussion of Case 17.4

This case seems to pit religion against science. A "reasonable" accommodation to a cultural or religious objection to death (as defined by standard neurological criteria) means setting reasonable time limits as to how long the circulation of a brain-dead patient will be supported. In some jurisdictions, any further maintenance of somatic function, if allowed at all, would be at the family's expense [57]. However, the idea that one might be able to "buy" a bed in the ICU to provide somatic support for a dead person seems repugnant and suggests a questionable commercialism. It is also a poor use of a scarce resource. Cultural interpretations of death should not be grounds for preventing measures to confirm death.

The bottom line is this: there are cultural differences in beliefs regarding illness and death that must be recognized by healthcare professionals. To understand and communicate with patients, these differences should not be dismissed as threats, superstitions or dogma, but instead treated in a respectful way. Ways of healing are varied and modern medicine may have much to learn from ancient traditions. When confronted with challenging cultural situations, physicians should seek help from "cultural navigators" and listen to the patient and the patient's family. Involving the police or courts, while necessary in some instances, should be considered a last resort to be called upon only when all else fails (see Chapter 9). It is important to remember that cross-cultural understanding goes both ways—we healthcare professionals can be wrong, our treatments may be ineffective, and other cultures can have much to teach us.

Or, as Karl Marx famously said, "The educator needs to be educated" [58].

V. Transcending Culture

Case 17.5   A Wound Too Terrible

A 14-year-old boy, Neseem R, has recently arrived in Canada as a refugee from a war-torn Middle Eastern country where both his parents were killed. His father's brother and his wife, landed immigrants in Canada for the past year, have adopted him and his only known surviving sibling, a younger sister. Neseem speaks surprisingly good English and seems mature. He has been unwell for some time as medical services were unavailable in his home country. Prompt attention in Canada has resulted in a diagnosis of a large, almost certainly incurable, glioblastoma multiforme, an aggressive form of brain cancer.

His uncle is devastated by the news. "It's like a wound upon wound in our family!" he cries out to the pediatricians who delivers the devastating news. "This is too terrible to bear!" He asks that Neseem not be told about the diagnosis, explaining that in their culture, children, when seriously ill, are looked after by their family. "I will make the decisions about my nephew's care," he states assertively. "Talk to me first!"

How should the pediatricians respond?

Local matters matter

Ethnography, the study of human conduct and mores, can help illuminate the cultural and moral complexities behind the everyday world of medical practice [59, 60]. Clinicians are not expected to be anthropologists or ethnographers, just as they need not be lawyers or philosophers. The ability to observe others and learn why certain patients or families conduct themselves as they do cannot replace bioethics or solve all of medicine's moral dilemmas, but is an invaluable skill for healthcare providers. In clinical encounters with patients, conscientious clinicians attempt to integrate the universal aspects of medicine with the unique views of the patients and their cultural backgrounds. This practice is grounded in the model of concordance or shared decision-making discussed in earlier chapters. It is not "mission impossible" but does take devoted interest and some time.

Transcending culture

For every cultural perspective, there are "facts," or circumstances, that can transcend the culture[61]. These may involve circumstances of commerce or exploration, scientific knowledge or works of philosophy and literature, or less serious aspects of everyday life, play, or entertainment[62]. They can be used in helpful ways to reflect, to understand, or to get out of one's own culture or to penetrate other cultures.

In past times—due to wars, famines, plagues, racism, rampant nationalism, paternalism, and imperialism—such pathways were not always reliable or accepted. Today, as these invidious practices and "isms" slowly fall away, there is more room for mutual respect and sharing among differing cultures. Respect and sharing can encourage dialogue and create a safe harbour, an "ethical space," for cooperative action and learning. The Internet now makes the worldwide sharing of ideas between cultures almost instantaneous. (There is a debate as to whether there can be a science of cultural history—"mimetics"—using memes instead of genes and genetics. On the face of it, this use of memes does seem implausible and may confuse the separation of nature from culture that stands out in the definition of culture used above[31]. However, we will leave it up to the reader to peruse this burgeoning avenue of interesting inquiry[63].)

Cultural relativism vs recognition

It has been said that "persons from different cultural, religious, and ethnic groups must be treated fairly, but…does not require that specific cultural practices always be tolerated equally"[64]. What is important in cross-culturally sensitive medicine is not so much that practitioners should be cognizant of, and give deference to, all the beliefs and practices of an unfamiliar culture; nor must they assume a stance that any one cultural perspective is as good as any other (the cultural relativist point of view). Rather, what is important is to encourage dialogue, to avoid dismissal of other systems of belief simply because they are different, and to negotiate a common ground, to search for the shared values of patient-based care.

Methods of communication and openness to other values are at the crux of culturally sensitive care. The idea of memes seems helpful as a way of thinking about cultures, not as monolithic blocks, but as composed of discrete digitalizable units. While the full meaning and significance of memes can be understood only as part of the larger culture, memes can retain some cultural independence—here we are specifically thinking of the memes of mutual respect and critical reflection—and can be used for a cultural critique.

There are principles and practices that will help foster sensitivity to other cultures and are relevant for professionals and trainees in all domains of healthcare. These are embodied in the following recommendations:

- Encourage patients and families to talk about themselves, and ensure they are listened to.
- Understand the faiths and beliefs of patients and families, and try to allow them to maintain some control even when they appear to be "unreasonable."
- Acknowledge and attempt to address strong emotions and your patients' and their families' suffering.
- Appreciate that you also have a duty to protect the welfare of the vulnerable and not allow harm to come to members of any culture.
- Recognize that, as a practitioner of the art and science of medicine in the twenty-first century, you may not have all the answers [35].

The Socratic view, expressed over two thousand years ago, that "the beginning of wisdom lies in knowing that you know nothing" still seems very applicable today.

Discussion of Case 17.5

The main issue in this case is the conflict between not harming Neseem R by violating the ideas and mores of his culture, while respecting his dignity as a person. First, you should try to explore the family's cultural values and prior experiences and their rationale for the uncle's request (by asking, "We can see how much you want to protect your nephew. What do you think might happen if we talked to Neseem directly about his illness?") Exploring shared values with regard to the child's best interests (a cultural meme!) may help align his adoptive parents with the healthcare team. This may open the door to conversations about the potentially positive consequences of truthtelling (another meme), such as explaining to Neseem what his treatment options are, what he might expect from them, and what his future sadly holds.

The team must also explore with his adoptive parents what will happen if Neseem asks his care team directly about his prognosis or disease (by saying, "It is important that Neseem knows he can trust us, so we would like to answer him honestly if he asks us"). Dealing with such contingencies can help prevent anxiety in staff and trainees who potentially may be asked uncomfortable questions by Naseem when they are on call [65]. One problem with not sharing the truth with the patient is that one deception readily leads to another

continued

(see Chapter 6). It's not hard to lie, but it is hard to do so only once. The family needs to be told that there are limits to subterfuge and that the care team cannot be expected to lie to Neseem if he asks about his condition, explaining this is not acceptable behaviour for clinicians in Canada. This is something Neseem may already understand given his greater fluency in English. An initial lack of veracity with the patient needs to be followed swiftly by a strategy of compassionate disclosure.

Conclusion

There are no simple answers in some cross-cultural cases. But regardless of how complex or enormous cultural differences may appear, healthcare providers should avoid unconsidered, reflex responses—either/or solutions that entail either acquiescence to the patient's cultural values or imposing our own values on them—in favour of a more nuanced decision-making process. We should try to find ways to show respect for a patient's culture and at the same time protect the interests of the patient. These interests may change over time, and different family members may have different views even when they are all ostensibly part of the same culture.

Genomic medicine and the understanding or appreciation of cultural divergence has expanded the borders of medical knowledge and what medicine can achieve. We are trapped neither by our genes nor by our culture. In the final chapter, we will focus on the moral issues raised more broadly by medical research involving human participants.

Cases for Discussion

Case 1: A Reproductive Dilemma

You work as a healthcare professional in a clinic evaluating individuals and couples as to their suitability for IVF services. A young heterosexual couple, Mr and Ms J, with a history of infertility, linked to male and female factors, come for assessment. Both are deaf due to congenital hearing loss. Neither have a cochlear implant and converse in sign language. They request help with getting pregnant and assistance as well with ensuring that their child will be, like them, congenitally deaf by using PGD (Preimplantation Genetic Diagnosis). If pregnancy is successful, they intend to raise the child within the Deaf community, expressing their intention not to allow their child to receive a cochlear implant.

Questions for Discussion

1. Should PGD or other forms of antenatal testing be used to screen for conditions that satisfy parental wishes as regards future offspring?
2. What if both parents were high-functioning adults with Down syndrome who wanted help with reproduction?

Case 2: A Case of Personal Judgment

While working as a family physician in a large city, you are seeing increasing numbers of Hungarian Roma. One of your patients, Mercianna T, a 15-year-old Roma girl in the process of claiming refugee status, informs you she is recently pregnant by her 19-year-old boyfriend. She has dropped out of school and plans to raise the baby with the help of Ms W, her 48-year-old grandmother. Her mother died of TB when Ms T was quite young. Her grandmother, her main support, is not terribly happy about the pregnancy, but admits that she had her first child at 15 as well.

In Roma culture, you are told by a colleague working in this area, girls frequently marry by age 16 and have children at very young ages [64]. They frequently smoke and tend to shun medical care. And indeed, during the pregnancy Mercianna smokes, misses appointments, and is generally noncompliant with prenatal care and advice. When you talk to her about the risks to the fetus and the importance of prenatal care, she reacts dismissively. "Everything will be fine!" You are not so sanguine and wonder whether or not to involve the child protection agency, both for Mercianna and her baby-to-be.

Questions for Discussion

1. What is the ethical dilemma here? Is there more than one?
2. What should you do in this situation?
3. How would you deal with your worries and concerns about this pregnancy and Mercianna's welfare?
4. Are there limits to how far cultural acceptance should go?
5. What does cultural sensitivity involve in this case?

✦ 18 ✦

....

The Ethical Regulation
of Research

No one—and certainly not researchers—can claim a monopoly of relevant wisdom in discussions about what deserves attention in health research.

Ian Chalmers, 1995 [1]

Progress in modern medicine—the "greatest benefit to mankind [2]"—would not be possible without scientific research involving humans. Society expects medicine to win the war on various conditions such as cancer, stroke, schizophrenia, and even aging itself. However, the battles in this war have come, at times, with tremendous costs—not just to patients but to doctors and other healthcare professions as well.

I. Medicine's Legacy

The most egregious examples of misconduct in medical research were revealed during the Nuremburg trials of Nazi doctors following World War II. Implicated physicians engaged in unprecedented and extraordinarily heinous forms of non-consensual research on other humans. Prisoners of the Nazis—including children—were subjected to mutilating and frequently lethal "research experiments" by doctors who had not the slightest interest in their consent or their well-being [3]. The trials ultimately led to the creation of a set of guiding ethical principles and inviolable standards for medical research involving human subjects, known as the Declaration of Helsinki. This document's most fundamental standard is that research may occur *only* with the *voluntary consent* of participants.

In the 1960s, Beecher in the United States and Pappworth in the United Kingdom publicized numerous research trials in each country that flouted this basic requirement for ethical research [4]. Individuals were enrolled in risky protocols without their knowledge. Vulnerable persons, such as children and the mentally ill, were the subjects of experimentation without either their assent or substitute consent.

While these exposés took a professional toll on both men, their writings helped launch the explicit institutional ethical regulation of research.

Yet unethical research continued. The most infamous in the United States was the Tuskegee Syphilis Study. Poor black farm labourers, not told they had syphilis, were followed by physicians for decades to observe the natural progression of the disease—even though antibiotic treatment for syphilis became widely available midway through the study. This trial was halted in 1972, after 40 years, only after coming to public attention. Many years later, the few survivors received compensation and a Presidential apology [5].

In Canada the most notoriously unethical trials were the CIA-funded "psychic driving" experiments of Dr Donald Ewen Cameron at McGill in the 1950s and 1960s. Amnesia and psychic reprogramming were attempted with psychedelics, drug-induced comas, and repetitive electroconvulsive therapy [6]. Consent was never obtained from participants, many of whom suffered severe permanent psychological harms. The experiments were revealed in the 1980s, long after they had run their course.

Case 18.1   A Reversal of Fortune

Dr S is an internist with a particular interest in disorders of consciousness. One of her patients is Mr Z, a 35-year-old father of two, in a minimally responsive state for over a year following a burst cerebral aneurysm. Initially in a persistent vegetative state, he brightened a little several months after the bleed. Since then there has been no further change in his level of awareness. Mr Z's mother and his wife have been very attentive and hope each day will bring an improvement.

Dr S has heard of a new study using a type of transcranial stimulation on the brains of patients in various comatose states. She mentions this to Mr Z's spouse. "Oh, yes! We want him in the study right away! We know it will help him!" she replies.

Is this an ethically acceptable study?
Ought Mr Z to be enrolled in the trial? What reservations might Dr S have about doing so?

II. The Purpose of Research

The primary goal of medical research is not specifically to provide therapeutic benefit to each participant, but rather to expand our knowledge of disease and its treatment (and perhaps secondarily to help participants). Research is undertaken to determine, for example, if a new substance or procedure is more efficacious, better tolerated, or more likely to be accepted and complied with than the standard of care. Even if some benefit is shown, we may be uncertain about the significance of the findings, as the benefits may be small, the studied group may not be representative of all patients, and the real-world use of the studied substance or procedure may differ in substantial ways from its use in the controlled circumstances of a clinical trial.

Although much of what we do in medicine has not been subject to rigorous trials, the purpose of everyday clinical practice is meant to be therapeutic: clinicians recommend interventions with the goal of helping patients. It is considered unethical to withhold standard effective care—unless, of course, the standard of care is not effective for all patients. It may also have harms of its own or not taken for reasons of expense, inconvenience, or intolerance.

Discussion of Case 18.1

It is hard to decide without further details whether the study is acceptable or not. What kind of stimulation will be used? Is there any possibility of harm (not likely, but who knows)? Has this method been used in humans before? Will there be a control group? A placebo arm? What kind of outcomes might be expected? Is there any possibility of a commercial application of the study? If so, is the researcher in a conflict of interest?

Dr S should be concerned that Mr Z's relatives may have fallen prey to the "therapeutic misconception," the idea that the trial is being done to help patients like Mr Z.? This simply is not the case and cannot be promised. Of course, Mr Z has little left to lose. As well, the study is probably innocuous and might help other patients with similar conditions in the future. Was he the type of person who would help others? If so, this might provide some rationale for enrolling him in a study to which he cannot consent. Dr S should try to help his family appreciate that, despite his participating in this trial, there is unlikely to be any reversal of the patient's ill fortune.

Clinical trials and the principle of equipoise

What justifies mounting a scientific trial? The existence of "equipoise" provides the ethical rationale for almost all clinical research trials. This term, coined by Benjamin Freedman in the 1980s, refers to those circumstances of genuine uncertainty about the best treatment for a given condition[7]. For example, in order to justify a trial comparing standard of treatment, drug A, to a test substance, drug B, in the treatment of hypertension, a researcher must believe that

1. drug A, the current standard of care, is ineffective or not well tolerated for at least some people; and
2. there is some good evidence to suppose that the test substance, drug B, will work; and
3. there is uncertainty as to which drug, A or B, is best suited for safely treating hypertension.

In other words, a researcher can only justify comparing drug A to drug B in the absence of clear evidence favouring one over the other.

This is not always as straightforward as it might seem, however. What and where is the standard of care? Medicine is not a homogenous enterprise and there are often different approaches to a particular problem. So from where does the doubt about a standard of care have to arise? The researcher alone? The researcher's immediate colleagues? The most advanced hospitals in the world? Society as a whole? What if patients suffering from a difficult illness are convinced, despite evidence to the contrary, that a poorly studied treatment will help them (such as "Liberation Therapy" for MS)? For such patients, often skeptical of mainstream medicine, there is no equipoise.

Thus, when it comes to equipoise there may be disagreement as to whether it exists in the first place or, if it does exist, where it is and what evidence would be required to resolve it.

Of course, also to be considered is the stance of the large pharmaceutical companies. Evidence is frequently malleable or interpreted differently by different observers. The pharmaceutical industry does not seek out just any new molecule. Rather, they fund research into pharmaceuticals that will suit their business interests. They may stop trials when it suits them or fund those drugs that allow them a niche in the marketplace. Although they cannot be entirely faulted for such practices (after all, they are in the profit-making business), their interests do skew research priorities.

When would it be unethical to propose a trial? How beneficial must a drug be for it to become the standard of care? Or how uncertain must the evidence be regarding a drug's benefit to justify withholding it from subjects in a trial? What balance of harm versus benefit justifies starting or halting a trial? Who is the judge of this? May participants offer to enrol themselves in risky research?

The regulation of research can be quite paternalistic and a trial may be carried out (its design, its execution) without input from participants. This angers some would-be participants who are "protected" from harm by well-meaning researchers but want a greater voice in the conduct of trials[8]. Although whether and how participants could play a role in research oversight is an issue for debate, it is clear that research participants are no longer to be considered passive "subjects" for research[9].

Unfortunately, in the real world of research science, the rules of ethical inquiry are frequently not followed: adverse events are underreported, drug effectiveness overrated, results incompletely reported, negative studies left to languish, and study outcomes changed to reflect better the performance of a new drug. Most disturbing is that without complete and honest reporting of *all* trial results (both negative and positive), the authorities responsible for the ethical conduct of research and those responsible for drug approvals, are unable to do their jobs properly [10]. The editors of the world's most reputable medical journals have in recent years come together to establish more rigorous rules for publishing in their journals [11]. This is a step in the right direction, yet reports of poorly executed and dangerous studies continue [12, 13].

III. Consent for Research

The rigour and readability of Informed Consent Forms (ICFs) used in research has also been challenged. Their complex language and excessive length can frequently obscure the true rationale for a given study, leaving potential participants perplexed or anxious. We can describe the components of a good ICF but, quite frankly, the devil is sometimes obscured by the details of these forms. See Box 18.1 for some important questions that need to be answered in order for research participants to give consent. The trick is to provide *just* the right amount of detail.

Box 18.1

Research participants need to know the following before giving consent:

- Why are they being asked to participate in the trial?
- What is the trial's rationale? What new knowledge will be gained?
- What is the standard of care and what is required of participants?
- What are the precise risks of complications?
- Who will benefit from the trial?
- Who will have access to confidential participant data?

Case 18.2 Poles Apart

It is hypothesized that a new drug, "Tarquinia," is superior to lithium, the standard of care for maintenance therapy of bipolar disorder. A study is proposed whereby 100 participants with bipolar disorder who are stable on lithium will be enrolled in a randomized controlled trial (RCT), the gold standard for most research in medicine [14]. Participants will be randomly assigned to one of three groups: one to receive lithium, another to receive Tarquinia, and a third to receive a placebo. Would-be participants are told about the randomization, but neither they nor the researcher will know to which group they are assigned.

Would you have any ethical concerns about this trial?

Discussion of Case 18.2

Lithium is known to be an efficacious therapy for prevention of relapse in bipolar disorder. However, it does not work for everyone, can cause intolerable symptoms for some, and has the potential for serious side effects. Hence, there is a strong rationale to study a new drug with possibly equal efficacy but fewer adverse effects. The moral acceptability of the trial depends on the science behind the study: how good is the evidence behind the new substance? Assuming that preliminary studies show Tarquinia to be reasonably effective, then it is likely ethically acceptable to mount a study comparing it with lithium.

    However, the inclusion of a placebo arm in this study is very problematic. Given that lithium is the standard of care, it would generally be inappropriate to submit participants to the risk of a placebo. This would violate the principle of equipoise. Other questions that must be considered for such a study include the following: How well monitored will study participants be? Who is the best judge of the acceptability of the hazards a trial might pose to participants? Is it a group of peers such as scientific review board? The answer to this is yes, but participants in the deliberations of such boards must not be in a conflict of interest (more on that below), and the group should include non-physicians, ethicists, lawyers, and community representatives.

Research trials and placebos

Box 18.2

"It's obviously wrong to put patients in a trial where half of them will be given a placebo, if there is a currently available option which is known to be effective, because you are actively depriving half of your patients of treatment for their disease." [15]

RCTs have more than one "arm"—each comprised of participants with similar characteristics. Study participants are randomly assigned to one of the arms with one arm (or more) getting the test substance while the other arm is given a look-alike placebo.

It is common, for example, in trials of new antidepressants for half of the subjects to get no drug at all and the other half the test drug. The placebo response rate is high for psychiatric conditions, hence, it is argued, the need for a trial design comparing the new drug against a background of no drug—just close supervision and monitoring. This type of trial will tell you if the test substance is better than nothing (the placebo arm).

However, such a trial should be considered acceptable only if there is no standard effective treatment for the studied condition or if the standard treatment is poorly tolerated or unwanted by many. But, where the standard care is beneficial (as antidepressants often are for depression or lithium for bipolar illness) and withheld, there must be careful supervision of the participants, for example by seeing them frequently.

In other RCTs all participants receive known effective treatment. While one group gets the test substance and the other receives a placebo, everyone receives the same basic or standard treatment. For example, in a trial of a new diuretic for hypertension, it would not be acceptable to stop all of the participants' antihypertensive drugs in order to compare the effects of the diuretic against a placebo. Instead, *everyone* in the trial must receive the normal treatment for hypertension (the standard of care drugs, for example). *In addition*, one group would get, by random assignment, the new drug while others would be given the placebo (a look-alike drug with no real efficacy).

Such trials can be expensive. New drugs are likely to be only marginally better than the standard of care. Hence, it takes the enrolment of many participants over prolonged periods of time to show evidence of hard outcomes, such as reduced rates of death or stroke. It takes fewer patients and less time if, however, the test drug is compared against placebo rather than against the standard of care—assuming the standard of care has *some* efficacy.

In practice, clinicians are most interested in direct (head-to-head) comparisons of a new drug with the standard of care [16]. Does a new anti-hypertensive perform better than the accepted alternatives? Testing it against placebo will not tell you this. The gain in effectiveness by the new drug can be determined only if the comparator group receives the standard of care. Currently, researchers may carry out studies that deny some participants an effective standard of care only if they can show that those not receiving it will not be harmed, there is a guarantee of close clinical vigilance of all participants in the trial, and participants give their informed consent to the trial.

For RCTs, therapeutic benefits cannot be guaranteed for participants because of the possibility they may be assigned to the placebo arm or because the test substance (the "active arm") may not end up working. Despite this, participants may enter a trial for the chance of benefit, with the hope they will not be randomized to the placebo arm. They may be motivated to do so for altruistic reasons and/or because the existing standard of care for their condition may not be sufficiently efficacious or is associated with adverse effects they prefer to avoid.

IV. The Tissue Issue

Without their knowledge, patients can be made the subject of research, although this was more common in the past than now. In *The Immortal Life of Henrietta Lacks*, Rebecca Skloot documents the sad tale of an impoverished woman who eventually died of cervical cancer in the early 1950s. Without Ms Lack's consent—recall this was from a time in medicine when, without the knowledge of patients or families, excised tissues and organs, both ante and post mortem, would be retained "for later use"[17]—her doctors used her tumour cells to create an "immortal" line of the cancer cells[18]. The "HeLa" cells, as they are called, have proven to be enormously valuable, widely used by many researchers on a variety of topics including cancers of all types. Neither Ms Lacks nor her family received any acknowledgement or benefits—health-related, financial, or otherwise. For many years, the Lacks family was without even basic health insurance. It took decades and Rebecca Skloot's book for Ms Lack's family to finally obtain any recognition for her (unwitting) contribution to medical science.

Does the nonclinical use of blood samples or patient tissue excised during surgery require patient consent? The answer to this is, generally, yes. While ordinary consent is obviously necessary for any surgery on a patient, a separate consent form, authorized by a research ethics board, must be completed if patient tissue will be used for nonclinical purposes[19]. Patients must be informed about the aims of the research and how the tissue will be used. For example, will it be used for commercial purposes? To study a specific disease? For how long will it be kept? Will it be shared? In the case of Ms Lacks, although the tissue was removed for clinical reasons, consent for its research use was never obtained (such consent was probably never even considered at the time). When the hidden use of pathology samples does come to light, it can seem to be illicit, sully the profession's reputation, and fuel the public ire directed against medical research[17]. It is obviously much better for everyone to have all research out in the open.

Case 18.3 An Unexpected Association

A 27-year-old woman, Ms T, has responded to treatment for T-cell lymphoma and has now been disease free for three years. As part of the treatment for her condition, she participated in a clinical trial of a new anti-lymphoma agent,

continued

which she tolerated well. Ms T also donated samples of her blood that were anonymized (to protect her privacy) and used solely for future research for "purposes connected with her condition."

Since that trial, new genome-wide studies have unexpectedly revealed an increased risk for hormonally dependent breast cancer in the first-degree relatives of patients, like Ms T, who responded well to the anti-lymphoma drug. The researchers involved in a proposed new trial now want to contact Ms T's relatives in order to study their health and genomes. They can do so only if they de-anonymize her results.

Should the institutional ethics board charged with overseeing the trial allow the researchers to "break the code" and contact members of at-risk families?

Discussion of Case 18.3

In this case, it is unclear to what Ms T consented. Was it her understanding that her stored blood could be retained indefinitely and potentially used for any "legitimate" research purposes? Or did she think her samples would be used only for lymphoma-related research and destroyed within a fixed period of time? Was Ms T told she or her family might need to be re-contacted if findings pertinent to her and her family's health were subsequently discovered? Or did she assume that, once anonymized, any future contact with her by the researchers was forbidden?

The broader the consent obtained from Ms T, the fewer restrictions there would be on any further research use of her samples. This is advantageous in many ways—for society, for future patients—but does infringe upon her right to privacy and the right to be left alone. It also opens the door more widely for the use of that information for commercial purposes—something perhaps not considered by the participants in the original trial.

US courts have found research participants not to have a right to ownership over tissue samples—they are considered "gifts" to the institution (for example, the university, the hospital, the biobank) that harbours them and cannot be revoked[20]. They belong neither to the patient nor to the researcher. In Canada, the issue is foggier—litigation is scanty but one court likewise found that retained or donated tissue belongs to the hospital[21]. In another leading US case, in 2007[22], a bank of thousands of prostate tissue samples collected by a physician over many years was considered by the court to be the property of the university where he worked. It was argued that giving over rights of ownership to the physician-researcher or his patients carried the risk of rampant commercialization. The judge in his ruling expressed an anti-commercial sentiment (see Box 18.3).

Box 18.3

....

"If left unregulated and to the whims of [donors], these highly prized bio-logical materials would become nothing more than chattel going to the highest bidder . . . . Selling excised tissue or DNA on eBay would become as commonplace as selling your old television on eBay."

....

Catalona v Washington University, 2006[23]

Although this may be a legitimate concern, it can be taken in two ways. A less charitable interpretation is that the original sponsoring institution was in a conflict of interest, having a strong pecuniary interest in retaining the samples for its own commercial purposes and wishing to use them no matter what the participants were told or expected. The traffic in human tissue is big business these days as this tissue contains a tremendous amount of information—our genome—about who we are (see Chapter 17). This advance in our understanding makes the traditional view[24], that individuals have no interest in tissue once extracted, an outmoded one.

One solution to these complexities would be to obtain in advance an explicit "tiered consent" from patients/research participants which specifies the precise circumstances of re-use of stored samples and when participants may be re-contacted (see Box 18.4)[25]. A blanket approval of either yes or no for the re-use of participants' samples is less helpful.

Box 18.4

....

Tiered consent forms could include language such as the following:

- "With your permission we would like to store your blood/tissue from this study for future research. You do not have to agree to this, but it is important for us to know how we might use your samples in the future."
- "Regarding my blood/tissue collected for my illness in this study, I request that this (please choose one or more of the following options):
  a. only be used for research concerning the illness I have.
  b. may be used for research concerning any health problems.
  c. may be used in future only if I am contacted first.
  d. may not be used at all beyond this study.
  e. may/may not be used for commercial purposes."

In addition to individual consent, should there be some form of local community/individual control over how this information about banked tissue, DNA, or blood samples is to be used and by whom? It has been suggested that "[t]issues are held in trust for the donors by a trustee who oversees uses in accordance with the wishes of the beneficiaries of the trust; in this case the general public"[26]. Tissues—that would extend to any patient samples such as their blood, DNA, or genome—held in trust would enable public benefit without exploiting individuals or their cultures.

V. Some Questions and Answers Regarding Research

In this section we will address some of the more common questions regarding research review.

Must all research receive ethics review?

In all cases a duly constituted Research Ethics Board (REB) or Institutional Review Board (IRB) is required to review and approve any research before it is undertaken. Community involvement in such a board is essential for maintaining transparency and helping lay people understand the rationale behind the research. Good oversight can help discourage bad science[27]. For multi-centred trials, there are now networks of REBs/IRBs accepting reviews done at participating institutions. This helps prevent duplicative reviews and so can make it easier to do multi-site research without cutting ethical corners. However, it does require institutions to know and trust each other's review process. The global accreditation of research ethics boards is currently being pursued as a way of harmonizing the review process between sites[28].

How do we know the research isn't fraudulent?

Quite frankly, we don't. There is very little oversight of research once approved by an REB. However, there is oversight by, for example, a researcher's peers, sponsors, and journal editors. Fraudulent researchers risk their reputation and livelihood. Deliberate fraud does occur but is uncommon. Much more common than deliberate fraud are the inventive and resourceful ways in which researchers or the research sponsors (typically, the pharmaceutical industry) can represent data or change a study's objectives to make a drug appear more attractive[29]. Thus, changing a study's outcome from hard end-points, such as death, to softer ones, such as tumour shrinkage or reductions in tumour serum markers, can make an anti-cancer drug appear more efficacious than it really is. However, such a *post hoc* manipulation of study objectives, data, and outcomes can seriously compromise the integrity of a great deal of research and undermine trust in such research by both the medical community and the public.

Is consent always necessary?

Although the answer is generally yes, there are exceptions. Consent is not needed for non-interventional research such as retrospective chart reviews or research involving the secondary manipulation of large anonymized data sets, so long as privacy is protected, and the collected data is not considered sensitive or intimate.

Consent may also be waived or deferred for research conducted on patients in emergency settings. While this type of research strictly goes against the Nuremberg consent requirement, it is considered acceptable if certain conditions are met:

1. time must be of the essence; that is, there is a narrow window of opportunity to prevent serious harm;
2. the patient is incapable and cannot give consent or cannot do so in the window of time;
3. the standard of care is of very limited efficacy (there must be equipoise);
4. the trial can be reasonably supposed to help or address the patient's condition; and
5. the trial is not considered to be more harmful than the standard of care.

This is the rationale underlying studies of CPR in ambulatory settings and of the use of thrombolytic and neuroprotective drugs in acute stroke. For example, in the case of a study of community cardiac arrest, the outcomes are so dismal and the risk of death so high (especially in an out-of-hospital setting) as to justify certain research interventions that might reasonably be expected to improve survival. For example, if a test intervention is unlikely to make would-be participants worse off—such as a new way of doing CPR—and, if seeking consent would undermine the possibility of demonstrating the intervention's effectiveness, the normal consent process can be waived, assuming the study has proper trial monitoring. Trial subjects and their families, needless to say, should be told of the trial and its impact, where possible, and as soon as feasible.

May children or incapable patients participate in research?

The answer is yes. The risks of any proposed study must be assessed by an REB to be no more than minimal, as young children or incapable patients cannot give valid consent. As well, parental or a substitute decision-maker's consent obviously would be required.

Although adults may altruistically assume risks for the benefit of others, children are unable to do so[30]. Patients with reduced capacity are considered a "vulnerable" group as they cannot consent to the particulars of a trial and ought never be enrolled for reasons of convenience (for example, by virtue of living in a residential or long-term care facility) as they may not be able to dissent from a trial.

Nevertheless, if the research pertains to conditions affecting children or incapable adults, it may be quite appropriate (with safeguards and oversight in place) to include them in a trial; otherwise it may be impossible to generalize the results from other trials enrolling only adults or capable patients.

Must researchers caution participants about new findings during a study?

The answer is generally yes—especially if these are relevant to a participant's well-being (for example, an unanticipated finding on a study X-ray or genomic "incidental findings"), or if they concern the safety or usefulness of an ongoing trial. Relevant information should be promptly conveyed to participants, the trial halted or put on hold, or a new consent obtained.

May a researcher accept recompense from the trial sponsor?

Yes, but the value of such recompense must be disclosed to the reviewing ethics board and to participants in the trial. Payment should be only for work done and not so excessive as to be seen to sway a researcher's judgment. Any involvement of the researcher with the sponsor of a trial outside the context of the trial, for example, as an advisor to the sponsor, puts them in a conflict of interest (see Chapter 10) and must be disclosed as well to the overseeing REB and to research participants.

Can research participants be paid for their participation in a study?

Compensation for the work and burdens of research is considered fair for research participants, providing it is not so generous as to induce them to trade off risk for money. Reasonable recompense for the inconveniences of participating in the research (such as parking, lunch, travel) and provision of some incentives to stay in a trial are also acceptable. Just where to draw the line between an incentive and a reasonable compensation is sometimes unclear, but research ethics committees have as one of their mandates a duty to consider this in evaluating the ethical acceptability of a trial [31, 32].

How do we assure the privacy of participants?

This concern is especially important given the capacity of modern institutions, such as banks, governments, and social media to obtain, store, and use vast banks of very personal information. This is true for medicine as well, as genomic data for individuals and communities and other large data sets are being increasingly used (see Chapter 7).

Case 18.4   Are You Coming Home Soon, Dad?

A medical researcher, Dr D, is running a study looking at the possible benefits of a new type of medication for diabetes. In order to spend more time with his family, he arranges to work on his research at home. The plan is to enjoy family dinners and work on his research after the kids have been tucked in. He puts all the information from the study onto his laptop, including patient names, their dates of birth, diagnoses, and test results.

The research is going well and so is his family life. Then, one day Dr D stops off at the grocery store on his way home to buy some bread and milk. When he returns to the car, he discovers his laptop is no longer on the back seat where he'd left it. Only after he searches the car to make sure the computer didn't fall and slide under the front seat does it hit him: his laptop has been stolen.

What should Dr D do?

Discussion of Case 18.4

Dr D needs to immediately inform the appropriate authorities in his hospital about the loss of patient data. Depending on the particular jurisdiction, there may also be an obligation to inform the research subjects of this incident (in some jurisdictions, such as Ontario, this notification is mandatory).

Going forward, Dr D needs to be vigilant about protecting patient information. There are several ways to help ensure privacy of research data, including separating identifiable information from study data, using only randomly generated study identification numbers for event reporting, avoiding inclusion of unique patient identifiers such as initials or birthdates, ensuring no research files leaving the office contain identifiable personal information, and using encryption and password protection protocols.

Privacy in research cannot, quite frankly, be guaranteed. Once health information leaves the institution of origin—especially if sent to another country—attempts at limiting the information's use and disclosure will be lost. One can only hope that the receiving country will have good information privacy protections. In case it does not, any information to be transmitted elsewhere should only be in the form of anonymized, not personalized, health information. All information must be encrypted and stored on a secure server. Anyone working with personalized data must be trained in privacy practices and held to strictly enforced oaths of confidentiality.

What about quality improvement studies?

Quality improvement (QI) is technically not "research" (the risks are zero or minimal, there is no participant randomization or hypothesis testing, and any data is de-identified) and so does not usually require ethics review. For example, the retrospective evaluation of the success of a new program of diabetes education would not require research review. It would require ethics review if the QI project had compared two different educational interventions[33]. However, as the line between research and QI is not always clear, it is prudent, when uncertain, to seek the opinion of the local research review board as to whether review is needed.

Must a research review board review all research with the same depth?

Not necessarily: research review ought to be proportionate to the risks involved. However, there must be extra careful scrutiny, for example, of research involving

- vulnerable subjects,
- risks of surgery undertaken in emergencies or sham surgery,
- novel test substances with uncertain side-effect profiles, and
- "first in human" trials (trials testing a new drug or device in humans for the first time).

Must research be carried out throughout the world according to the same standards?

This is a topic of great concern as much research has been transferred to "underdeveloped" countries where research and human lives are often cheaper.

Case 18.5 An Unfair Trial

Radha, a three-year-old girl in rural India, is playing at home when she suddenly suffers a seizure. She is stabilized after her parents rush her to the hospital in the nearest town. The doctor explains she most likely has a seizure disorder, but that further testing, including a CAT scan of her brain, is needed to rule out other causes. When her parents tell him they cannot afford the tests, he asks if they would consent to enrolling Radha in a pharmaceutical company-sponsored study comparing two types of anti-seizure drugs. If so, the study sponsors will pay for her hospitalization, the investigations, and drugs as well, should she need them. She will be required to come to the hospital every month, but the pharmaceutical company will pay for transport.

Radha's parents readily agree. Tests reveal she has an epileptogenic focus. She does well in the trial. When the study ends 18 months later, her parents are informed that they will no longer receive free medicine and the local clinic does not carry either of the test medications. Lacking effective medication, her seizures will almost certainly recur, with negative impact on her long-term neuropsychological development. Indeed, one week later, Radha suffers another seizure.

What is wrong with this trial?
What ethical concerns about medical research does it raise?

International standards

No matter what the milieu or culture, the same standards of research must hold[34]. There are ICH–GCP ("International Conference on Harmonization of technical requirements for registration of pharmaceuticals for human use"—"Good Clinical Practice") guidelines that set out international standards for human research[35]. Burdensome as they may sometimes be[36], the standards of research review boards exist to prevent the abuses of human rights identified by Beecher and Pappworth over 50 years ago. Clearly, some standards, such as free and informed consent, are harder to implement in regions with high rates of impoverishment, illiteracy, and paternalistic or authoritarian attitudes and practices.

Where research appears to be conducted for the benefit of others, there must be genuine social value, participants must be fairly selected, and the risks ought to be minimized. "Mutual aid" is an important principle that can be applied to clinical research and justify participation in research that may not directly help individual participants[37]. In fact, without such altruism, much medical research would not occur. Unfortunately, the altruism of many participants is not always matched by the ethical standards of a trial's sponsor.

Discussion of Case 18.5

Just about everything was wrong with this trial. It typifies the problems of conducting research in the developing world[38]. The parents' decision to join the trial was motivated by financial factors—not unusual in poor regions—but the

continued

researchers did not inform the parents how limited the free ride would be and failed to plan for the trial's end. This too is not unusual; research participants are frequently used to "try out" medications they will not be able to obtain at the trial's completion, no matter how beneficial the test substances might be. This seems unjust, as participants risk their well-being for the benefit of others but, even if lucky enough to benefit in the short term, fail to reap gains in the long run.

Impoverished participants may be less used to asking questions of researchers and may be happy with whatever assistance they can get. They cannot be blamed for that; it is the researcher's responsibility to protect the rights and welfare of subjects wherever the research is conducted. The ICH–GCP guidelines are known in countries such as India [39] and throughout the world [40]. Failure to follow them may stem from lack of effective local oversight [41].

Conclusion

In this chapter, we have briefly touched on the complicated area of ethics in medical research. There are Internet sites where the most recent updates and guidelines for human research may be found for Canada [42], India [43], the UK [44], Australia [45], the US [46, 47], and for global efforts [48, 49]. Patients who wish to be participants in trials can now search online for studies relevant to them by going to sites such as www.ClinicalTrials.gov, a US database for thousands of publicly and privately funded studies worldwide.

Cases for Discussion

Case 1: The New Drug on the Block

A research study proposes to use a new drug, "Superbia," for the maintenance of positive symptom regression in schizophrenia. Preliminary research suggests that Superbia may have a better patient tolerability profile and possibly be safer as there appears to be a lower risk of agranulocytosis, a serious side effect of one of the currently accepted antipsychotic drugs. In this 48-week study, one-third of the 200 patients to be enrolled at 30 sites will be randomized to continue their current regimen, one-third randomized to Superbia, and the remainder to placebo.

All participants will be seen every two weeks initially, then every four to six weeks, with some visits conducted by telephone. Regular blood tests will be done throughout the study to look for evidence of reduced white cells, liver inflammation, and kidney damage.

Other side effects noted with Superbia, as with other maintenance drugs, include high blood pressure, dizziness, headaches, fatigue, dry mouth, nausea, rashes, numbness in the body, a fuzzy feeling in the head, and diarrhea. Additional side effects—previously unidentified, it is noted—may also occur.

Doses 15 times as high as those used in this study resulted in weight loss, inflammation of the gastrointestinal tract, and red, swollen gums in rats and dogs. No deaths have been reported to date with Superbia. Patients who deteriorate during this study will be withdrawn from the study and offered "rescue" antipsychotics.

Questions for Discussion

1. What concerns might you have about this trial?
2. Discuss what improvements could be made in the trial to make it more appropriate.

Case 2: A Modest Proposal

Dr U has had a longstanding interest in chronic kidney disease, hypertension, and non-insulin-dependent diabetes. All three conditions, he knows, are prevalent in the Indigenous communities in the North. He has acted as a long-distance consultant to various northern communities and has been frustrated by his poor success rate in preventing renal failure in this population. Dr U is unsure how much of the burden of the disease is due to nature and how much due to the environment. He proposes a study that will compare the genomes of Indigenous patients in various communities and Indigenous people in the city.

All he needs, he speculates, are buccal swabs from individuals and data that would link these to an individual's family and medical history.

He hopes then to piggyback on to this a promising new anti-hypertensive drug.

Questions for Discussion

1. What concerns ought Dr U have about his proposed study?
2. What authorization should he seek?

Conclusion

Setting Our Sights

All things living are in search of a better world.

Karl Popper, 1995 [1]

There are many national and international efforts underway to arrive at a global understanding of medical professionalism [2]. Although A Physician Charter for the New Millennium [3] may have initially spurred on other medical associations, it is not the final word on professionalism. For example, physicians in China have emphasized the need for a greater focus on social justice [4, 5]. Arab physicians look for greater congruency between the personal moral sphere and the professional arena of life [6]. Despite differences in culture, religion, and politics, healthcare professionals throughout the world share similar goals: the prevention of premature death and the treatment and prevention of illness and human suffering. These are the good outcomes the virtuous clinician strives to achieve by "doing right" in medicine.

In approaching ethical issues, it's easy to be confused by the cacophony of language and everyday morals. Some think we are forever circumscribed and held hostage by our languages and cultures and, consequently, are left only with moral and cultural relativism—"be true to yourself/your culture/your religion/your country." As we have demonstrated in this book, we do not subscribe to this view.

Yes, all languages and cultures may be limited in scope, with embedded values and often different world-views. And, yes, it is good that people should feel allegiance to their families and cultures. But when clashes of values or commitment occur, the solution isn't to seek a value-free language or throw up one's hands in despair. Rather, it is to engage in dialogue with others over the common problems we face as people—whether patients, healthcare providers, or citizens. Ernest Gellner, a twentieth-century anthropologist, arguing against the relativism ever present in his field, wrote, "[E]ven if no absolute point of view is possible, fairly comfortable resting places . . . will do instead . . . . We cannot but adopt some vantage point, even if only to express some doubt or to recognize some uncertainty"[7].

Here lies the value of what is known as critical rationalism: the ability to stand back from one's beliefs, to be self-aware, to be mindful, to admit one might be wrong, and to learn from one's errors[8].

Cultures can differ in fundamental ways with regard to basic rules and values and yet still work together to achieve very practical results, such as sustainably managing scarce resources to access clean water or food supplies[9]. Successful cooperation occurs, in part, because of a focus on shared local problems and because of mutual respect, despite differences in outlook and culture. For example, founded in 2002, the Global Fund to Fight AIDS, Tuberculosis, and Malaria is a partnership between governments, civil society, the private sector, and people affected by the diseases. This fund raises and invests nearly $4 billion USD a year to support programs run by local experts in countries and communities most in need. "A fantastic vehicle for scaling up the treatments and preventative tools"[10], the organization employs staff from all professional backgrounds and more than 100 different countries.

International aid organizations, such as NGOs like OXFAM or MSF (Médecins Sans Frontières), would not exist if very different cultures did not share a common belief in the value of human life[11]. As a result, the lives of millions of people have changed for the better, not only in small, but also in large, tectonic plate–shifting ways. We don't want to overstate it, but those advances—the reduction in abject poverty levels and the treatment of childhood diarrhea, for example—continue at rates unparalleled in human history[12]. The question is how the tolerance and altruism required for fair and just medical care can be extended around the world to address other medical conditions.

In 2016 Rosenthal and Verghese wrote eloquently in *The New England Journal of Medicine* that "the majority of what we define as [the physician's] 'work' takes place away from the patient, in workrooms and on computers . . . . We've distanced ourselves from the personhood, the embodied identity, of patients"[13]. They recommended the healthcare system be improved to make it a more humane environment for those who work in it; in order to achieve this, we need to spend "more time with each other and with our patients." Certainly, this would be a step in the right direction. Physician burnout—one consequence of how medicine is practised in the modern era—will have to be prevented by ethically reconfiguring healthcare in ways that can restore "meaning and sanity" for physicians and other professionals[14].

Due, in part, to the international equalizing trend of the Internet, patients are less dependent on professionals for information and have more choices than ever. Transparency and access to information are key in making informed decisions and increasingly put power in the hands of patients[15].

This is not the end of professionalism, as some have claimed [16]. Healthcare is *not* a zero-sum game: we all gain when patients and professionals work together in partnership to improve and re-model healthcare. This trajectory makes it less likely (but not impossible, unfortunately) that medicine can ever again serve evil ends, as it has done in the not too distant past.

The siege mentality

Many healthcare professionals view their future, and their patients' futures, with dismay, feeling theirs is a profession under siege [17]. Indeed, attacks upon healthcare workers do seem to be escalating in some parts of the world [18], and drug addiction [19] and mental despair [20] are altogether too common among medical practitioners [21]. Medicine can be a demanding and dangerous enterprise [22]. Politicians do not make it any easier and are wont to use healthcare as a political football with all the negative consequences this can have for the continuity and comprehensiveness of care. Patients and families, too, are restive and critical and know all is not right with healthcare [23].

Hard Times, Dickens's nineteenth-century novel [24], seems apt for our times as well: "hard times are here and also lie ahead." Nonetheless, hard times can be a catalyst for development and improvement [25]. In any time, an emphasis on the key ethical principles and professional values, such as altruism, humility, honesty, transparency, trust, and mutual respect, can enhance the relationships between practitioner, patient, and other healthcare workers, and can make for a more satisfying practice [26].

Box C.1

"While it has been frequently suggested that the aim of professionalism and ethics preparation is not to midwife virtue or to assure sound moral character, medical students and residents themselves believe it may confer positive qualities and preservation of compassion." [26]

Studies suggest healthcare professionals experience less burnout and cynicism if they remain in touch with the meaning and significance of what they do [27]. Medical trainees can benefit from ethics awareness and from self-reflection, as well [28]. The joys and challenges of medical work can prevail over its discouragements if practitioners "re-moralize" their practice: connecting with patients and recognizing them as unique persons with fascinating stories, and remembering our good fortune in being able to make remarkable and unforgettable differences in their lives[29]. In order to avoid the anomie and melancholy that can sometimes accompany the burdens of practice, all healthcare professionals need to "devote time and resources to promoting self-care"[30].

Box C.2

Suggested Readings

Alderson P. *Children's Consent to Surgery*[32]. The best book to qualitatively explore children's consent to surgery.

Balint M. *The Doctor, His Patient and the Illness*[33]. The classic text on psychosomatic illness and the role of the doctor.

Beauchamp T and Childress J. *Principles of Biomedical Ethics*, 7th ed[34]. The modern statement on philosophical bioethics.

Berger J and Mohr J. *A Fortunate Man*[35]. An elegy to the life and lost times of the solo practitioner.

Breen KJ, Cordner SM, Thomson CJH. *Good Medical Practice: Professionalism, Ethics, and the Law*, 4th ed[36], from the Australian Medical Council. A comprehensive overview of professional ethics from Down Under.

Gawande A. *Being Mortal: Medicine and What Matters at the End*[37]. An elegant statement of a physician's grappling with mortality.

Gottlieb A. *The Dream of Enlightenment: The Rise of Modern Philosophy*[38]. A history of philosophy from Descartes and Hobbes to Hume and Rousseau.

Ingelfinger F. Arrogance[39], *The New England Journal of Medicine*. A dying doctor looks for professional help and eschews autonomy.

Jameson L. *The Empathy Exams: Essays*[40]. Not to be missed, a modern meditation on the importance of empathy.

Somerville A. *Medical Ethics Today: The BMA's Handbook of Ethics and Law. 3rd ed*[41]. Professional ethics as seen from the British Medical Association.

Verghese A. Cutting for stone. (Vintage Books Canada. Toronto 2010). An elegant exploration of the Hippocratic oath not to cut for stone set in modern Ethiopia.

Williams J. *Medical Ethics Manual*[42]. Ethics as seen from the World Medical Association.

Ethical sensitivity can help patients and clinicians alike by enabling them to recognize and strive for the best possible outcomes not only in good times but also in hard times, when resources are scarce, practices criticized, and outcomes uncertain. Assiduous attention to professionalism and ethical concerns can help those involved do their best to do what seems right and to feel confident they have done so. This enriches us all.

Hard times, perhaps, but also exciting times when we are able to combine science with humanism to renew medicine, "the greatest benefit to mankind"[31].

Notes

Preface

1. O'Toole G. Quote investigator (Internet). The future is not what it used to be; 2012 Dec 6 [cited 2018 Oct 16]; [about 5 screens]. Available from: https://quoteinvestigator.com/2012/12/06/future-not-used/
2. Jagsi R. Sexual harassment in medicine: #MeToo. N Engl J Med. 2018;378(3):209–11. DOI: 10.1056/NEJMp1715962
3. Annas GJ. Doctors, patients, and lawyers: two centuries of health law. N Engl J Med. 2012;367(5):445–50. DOI 10.1056/NEJMra1108646
4. Wilson C. Moral animals: ideals and constraints in moral theory. Oxford: Oxford University Press; 2004.

Acknowledgements

1. Marx K, Engels F. Marx/Engels selected works. Moscow: Progress Publishers; 1969. Third thesis on Feuerbach; p. 27.
2. Flaubert G. Sentimental education. Oxford: Oxford University Press; 2016.

Introduction

1. Rhoades DR, McFarland KF, Finch WH, et al. Speaking and interruptions during primary care office visits. Fam Med. 2001;33(7):528–32. PMID: 11456245.
2. Westbrook JI, Duffield C, Li L, et al. How much time do nurses have for patients? A longitudinal study quantifying hospital nurses' patterns of task time distribution and interactions with health professionals. BMC Health Serv Res. 2011;11(1):319. DOI: 10.1186/1472-6963-11-319
3. Hébert P. Do what you are passionate about: reflections for an incoming medical class. UTMJ. 2018;95(1):6–8. Available at: http://utmj.org/index.php/UTMJ/article/view/339/296
4. Cooke M, Irby DM, O'Brien BC. Educating physicians: a call for reform of medical school and residency. San Francisco (CA): Jossey-Bass; 2010. (Jossey-Bass/Carnegie Foundation for the Advancement of Teaching; 16).
5. Birnbaum F, Lewis DM, Rosen R, et al. Patient engagement and the design of digital health. Acad Emerg Med. 2015;22(6):754–6. DOI: 10.1111/acem.12692
6. Harris S. The moral landscape: how science can determine human values. New York: Free Press; 2010. p. 2.
7. Nussbaum M. Upheavals of thought: the intelligence of emotions. Cambridge: Cambridge University Press; 2001. p. 432–3.
8. Toews M. All my puny sorrows. Toronto (ON): Knopf Canada; 2014.
9. Tolstoy LN. Anna Karenina. Edmonds R, translator. Harmondsworth: Penguin Books; 1969.
10. Richie D. Red Beard. The Current [Internet]. 1989 Nov 20; [about 4 screens]. Available from: https://www.criterion.com/current/posts/922-red-beard
11. Peterkin AD, Skorzewska A. Health humanities in post-graduate medical education. Toronto (ON): Oxford University Press; 2018.
12. PLOS [Internet]. San Francisco (CA): Public Library of Science. Open access [about 2 screens]. Available from: https://www.plos.org/open-access/
13. IBM Watson Health [Internet]. Armonk (NY): IBM; [cited 2017 Jan 12]. Available from: https://www.ibm.com/watson/health/
14. Obermeyer Z, Lee TH. Lost in thought: the limits of the human mind and the future of medicine. N Engl J Med. 2017;377(13):1209–11. DOI: 10.1056/NEJMp1705348
15. Parfit D. On what matters. Vol. 1. Oxford: Oxford University Press; 2011.
16. Simpkin AL, Schwartzstein RM. Tolerating uncertainty: the next medical revolution? N Engl J Med. 2016;375(18):1713–15. DOI: 10.1056/NEJMp1606402
17. Gupta M. Is evidence-based psychiatry ethical? Oxford: Oxford University Press; 2014.
18. Constand MK, MacDermid JC, Dal Bello-Haas V, et al. Scoping review of patient-centered care approaches in healthcare. BMC Health Serv Res. 2014;14:271. DOI: 10.1186/1472-6963-14-271
19. Barry MJ, Edgman-Levitan S. Shared decision-making: the pinnacle of patient-centered

care. N Engl J Med. 2012;366(9):780–1. DOI: 10.1056/NEJMp1109283

20. Feyerabend P. Against method. London: New Left Books; 1975.

21. World Medical Association. World Medical Association Declaration of Helsinki: ethical principles for medical research involving human subjects. JAMA. 2013;310(20):2191–4. DOI: 10.1001/jama.2013.281053

22. Hoffman SJ. Ending medical complicity in state-sponsored torture. Lancet. 2011;378(9802):1535–7. DOI: 10.1016/S0140-6736(11)60816-7

23. Gross ML. Military medical ethics. Camb Q Healthc Ethics. 2013;22(1):92–109. DOI: 10.1017/S0963180112000424

24. Hedges C. The world as it is: dispatches on the myth of human progress. New York: Nation Books; 2013.

25. Popper K. In search of a better world: lectures and essays from thirty years. 1st ed. London: Routledge; 1995. p. 83.

26. Dyrbye LN, Thomas MR, Massie FS, et al. Burnout and suicidal ideation among US medical students. Ann Intern Med. 2008;149(5):334–41. PMID: 18765703.

27. Dzau V, Kirch D, Nasca T. To care is human: collectively confronting the clinician-burnout crisis. N Engl J Med. 2018;378(4):312–14. DOI: 10.1056/NEJMp1715127

28. Malina D. Performance anxiety: what can health care learn from K–12 education? N Engl J Med. 2013;369(13):1269–74. DOI: 10.1056/NEJMms1306048

Chapter 1

1. Blackburn S. Being good: a short introduction to ethics. Oxford: Oxford University Press; 2002.

2. Perkins R. Medical ethics. Lecture notes, Period III curriculum, University of Toronto; 1967; Toronto (ON). Gift from the author.

3. Horn J. Away with all pests: an English surgeon in People's China, 1954–69. New York: Monthly Review Press; 1969.

4. Maskalyk J. Six months in Sudan: a young doctor in a war-torn village. Toronto (ON): Random House; 2009.

5. Hilfiker D. Not all of us are saints: a doctor's journey with the poor. Toronto (ON): Macmillan; 1994.

6. Carlet J, Collignon P, Goldmann D, et al. Society's failure to protect a precious resource: antibiotics. Lancet. 2011;378(9788):369–71. DOI: 10.1016/S0140-6736(11)60401-7

7. National Commission for the Protection of Human Subjects of Biomedical and Behavioral Research. The Belmont report: ethical principles and guidelines for the protection of human subjects of research. Washington (DC): Office for Human Research Protections; 1978.

8. The President's Commission for the Study of Ethical Problems in Medicine and Biomedical and Behavioral Research. Deciding to forego life-sustaining treatment: a report on the ethical, medical, and legal issues in treatment decisions. Washington (DC): The President's Commission for the Study of Ethical Problems in Medicine and Biomedical and Behavioral Research; 1983.

9. The President's Commission for the Study of Ethical Problems in Medicine and Biomedical and Behavioral Research. Making health care decisions: a report on the ethical and legal implications of informed consent in the patient–practitioner relationship. Vol. 1. Washington (DC): The President's Commission for the Study of Ethical Problems in Medicine and Biomedical and Behavioral Research; 1982.

10. Pelčić G. Bioethics and medicine. Croat Med J. 2013;54(1): ditto. PMID:23444239.

11. Drummond D. The Happy MD [Internet]. TheHappyMD.com. Antibiotics for a virus? How to just say no; [cited 2017 Dec 3]; [about 4 screens]. Available from: https://www.thehappymd.com/blog/bid/290777/Antibiotics-for-a-Virus-How-to-Just-Say-No

12. Girgis L. How to say no to unreasonable patient requests [Internet]. UBM Medica; 2017 Oct 5 [cited 2017 Dec 3]; [about 2 screens]. Available from: http://www.physicianspractice.com/how-say-no-unreasonable-patient-requests

13. Ulrich CM, Taylor C, Soeken K, et al. Everyday ethics: ethical issues and stress in nursing practice. J Adv Nurs. 2010;66(11):2510–19. DOI: 10.1111/j.1365-2648.2010.05425

14. Jha V, Martin DE, Bargman JM, et al. Ethical issues in dialysis therapy. Lancet. 2017;389(10081):1851–56. DOI: 10.1016/S0140-6736(16)32408-4.

15. Hurst SA, Perrier A, Pegoraro R, et al. Ethical difficulties in clinical practice: experiences of European doctors. J Med Ethics. 2007;33(1):51–7. DOI: 10.1136/jme.2005.014266

16. Vallurupalli M. Mourning on morning rounds. N Engl J Med. 2013;369(5):404–5. DOI: 10.1056/NEJMp1300969

17. Brewin T. Primum non nocere? Lancet. 1994;344(8935):1487. PMID:7968126.

18. Smith CM. Origin and uses of primum non nocere: above all, do no harm! J Clin Pharmacol. 2005;45(4):371–7. DOI:10.1177/0091270004273680

19. Illich I. Medical nemesis: the expropriation of health. Toronto (ON): Random House; 1976.

20. "Drugs are the third leading cause of death after heart disease and cancer." Gøtzsche P. Deadly medicines and organised crime: how big pharma has corrupted healthcare. London: Radcliffe Publishing; 2013. p. 1.

21. Esmail A. Physician as serial killer: the Shipman case. N Engl J Med. 2005;352(18):1843–4. DOI:10.1056/NEJMp048331

22. Lemieux-Charles L, McGuire WL. What do we know about health care team effectiveness? A review of the literature. Med Care Res Rev. 2006;63(3):263–300. DOI:10.1177/1077558706287003

23. von Gunten CF. Discussing do-not-resuscitate status. J Clin Oncol. 2001;19(5):1576–81. DOI:10.1200/JCO.2001.19.5.1576

24. Kleinman A. Presence. Lancet. 2017;389(10088):2466–7. DOI: 10.1016/S0140-6736(17)31620-3

25. Jameson L. The empathy exams: essays. Minneapolis (MN): Graywolf Press; 2014.

26. Hébert PC. Good medicine: the art of ethical care in Canada. Toronto (ON): Random House Canada; 2016.

27. Frankfurt H. The reasons of love. Princeton (NJ): Princeton University Press; 2009.

28. Nussbaum M. Anger and forgiveness: resentment, generosity, justice. New York: Oxford University Press; 2016.

29. Nussbaum MC. Political emotions. Cambridge (MA): Harvard University Press; 2013. p. 3.

30. Williams B. Morality: an introduction to ethics. New York: Harper Torchbooks; 1972.

31. Oser TK, Haidet P, Lewis PR, et al. Frequency and negative impact of medical student mistreatment based on specialty choice: a longitudinal study. Acad Med. 2014;89(5):755-61. DOI: 10.1097/acm.0000000000000207

32. Cohen G. What's wrong with hospitals? London: Penguin Books; 1964.

33. Silver HK, Glicken AD. Medical student abuse: incidence, severity, and significance. JAMA. 1990;263(4):527–32. PMID: 2294324.

34. Hicks LK, Lin Y, Robertson DW, et al. Understanding the clinical dilemmas that shape medical students' ethical development: questionnaire survey and focus group study. BMJ. 2001;322(7288):709–10. PMID:11264209.

35. Peres MFT, Babler F, Arakaki JNL, et al. Mistreatment in an academic setting and medical students' perceptions about their course in São Paulo, Brazil: a cross-sectional study. Sao Paulo Med J. 2016;134(2):130–7. DOI: 10.1590/1516-3180.2015.01332210

36. Siller H, Tauber G, Komlenac N, et al. Gender differences and similarities in medical students' experiences of mistreatment by various groups of perpetrators. BMC Med Educ. 2017;17(1):134. DOI: 10.1186/s12909-017-0974-4

37. Pellegrino E, Thomasma D. The virtues in medical practice. New York: Oxford University Press; 1993. p. 177.

38. Bursch B, Fried JM, Wimmers PF, et al. Relationship between medical student perceptions of mistreatment and mistreatment sensitivity. Med Teach. 2013;35(3):e998-1002. DOI: 10.3109/0142159X.2012.733455

39. Srivastava R. Speaking up: when doctors navigate medical hierarchy. N Engl J Med. 2013;368(4):302-5. DOI: 10.1056/NEJMp1212410

40. Fried JM, Vermillion M, Parker NH, et al. Eradicating medical student mistreatment: a longitudinal study of one institution's efforts. Acad Med. 2012;87(9):1191–8. DOI: 10.1097/ACM.0b013e3182625408

41. Lucey C, Levinson W, Ginsburg S. Medical student mistreatment. JAMA. 2016;316(21):2263–4. DOI: 10.1001/jama.2016.17752

42. Cook A, Arora VM, Rasinski K, et al. The prevalence of medical student mistreatment and its association with burnout. Acad Med. 2014;89(5):749–54. DOI: 10.1097/ACM.0000000000000204

43. Barrett J, Scott KM. Acknowledging medical students' reports of intimidation and humiliation by their teachers in hospitals.

J Paediatr Child Health. 2018;54(2):69–73. DOI:10.1111/jpc.13656

44. Cooke M, Irby D, Sullivan W, et al. American medical education 100 years after the Flexner Report. N Engl J Med. 2006;355(13):1339–44. DOI:10.1056/NEJMra055445

45. Kumar S. Burnout and doctors: prevalence, prevention and intervention. Healthcare. 2016;4(3):37. DOI: 10.3390/healthcare4030037

46. Muller D. Kathryn. N Engl J Med. 2017;376(12):1101–3. DOI: 10.1056/NEJMp1615141

47. This case is adapted from Burrows A. The man who didn't know he had cancer. JAMA. 1991;266(18):2550. PMID:1942391.

48. Based on a short story by Williams WC. The use of force [Internet]. EServer Fiction. Available at: http://fiction.eserver.org/short/the_use_of_force.html

Chapter 2

1. Parfit D. On what matters. Vol. 1. Oxford: Oxford University Press; 2011. p. 419.

2. Clarfield AM, Gordon M, Markwell H, et al. Ethical issues in end-of-life geriatric care: the approach of three monotheistic religions—Judaism, Catholicism, and Islam. J Am Geriatr Soc. 2003;51(8):1149-54. DOI: 10.1046/j.1532-5415.2003.51364.x

3. De Ville K. 'What does the law say?' Law, ethics, and medical decision making. West J Med. 1994;160(5):478-80. PMID: PMC1022504.

4. Hathout L. The right to practice medicine without repercussions: ethical issues in times of political strife. Philos Ethics Humanit Med. 2012;7(1):11. DOI: 10.1186/1747-5341-7-11

5. De Peyer R. Ireland abortion vote: how the death of Savita Halappanavar helped bring about referendum. Evening Standard [Internet]. 2018 May 25;World:[about 4 screens]. Available from: https://www.standard.co.uk/news/world/savita-halappanavar-how-an-indian-dentists-death-helped-bring-about-the-referendum-on-abortion-in-a3848356.html

6. Saadi A, Ahmed S, Katz M. Making the case for sanctuary hospitals. JAMA. 2017;318(21):2079-80. DOI:10.1001/jama.2017.15714

7. Sontag D. Deported in a coma, saved back in US. New York Times. 2008 Nov 8;9.

8. MacKenzie M, Bosk E, Zeanah C. Separating families at the border: consequences for children's health and well-being. N Engl J Med. 2017;376(24):2313–15. DOI: 10.1056/NEJMp1703375

9. Hart HLA. Positivism and the separation of law and morals. Harv Law Rev. 1958;71(4):593–629. DOI:10.2307/1338225

10. Rowan M. The latest chapter in the saga of a spiritless law: detaining Haitian asylum seekers as a violation of the spirit and the letter of international law. U Md Law J Race Relig Gender Class. 2003;3(2):371–404. Available from: https://digitalcommons.law.umaryland.edu/rrgc/vol3/iss2/8/

11. Bloche MG. The Supreme Court and the purposes of medicine. N Engl J Med. 2006;354(10):993–5. DOI: 10.1056/NEJMp068019

12. Kent CA. Medical ethics: the state of the law. Markham (ON): LexisNexis-Butterworths; 2005.

13. Pellegrino E, Thomasma D. The virtues in medical practice. Oxford: Oxford University Press; 1993.

14. Parfit D. On what matters. Vol. 1. Oxford: Oxford University Press; 2011. p. 375.

15. Aristotle. Nicomachean ethics. Ostwald M, translator. New York: Bobbs-Merrill; 1962. p. 33–5.

16. MacIntyre A. After virtue: a study in moral theory. 2nd ed. Notre Dame (IN): University of Notre Dame Press; 1984.

17. Kant I. The groundwork of the metaphysic of morals. Paton HJ, translator. New York: Harper Torchbooks; 1964. p. 88–9.

18. Bok S. Lying. Toronto (ON): Random House Books; 1979. p. 41–4.

19. Kant I. The groundwork of the metaphysic of morals. Paton HJ, translator. New York: Harper Torchbooks; 1964. p. 96.

20. Khurana T. Kant and colonialism: historical and critical perspectives. Notre Dame Philos Rev. 2015;08(42). Available from: https://ndpr.nd.edu/news/kant-and-colonialism-historical-and-critical-perspectives/

21. Rawls J. A theory of justice. Cambridge (MA): Harvard University Press; 1971.

22. Cohen GA. Rescuing justice and equality. Cambridge (MA): Harvard University Press; 2008. p. 5–7.

23. Mill JS. Utilitarianism. London: Longmans, Green and Company; 1901.

24. Sen A, Williams B. Utilitarianism and beyond. Cambridge (UK): Cambridge University Press; 1982.

25. Mill, JS. On Liberty. New York: Appleton-Century Crofts, Meredith Publishing; 1947.

26. Singer P. Ethics in the real world: 82 brief essays on things that matter. Princeton (NJ): Princeton University Press; 2016.

27. Sumner W. The hateful and the obscene: studies in the limits of free expression. Toronto (ON): University of Toronto Press; 2004.

28. Singer P. Rethinking life and death: the collapse of our traditional ethics. New York: St Martin's Press; 1994.

29. Mason E. Value pluralism [Internet]. In: Zalta EN, editor. The Stanford encyclopedia of philosophy. Spring 2018 ed. Stanford (CA): Metaphysics Research Lab, Stanford University; 2018. Available from: https://plato.stanford.edu/archives/spr2018/entries/value-pluralism/

30. Sen A. The idea of justice. Cambridge (MA): Harvard University Press; 2011.

31. Sen A. Inequality re-examined. Cambridge (MA): Harvard University Press; 1992.

32. Nussbaum MC. Frontiers of justice: disability, nationality, species membership. Cambridge (MA): Harvard University Press; 2006. p. 76–8. This list of the "minimal requirements" for human well-being is open-ended and being modified.

33. Nussbaum MC. Frontiers of justice: disability, nationality, species membership. Cambridge (MA): Harvard University Press; 2006. p. 75.

34. Kinghorn P, Coast J. Assessing the capability to experience a 'good death'. PLOS ONE. 2018;13(2):e0193181. DOI: 10.1371/journal.pone.0193181

35. Nussbaum MC. Upheavals of thought: the intelligence of emotions. New York: Cambridge University Press; 2001. p. 1.

36. Nussbaum MC. Upheavals of thought: the intelligence of emotions. New York: Cambridge University Press; 2001. p. 392.

37. Charon R. Narrative and medicine. N Engl J Med. 2004;350(9):862–4. DOI:10.1056/NEJMp038249

38. Divinsky M. Stories for life. Can Fam Physician. 2007;53(2):203–5. PMID:17872627.

39. Peterkin A. Practical strategies for practising narrative-based medicine. Can Fam Physician. 2012;58(1):63–4. PMID:22267625.

40. Meekosha H. The complex balancing act of choice, autonomy, valued life, and rights: bringing a feminist disability perspective to bioethics. IJFAB. 2010;3(2):1–8. DOI: 10.2979/fab.2010.3.2.1

41. Garland-Thomson R. Integrating disability, transforming feminist theory. NWSA J. 2002;14(3):1–32. Available from: http://www.jstor.org/stable/4316922

42. Sherwin S. Relational autonomy. In: Llewellyn JJ, Downie J, editors. Being relational: reflections on relational theory and health law. Vancouver (BC): UBC Press; 2012. p. 13–34.

43. Donchin A. Converging concerns: feminist bioethics, development theory, and human rights. Signs. 2004;29(2):299–324. DOI:10.1086/378104

44. Jonsen A, Toulmin S. The abuse of casuistry: a history of moral reasoning. Los Angeles (CA): University of California Press; 1988. p. 265.

45. Jonsen A, Toulmin S. The abuse of casuistry: a history of moral reasoning. Los Angeles (CA): University of California Press; 1988. p. 313.

46. Nussbaum M. Frontiers of justice. Cambridge (MA): Harvard University Press; 2007. p. 277.

47. Beauchamp T, Childress J. Principles of biomedical ethics. 7th ed. New York: Oxford University Press; 2013.

48. Gellner E. Thought and change. Chicago (IL): Midway Reprints, University of Chicago Press; 1964.

49. Parfit D. On what matters. Vol. 1. Oxford: Oxford University Press; 2011.

50. Kekes J. How should we live? A practical approach to everyday morality. Chicago (IL): University of Chicago Press; 2014. p. 168.

51. Hill J. A healthy dose of fallibilism. Taming the SRU. 2016 Aug 18 [cited 2018 Jan 20] Available from: http://www.tamingthesru.com/blog/grand-rounds/fallibilism

52. Gupta M, Upshur R. Critical thinking in clinical medicine: what is it? J Eval Clin Pract. 2012;18(5):938–44. DOI: 10.1111/j.1365-2753.2012.01897.x

53. Lévi-Strauss C. The savage mind. Chicago (IL): University of Chicago Press; 1966.

Chapter 3

1. Hume D. A treatise of human nature. Atkin H, editor. New York: Harper Collins Press; 1975. p. 43.
2. Lo B. Resolving ethical dilemmas: a guide for clinicians. 5th edition. Philadelphia (PA): Lippincott Williams & Wilkins; 2013.
3. Thomasma D. Training in medical ethics: an ethical workup. Forum Med. 1978;1(9):33–6. PMID: 10239719.
4. Jonsen A, Siegler M, Winslade W. Clinical ethics. 5th ed. New York: McGraw-Hill; 2002.
5. Sherwin S. Relational autonomy. In: Llewellyn JJ, Downie J, editors. Being relational: reflections on relational theory and health law. Vancouver (BC): UBC Press; 2012. p. 13–34.
6. Thanks to Dr Mary Rose MacDonald for making this point.
7. Sen A. Identity and violence: the illusion of destiny. New Delhi: Penguin Books India; 2007.
8. Rhodes KV, Frankel RM, Levinthal N, et al. "You're not a victim of domestic abuse, are you?" Provider–patient communication about domestic violence. Ann Intern Med. 2007;147(9):620–7. PMID: 17975184.
9. Liebschutz J, Rothman E. Intimate-partner violence—what physicians can do. N Engl J Med. 2012;367(22):2071–3. DOI: 10.1056/NEJMp1204278
10. Burnum J. Secrets about patients. N Engl J Med. 1991;324(16):1130–3. DOI: 10.1056/NEJM199104183241611
11. Styron W. Sophie's choice. New York: Random House; 2004.
12. Li H, Rosenzweig M, Zhang J. Altruism, favoritism, and guilt in the allocation of family resources: Sophie's Choice in Mao's mass send-down movement. J Political Econ. 2010;118(1):1–38. DOI: 10.1086/650315
13. Korones D. The long ride home. N Engl J Med. 2018;378(17):1569–71. DOI: 10.1056/NEJMp1801166
14. Callahan S. The role of emotion in ethical decision making. Hastings Cent Rep. 1988;18(3):9–14. PMID: 3397281.
15. Gardner A. A fateful winter's night. Sometimes doing the right thing is the hardest thing. Minn Med. 2014;97(11-12):26–7. PMID: 25651649.
16. Mill JS. On liberty. Wooster (OH): Appleton-Century-Crofts; 1947.
17. Attia E. Eating disorders. Ann Intern Med. 2012;156(7):ITC4-1. DOI: 10.7326/0003-4819-156-7-201204030-01004
18. Robb AS, Silber TJ, Orrell-Valente JK, et al. Supplemental nocturnal nasogastric refeeding for better short-term outcome in hospitalized adolescent girls with anorexia nervosa. Am J Psychiatry. 2002;159(8):1347–53. DOI: 10.1176/appi.ajp.159.8.1347
19. Levy-Barzilai V. Death wish: does an anorexic whose life is in danger have a right to starve herself to death? Ha'aretz [Internet]. 2001 Aug 17:[about 15 screens]. Available from: https://www.haaretz.com/1.5385498
20. Christodoulou M. Pro-anorexia websites pose public health challenge. Lancet. 2012;379(9811):110. PMID: 22256351.
21. Szasz TS. Ideology and insanity: essays on the psychiatric dehumanization of man. Syracuse (NY): Syracuse University Press; 1991. p. 52.
22. Burns-Cox C, Halpin D, Frost CS, et al. Ethical treatment of military detainees. Lancet. 2007;370(9604):1999–2000. DOI: 10.1016/S0140-6736(07)61853-4
23. Bruch H. The golden cage: the enigma of anorexia nervosa. Cambridge (MA): Harvard University Press; 2001.
24. Annas GJ. Hunger strikes at Guantanamo – medical ethics and human rights in a "legal black hole." N Engl J Med. 2006;355(13):1377. DOI: 10.1056/NEJMhle062316
25. Schneiderman LJ, Faber-Langendoen K, Jecker NS. Beyond futility to an ethic of care. Am J Med. 1994;96(2):110–4. PMID: 8109595.
26. Welsh J. Responding to food refusal. In: Goodman R and Roseman MJ, editors. Interrogations, forced feedings, and the role of health professionals: new perspectives on international human rights, humanitarian law, and ethics. Vol. 1. Cambridge (MA): Human Rights Program at Harvard Law School; 2009. p. 152.
27. Homer. The Odyssey. Wilson E, translator. New York: W. W. Norton & Co.; 2018. p. 302–13.
28. Strauss S. Death: one, Medicine: no score. CMAJ. 2007;177(8):903-4. DOI: 10.1503/cmaj.071282
29. Hébert P, C. Weingarten M. The ethics of forced feeding in anorexia nervosa. CMAJ. 1991;144(2):141–4. PMID: 1898869.

30. Palmer RL. Death in anorexia nervosa. Lancet. 2003;361(9368):1490. DOI:10.1016/S0140-6736(03)13221-7

31. Nussbaum MC. Upheavals of thought: the intelligence of emotions. Cambridge (UK): Cambridge University Press; 2003.

32. Hume D. A treatise of human nature. Selby-Bigge L, editor. Oxford: Oxford University Clarendon Press; 1967. p. 457.

33. Hume D. A treatise of human nature. Selby-Bigge L, editor. Oxford: Oxford University Clarendon Press; 1967. p. 618.

Chapter 4

1. The English Dictionarie, 1623. Oxford English dictionary [CD-ROM]. 2nd ed. Oxford: Oxford University Press; 2002. "autonomy, n."

2. Sen A. Identity and violence: the illusion of destiny. New Delhi: Penguin Books India; 2007.

3. Wolpaw DR. Seeing eye to eye. N Engl J Med. 2011;365(22):2052–3. DOI: 10.1056/NEJMp1108469

4. Baker LH, O'Connell D, Platt FW. "What else?" Setting the agenda for the clinical interview. Ann Intern Med. 2005;143(10):766–70. PMID: 16287811.

5. Coulehan JL, Platt FW, Egener B, et al. "Let me see if I have this right . . .": words that help build empathy. Ann Intern Med. 2001;135(3):221–7. PMID: 11487497.

6. Walker J, Leveille SG, Ngo L, et al. Inviting patients to read their doctors' notes: patients and doctors look ahead: patient and physician surveys. Ann Intern Med. 2011;155(12):811–9. DOI: 10.7326/0003-4819-155-12-201112200-00003

7. Killoran M, Moyer A. Surgical treatment preferences in Chinese-American women with early-stage breast cancer. Psychooncology. 2006;15(11):969–84. DOI: 10.1002/pon.1032

8. See also: Morrow M, Winograd J, Freer P, et al. Case 8-2013: a 48-year-old woman with carcinoma in situ of the breast. N Engl J Med. 2013;368(11):1046–53. DOI: 10.1056/NEJMcpc1214221. The latter case is of a woman who wanted, and received, bilateral mastectomy, not the unilateral BCS that was initially offered.

9. Joseph K, Vrouwe S, Kamruzzaman A, et al. Outcome analysis of breast cancer patients who declined evidence-based treatment. World J Surg Oncol. 2012;10:118. DOI: 10.1186/1477-7819-10-118. See also: El-Charnoubi W, Svendsen J, Tange U, et al. Women with inoperable or locally advanced breast cancer—what characterizes them? A retrospective review of 157 cases. Acta Oncol. 2012;51(8):1081–5. DOI: 10.3109/0284186X.2012.707788

10. Oxford English dictionary [CD-ROM]. 2nd ed. Oxford: Oxford University Press; 2002. "autonomy, n."

11. Kant I. The groundwork of the metaphysic of morals. Paton HJ, translator. New York: Harper Torchbooks, Harper and Row; 1958. p. 132.

12. Kaufman W. Without guilt and justice: from decidophobia to autonomy. New York: PH Wyden; 1973. p. 273.

13. Schneider C. The practice of autonomy: patients, doctors, and medical decisions. New York: Oxford University Press; 1998.

14. Bartley W III. The retreat to commitment. 2nd ed. La Salle (IL): Open Court; 1984.

15. Frankfurt H. The reasons of love. Princeton (NJ): Princeton University Press; 2004. ft. 5, p. 20.

16. Descartes R. Discourse on method: discourse 4. Sutcliffe F, translator. Baltimore (MD): Penguin Books; 1968. p. 53.

17. Malette v Shulman, [1987] 63 OR 2d 243 (ONHCJ).

18. Malette v Shulman, [1990] 72 OR 2d 417 (ONCA).

19. Fleming v Reid, [1991] 4 OR 3d 74 (ONCA).

20. Holt GE, Sarmento B, Kett D, et al. An unconscious patient with a DNR tattoo. N Engl J Med. 2017;377(22):2192-3. PMID: 29171810.

21. Migden DR, Braen GR. The Jehovah's Witness blood refusal card: ethical and medicolegal considerations for emergency physicians. Acad Emerg Med. 1998;5(8):815–24. PMID:9715245.

22. Brauer S, Biller-Andorno N, Andorno R, workshop convenors. Country reports on advance directives. ESF exploratory workshop: advance directives: towards a coordinated European perspective?; 2008 Jun 18-22; Zurich, Switzerland. Zurich: Institute of Biomedical Ethics, University of Zurich; 2008. Available from: https://www.ethik.uzh.ch/dam/jcr:00000000-14d5-886d-ffff-ffff1488f30/Country_Reports_AD.pdf

23. Brockwell H. Why can't I get sterilized in my 20's? The Guardian [Internet]. 2015 Jan 28;Opinion:[about 3 screens]. Available from: https://www.theguardian.com/commentisfree/2015/jan/28/why-wont-nhs-let-me-be-sterilised

24. Pearson C. Meet the 20-somethings who want to be sterilized. Huffington Post [Internet]. 2014 Oct 24;Women:[about 9 screens]. Available from: https://www.huffingtonpost.ca/entry/female-sterilization-young-women_n_5882000

25. Thanks to Dr Chryssa McAllister for emphasizing this point.

26. Lunau K. Tying the knot. Maclean's. 2007 Nov 12;Health:51. Available from: https://archive.macleans.ca/article/2007/11/12/tying-the-knot

27. Based loosely on: Allan v New Mount Sinai Hospital, [1980] 28 OR 2d 356 (HC).

28. Allan v New Mount Sinai Hospital, [1980] 28 OR 2d 356 (HC).

29. Sneiderman B, Irvine J, Osborne P. Canadian medical law. 3rd ed. Toronto (ON): Thomsen Carswell; 2003. p. 23.

30. Based loosely on: Allan v New Mount Sinai Hospital, [1980] 28 OR 2d 356, 364 (HC).

31. Brock DW, Wartman SA. When competent patients make irrational choices. N Engl J Med. 1990;322(22):1595–9. DOI: 10.1056/NEJM199005313222209

32. McIntyre L. Post-truth. Cambridge (MA): MIT Press; 2018.

33. Feyerabend P. Against method. London: New Left Books; 1975.

34. Canadian Institute for Health Information. Drug use among seniors in Canada, 2016. Ottawa (ON): CIHI; 2018.

35. Bogunovic OJ, Greenfield SF. Practical geriatrics: use of benzodiazepines among elderly patients. Psychiatr Serv. 2004;55(3):233–5. DOI: 10.1176/appi.ps.55.3.233

36. Farrell L. The threat. BMJ. 2006;332(7554):1399. DOI: 10.1136/bmj.332.7554.1399-a

37. Reuben DB, Tinetti ME. Goal-oriented patient care: an alternative health outcomes paradigm. N Engl J Med. 2012;366(9):777-9. DOI: 10.1056/NEJMp1113631.

38. Heeren T, Derksen P, van Heycop Ten Ham BF, et al. Treatment, outcome and predictors of response in elderly depressed in-patients. Br J Psychiatry. 1997;170(5):436–40. PMID: 9307693.

39. Reyes-Ortiz CA. Diogenes syndrome: the self-neglect elderly. Compr Ther. 2001;27(2):117. PMID: 11430258.

40. Wikipedia [Internet]. Wikimedia Foundation, Inc.; 2018. Diogenes and Alexander; 2018 Oct 26 [cited 2018 May 31]; [about 6 screens]. Available from: https://en.wikipedia.org/wiki/Diogenes_and_Alexander

41. Mitchell AJ, Lord O, Malone D. Differences in the prescribing of medication for physical disorders in individuals with and without mental illness: a meta-analysis. Br J Psychiatry. 2012;201(6):435. DOI: 10.1192/bjp.bp.111.094532

42. Groves J. Taking care of the hateful patient. N Engl J Med. 1978;298(16):883-887. DOI: 10.1056/NEJM197804202981605

43. Hardy R, Kell C. Understanding and working with the concept of denial and its role as a coping strategy. Nurs Times. 2009;105 (32-33):22–4. PMID: 19736742.

44. Foster C. Putting dignity to work. Lancet. 2012;379(9831):2044–5. PMID: 22666882. DOI: https://doi.org/10.1016/S0140-6736(12)60885-X

45. Siegler M. Critical illness: the limits of autonomy. Hastings Cent Rep. 1977;7(5):12–15. PMID: 914506.

46. Srivastava R. Dealing with uncertainty in a time of plenty. N Engl J Med. 2011;365(24):2252–3. PMID: 22168641.

47. Bardes CL. Defining "patient-centered medicine." N Engl J Med. 2012;366(9):782–3. DOI: 10.1056/NEJMp1200070

48. Hébert PC, Selby D. Should a reversible, but lethal, incident not be treated when a patient has a do-not-resuscitate order? CMAJ. 2014;186(7):528–30. DOI: 10.1503/cmaj.111772

Chapter 5

1. Schloendorff v Society of New York Hospital, 105 NE 92 (NYCA 1914).

2. Friedman DA. Informed dissent: a new corollary to the informed consent doctrine? Chi-Kent Law Rev. 1981;57(4):1119–44. PMID: 11658347.

3. Evans KG. Consent: a guide for Canadian physicians [Internet]. Ottawa (ON): CMPA; 2016 [cited 2017 Nov 2017]. Available from: https://www.cmpa-acpm.ca/en/advice-publications/handbooks/consent-a-guide-for-canadian-physicians#implied%20consent

4. Hopp v Lepp, [1980] 2 SCR 192.
5. Salgo v Leland Stanford Jr. University Board of Trustees, 154 Cal. App. 2d 560 (Cal. Ct. App. 1957).
6. Kroft D. Informed consent: a comparative analysis. J Int Law Pract. 1997;6:457.
7. Beauchamp TL. Informed consent: its history, meaning, and present challenges. Camb Q Healthc Ethics. 2011;20(4):515-23. PMID: 21843382.
8. Canterbury v Spence, 464 F.2d 772 (D.C. Cir. 1972).
9. Reibl v Hughes, [1980] 2 SCR 880.
10. Shinal v Toms, 162 A.3d 429 (Pa. 2017).
11. Fernandez Lynch H, Joffe S, Feldman EA. Informed consent and the role of the treating physician. N Engl J Med. 2018;378(25):2433-8. PMID: 29924950.
12. Arndt v Smith, [1997] 2 SCR 539.
13. Farnsworth MG. Evaluation of mental competency. Am Fam Physician. 1989;39(6):182-90. PMID: 2729043.
14. Ziegler DK, Mosier MC, Buenaver M, et al. How much information about adverse effects of medication do patients want from physicians? Arch Intern Med. 2001;161(5):706-13. PMID: 11231703.
15. Woloshin S, Schwartz LM. Communicating data about the benefits and harms of treatment: a randomized trial. Ann Intern Med. 2011;155(2):87-96. PMID: 21768582.
16. Schwartz LM, Woloshin S, Welch HG. Using a drug facts box to communicate drug benefits and harms: two randomized trials. Ann Intern Med. 2009;150(8):516-27. PMID: 19221371.
17. The Royal Australian & New Zealand College of Psychiatrists. Professional practice guideline 10: Antipsychotic medications as a treatment of behavioural and psychological symptoms of dementia [Internet]. Melbourne (AU): RANZCP; 2016. Available from: https://www.ranzcp.org/Files/Resources/College_Statements/Practice_Guidelines/pg10-pdf.aspx
18. Brummel-Smith K. It's time to require written informed consent when using antipsychotics in dementia. BJMP. 2008;1(2):4-6.

Chapter 6
1. Durrell L. The Alexandria quartet: Clea. New York: E.P. Dutton & Co.; 1961.
2. Friedman DA. Informed dissent: a new corollary to the informed consent doctrine?

Chi-Kent Law Rev. 1981;57(4):1119-44. PMID: 11658347.
3. Conti AA. From informed consent to informed dissent in health care: historical evolution in the twentieth century. Acta Biomed. 2017;88(2):201-3. PMID: 28845838.
4. Bélanger-Hardy L. Informed consent in medical care. In: Erdman J, Gruben V, Nelson E, editors. Canadian health law and policy. 5th ed. Toronto (ON): LexisNexis Canada Inc.; 2017. p. 329-49.
5. Evans KG. A medico-legal handbook for Canadian physicians. Ottawa (ON): Canadian Medical Protective Association; 1990.
6. Oxford English dictionary [CD-ROM]. 2nd ed. Oxford: Oxford University Press; 2002.
7. Daniels v Heskin, IR 73 (Supreme Court of Ireland 1954).
8. Oken D. What to tell cancer patients. A study of medical attitudes. JAMA. 1961;175:1120-8. PMID: 13730593.
9. Novack DH, Plumer R, Smith RL, et al. Changes in physicians' attitudes toward telling the cancer patient. JAMA. 1979;241(9):897-900. PMID: 762865.
10. Delvecchio Good MJ, Good BJ, Schaffer C, et al. American oncology and the discourse on hope. Cult Med Psychiatry. 1990;14(1):59-79. PMID: 2340733.
11. Samp RJ, Curreri AR. A questionnaire survey on public cancer education obtained from cancer patients and their families. Cancer. 1957;10(2):382-4. PMID: 13426996.
12. President's Commission for the Study of Ethical Problems in Medicine and Biomedical and Behavioral Research. Congressional Record. 1978;124(168):H13571-3. PMID: 11661779.
13. Elson P. Do older adults presenting with memory complaints wish to be told if later diagnosed with Alzheimer's disease? Int J Geriatr Psychiatry. 2006;21(5):419-25. PMID: 16676286.
14. Silverstein MD, Stocking CB, Antel JP, et al. Amyotrophic lateral sclerosis and life-sustaining therapy: patients' desires for information, participation in decision making, and life-sustaining therapy. Mayo Clin Proc. 1991;66(9):906-13. PMID: 1921500.
15. Ajaj A, Singh MP, Abdulla AJ. Should elderly patients be told they have cancer? Questionnaire survey of older people. BMJ. 2001;323(7322):1160. PMID: 11711408.

16. Nyberg D. The varnished truth. Chicago (IL): University of Chicago Press; 1993.

17. Groopman J. The anatomy of hope. New York: Random House; 2005.

18. Elian M, Dean G. To tell or not to tell the diagnosis of multiple sclerosis. Lancet. 1985;2(8445):27–8. PMID: 2861463.

19. Fallowfield LJ, Hall A, Maguire P, et al. Psychological effects of being offered choice of surgery for breast cancer. BMJ. 1994;309(6952):448. PMID: 7920129.

20. Anonymous. Once a dark secret. BMJ. 1994;308(6927):542. DOI: 10.1136/bmj.308.6927.542

21. Mongan NP, Tadokoro-Cuccaro R, Bunch T, et al. Androgen insensitivity syndrome. Best Pract Res Clin Endocrinol Metab. 2015;29(4):569–80. PMID: 26303084.

22. Bok S. Lying: moral choice in public and private life. Toronto (ON): Random House; 1979.

23. Berger JT. Ignorance is bliss? Ethical considerations in therapeutic nondisclosure. Cancer Invest. 2005;23(1):94–8. PMID: 15779872.

24. Bowling A, Ebrahim S. Measuring patients' preferences for treatment and perceptions of risk. Qual Health Care. 2001;10 Suppl 1:i2-8. PMID: 11533430.

25. Egbert LD, Battit GE, Welch CE, et al. Reduction of postoperative pain by encouragement and instruction of patients. A study of doctor–patient rapport. N Engl J Med. 1964;270:825–7. PMID: 14108087.

26. Luck A, Pearson S, Maddern G, et al. Effects of video information on precolonoscopy anxiety and knowledge: a randomised trial. Lancet. 1999;354(9195):2032–5. PMID: 10636368.

27. Woloshin S, Schwartz LM, Welch HG. The effectiveness of a primer to help people understand risk: two randomized trials in distinct populations. Ann Intern Med. 2007;146(4):256–65. PMID: 17310049.

28. Kaplan SH, Greenfield S, Gandek B, et al. Characteristics of physicians with participatory decision-making styles. Ann Intern Med. 1996;124(5):497–504. PMID: 8602709.

29. Bursztajn H, Feinbloom R, Hamm R, et al. Medical choices, medical chances: how patients, families, and physicians can cope with uncertainty. New York: Dell Publishing; 1981.

30. Cabot RC. The use of truth and falsehood in medicine: an experimental study. JAMA. 1903;XL(15):994. DOI:10.1001/jama.1903.02490150046006

31. Etchells E, Sharpe G, Walsh P, et al. Bioethics for clinicians: 1. Consent. " CMAJ. 1996;155(2):177–80. PMID: 8800075.

32. Beauchamp TL, Childress JF. Principles of biomedical ethics. 5th ed. New York: Oxford University Press; 2001.

33. Reibl v Hughes, [1980] 2 SCR 880.

34. Hopp v Lepp, [1980] 2 SCR 192.

35. Picard E, Robertson G. Legal Liability of Doctors and Hospitals in Canada. 3rd ed. Toronto, Carswell Thomson, 1996.

36. Sharpe G. The law and medicine in Canada. 2nd ed. Toronto (ON): Butterworths; 1987. p. 57.

37. Evans KG. Consent: A guide for Canadian physicians [Internet]. Ottawa (ON): CMPA; 2016 [cited 2017 Nov]. Available from: https://www.cmpa-acpm.ca/en/advice-publications/handbooks/consent-a-guide-for-canadian-physicians#implied%20consent

38. Miola J. Autonomy rued OK? Al Hamwi v Johnston and another. Med Law Rev. 2006;14(1):108–14. PMID: 16787909.

39. Cojocaru v British Columbia Women's Hospital and Health Centre, 2013 SCC 30, [2013] 2 SCR 357.

40. Re T. 4 All ER 649 (CA 1992).

41. Buchanan A. Mental capacity, legal competence and consent to treatment. J R Soc Med. 2004;97(9):415-20. PMID: PMC1079581.

42. Dykeman MJ, Dewhirst K. Voluntariness. In: Singer PA, Viens AM, editors. The Cambridge textbook of bioethics. Cambridge (UK): Cambridge University Press; 2008. p. 31–5.

43. Kahneman D. Thinking, fast and slow. Toronto (ON): Doubleday Canada; 2011.

44. McNeil BJ, Pauker SG, Sox HC Jr, et al. On the elicitation of preferences for alternative therapies. N Engl J Med. 1982;306(21):1259–62. PMID: 7070445.

45. Ingelfinger FJ. Arrogance. N Engl J Med. 1980;303(26):1507–11. PMID: 7432420.

46. Sherlock R. Reasonable men and sick human beings. Am J Med. 1986;80(1):2–4. PMID: 3942152.

47. Veatch RM. Abandoning informed consent. Hastings Cent Rep. 1995;25(2):5–12. PMID: 7782200.

48. Boyd K. The impossibility of informed consent? J Med Ethics. 2015;41(1):44–7. PMID: 25516933.

49. McKneally MF, Martin DK, Ignagni E, et al. Responding to trust: surgeons' perspective on informed consent. World J Surg. 2009;33(7):1341–7. PMID: 19381720.

50. McKneally MF, Martin DK. An entrustment model of consent for surgical treatment of life-threatening illness: perspective of patients requiring esophagectomy. J Thorac Cardiovasc Surg. 2000;120(2):264–9. PMID: 10917940.

51. McKneally MF, Ignagni E, Martin DK, et al. The leap to trust: perspective of cholecystectomy patients on informed decision making and consent. J Am Coll Surg. 2004;199(1):51–7. PMID: 15217630.

52. O'Neill O. Some limits of informed consent. J Med Ethics. 2003;29(1):4–7. PMID: 12569185.

53. Aja B. The effects of pain on informed consent [Internet]. Nurse Anesthesia Capstones. 2017 [cited 2017 Dec 11];10. Available from: https://dune.une.edu/na_capstones/10

54. Brewster GS, Herbert ME, Hoffman JR. Medical myth: analgesia should not be given to patients with an acute abdomen because it obscures the diagnosis. West J Med. 2000;172(3):209–10. PMID: PMC1070812.

55. Ciarlariello v Schacter [1993] 2 SCR 119.

56. Nightingale v Kaplovitch, [1989] OJ No. 585 (QL HC).

57. Macdonald L, Sackett D, Haynes R, et al. Labelling in hypertension: a review of the behavioural and psychological consequences. J Chronic Dis. 1984;37(12):933–42.

58. Jenkins V, Fallowfield L, Saul J. Information needs of patients with cancer: results from a large study in UK cancer centres. Br J Cancer. 2001;84(1):48–51. DOI: 10.1054/bjoc.2000.1573

59. Sato R, Beppu H, Iba N, et al. The meaning of life prognosis disclosure for Japanese cancer patients: a qualitative study of patients' narratives. Chronic Illn. 2012;8(3):225–36. DOI: 10.1177/1742395312448940

60. Schattner A. What do patients really want to know? QJM. 2002;95(3):135–6. PMID: 11865167.

61. Brown JB, Boles M, Mullooly JP, et al. Effect of clinician communication skills training on patient satisfaction. A randomized, controlled trial. Ann Intern Med. 1999;131(11):822–9. PMID: 10610626.

62. El-Wakeel H, Taylor GJ, Tate JJ. What do patients really want to know in an informed consent procedure? A questionnaire-based survey of patients in the Bath area, UK. J Med Ethics. 2006;32(10):612–6. PMID: 17012508.

63. Jonsen A, Siegler M, Winslade W. Clinical ethics. 5th ed. New York: McGraw-Hill; 2002.

64. Mann AH. Factors affecting psychological state during one year on a hypertension trial. Clin Invest Med. 1981;4(3-4):197–200. PMID: 7039900.

65. Temple WJ. Inspiring hope—A physician's responsibility, translating the science into clinical practice. J Surg Oncol. 2018;117(4):545-550. DOI: 10.1002/jso.24887

66. Chochinov HM, Tataryn DJ, Wilson KG, et al. Prognostic awareness and the terminally ill. Psychosomatics. 2000;41(6):500–4. PMID: 11110113. See: De Lima Thomas J. When patients seem overly optimistic. AMA Virtual Mentor. 2012;14(7):539–44. DOI: 10.1001/virtualmentor.2012.14.7.ecas2-1207

Chapter 7

1. Lyttelton G. The Works of Lord George Lyttelton. Dublin; J Williams; 1775. p. 202. Available from: https://catalog.hathitrust.org/Record/007666225

2. Siegler M. Confidentiality in medicine: a decrepit concept. N Engl J Med. 1982;307:1518–21. DOI: 10.1056/NEJM198212093072411

3. Gibson E. Publication of case reports: Is consent required? Paediatr Child Health. 2008;13(8):666–7. PMID: PMC2606070.

4. Appelbaum PS. Privacy in psychiatric treatment: threats and responses. Am J Psychiatry. 2002;159(11):1809–18. PMID: 12411211.

5. Warren SD, Brandeis LD. The right to privacy. Harv Law Rev. 1890;4(5):193-220.
6. Igo S. The known citizen: a history of privacy in modern America. Cambridge (MA): Harvard University Press; 2018.
7. Yao-Huai L. Privacy and data privacy issues in contemporary China. Ethics Inf Technol. 2005;7(1):7–15. DOI: 10.1007/s10676-005-0456-y
8. Meyer R. The Cambridge Analytica scandal, in 3 paragraphs. The Atlantic [Internet]. 2018 Mar 20;Technology:[about 3 screens]. Available from: https://www.theatlantic.com/technology/archive/2018/03/the-cambridge-analytica-scandal-in-three-paragraphs/556046/
9. Friedersdorf C. Edward Snowden or the NSA: who violated your privacy more? The Atlantic [Internet]. 2014 July 8; Politics:[about 4 screens]. Available from: https://www.theatlantic.com/politics/archive/2014/07/edward-snowden-or-the-nsa-who-violated-your-privacy-more/374066/
10. Wikipedia [Internet]. Wikimedia Foundation, Inc.; 2018. Privacy laws of the United States; 2018 Nov 29 [cited 2018 Jan]; [about 7 screens]. Available from: https://en.wikipedia.org/wiki/Privacy_laws_of_the_United_States
11. Gibson E. Health information: privacy, confidentiality and access. In: Erdman J, Gruben V, Nelson E, editors. Canadian health law and policy. 5th ed. Toronto (ON): LexisNexis Canada; 2017. p. 207–27.
12. McInerney v MacDonald, [1992] 2 SCR 138.
13. Doctor probed for improper health record access. CBC News [Internet]. 2011 Dec 1 [cited 2018 May 22];Edmonton:[about 2 screens]. Available from: http://www.cbc.ca/news/canada/edmonton/doctor-probed-for-improper-health-record-access-1.1045719
14. Proctor J. Former Island Health nurse suspended over privacy breach. CBC News [Internet]. 2018 Jan 5 [cited 2018 May 23];British Columbia:[about 2 screens]. Available from: http://www.cbc.ca/news/canada/british-columbia/island-health-privacy-breach-1.4473934
15. Privacy-breach discipline against 24 of 48 healthcare workers withdrawn. CBC News [Internet]. 2016 Jan 15 [cited 2018 May 23];Calgary:[about 3 screens]. Available from: http://www.cbc.ca/news/canada/calgary/privacy-breach-discipline-dropped-una-ahs-1.3405283
16. CMPA: empowering better health care [Internet]. Ottawa (ON): Canadian Medical Protective Association. Subpoenas: what are a physician's responsibilities?; 1995 Mar [revised 2008 Apr, 2009 Dec, cited 2018 Jan]; [about 2 screens]. Available from: https://www.cmpa-acpm.ca/en/advice-publications/browse-articles/1995/subpoenas-what-are-a-physician-s-responsibilities
17. Beck P. The confidentiality of psychiatric records and the patient's right to privacy [Internet]. Ottawa (ON): Canadian Psychiatric Association; 2000 [cited 2018 Jan]. Available from: https://ww1.cpa-apc.org/Publications/Position_Papers/Records.asp
18. Spielberg AR. On call and online: socio-historical, legal, and ethical implications of e-mail for the patient–physician relationship. JAMA. 1998;280(15):1353-9. PMID: 9794317.
19. Brown J. How to master electronic communication with patients. Med Econ. 2013;90(7):60–7. PMID: 24066458.
20. Bergen M. Google will stop reading your emails for Gmail ads. Bloomberg [Internet]. 2017 June 23;Technology. Available from: https://www.bloomberg.com/news/articles/2017-06-23/google-will-stop-reading-your-emails-for-gmail-ads
21. CMPA: empowering better health care [Internet]. Ottawa (ON): Canadian Medical Protective Association. Using email communication with your patients: legal risks; 2005 Mar [revised 2015 May, cited 2017 Oct 14]. https://www.cmpa-acpm.ca/en/advice-publications/browse-articles/2013/using-electronic-communications-protecting-privacy
22. Shah DR, Galante JM, Bold RJ, et al. Text messaging among residents and faculty in a university general surgery residency program: prevalence, purpose, and patient care. J Surg Educ. 2013;70(6):826–34. PMID: 24209663.
23. Kuhlmann S, Ahlers-Schmidt CR, Steinberger E. TXT@WORK: pediatric hospitalists and text messaging. Telemed J E Health. 2014;20(7):647–52. PMID: 24784021.
24. Drolet BC. Text messaging and protected health information: what is permitted?

JAMA. 2017;317(23):2369–70. PMID: 28492922.

25. Butt HR. A method for better physician–patient communication. Ann Intern Med. 1977;86(4):478–80. PMID: 848814.

26. Rieger KL, Hack TF, Beaver K, et al. Should consultation recording use be a practice standard? A systematic review of the effectiveness and implementation of consultation recordings. Psychooncology. 2017;25:25. PMID: 29178602.

27. Hack TF, Ruether JD, Weir LM, et al. Promoting consultation recording practice in oncology: identification of critical implementation factors and determination of patient benefit. Psychooncology. 2013;22(6):1273–82. PMID: 22821445.

28. Tsulukidze M, Durand MA, Barr PJ, et al. Providing recording of clinical consultation to patients–a highly valued but underutilized intervention: a scoping review. Patient Educ Couns. 2014;95(3):297–304. PMID: 24630697.

29. Elwyn G. "Patientgate": digital recordings change everything. BMJ. 2014;348:g2078. PMID: 24620357.

30. Elwyn G, Barr PJ, Grande SW. Patients recording clinical encounters: a path to empowerment? Assessment by mixed methods. BMJ Open. 2015;5(8): e008566. DOI: 10.1136/bmjopen-2015-008566

31. Chesanow N. Should patients be permitted to record doctor visits? [Internet]. Medscape, WebMD LLC; 2015 Feb 17 [cited 2017 Oct 18]. Available from: https://www.medscape.com/viewarticle/838207

32. Tsulukidze M, Grande SW, Thompson R, et al. Patients covertly recording clinical encounters: threat or opportunity? A qualitative analysis of online texts. PLOS ONE. 2015;10(5):e0125824. DOI: 10.1371/journal.pone.0125824

33. Elwyn G, Barr PJ, Castaldo M. Can patients make recordings of medical encounters?: What does the law say? JAMA. 2017;318(6):513–4. PMID: 28692707.

34. Legaltree [Internet]. British Columbia: Legaltree Law Corporation; 2007–2018. Is it legal to record a private conversation? Wiretapping and the one-party consent exception to the rule against interception; 2008 May 6 [cited 2018 May 23]; [about 8

screens]. Available from: https://legaltree.ca/node/908

35. Rudner S. Should I record the conversation? [Internet]. Toronto (ON): Canadian HR Reporter, Thomson Reuters; 2017 Jul 14 [cited 2018 May 23]; [about 2 screens]. Available from: https://www.hrreporter.com/columnist/canadian-hr-law/archive/2017/07/14/should-i-record-the-conversation

36. Allen J. The hospital medical director [Internet]. Columbus (OH): James Allen; 2018. When patients want to video physician encounters; 2017 May 31 [cited 2017 Oct 18]; [about 4 screens]. Available from: https://hospitalmedicaldirector.com/when-patients-want-to-video-physician-encounters/

37. Halls v Mitchell, [1928] SCR 125.

38. The College of Physicians and Surgeons of Ontario. Mandatory and permissive reporting [Internet]. Toronto (ON): CPSO; 2000 Nov [updated 2017 Oct]. Available from: https://www.cpso.on.ca/policies-publications/policy/mandatory-and-permissive-reporting#impaired

39. Health Protection and Promotion Act, R.S.O. 1990, c. H.7.

40. R v Mabior, 2012 SCC 47, [2012] 2 SCR 584.

41. Department of Justice Canada. Fact sheet: HIV non-disclosure and the criminal law [Internet]. Ottawa (ON): Department of Justice Canada; 2017 Dec [cited 2018 May 23]. Available from: https://www.canada.ca/en/department-justice/news/2017/12/fact_sheet_hiv_non-disclosureandthecriminallaw.html

42. CMPA: empowering better health care [Internet]. Ottawa (ON): Canadian Medical Protective Association. Protecting children: reporting child abuse; 2012 Mar [cited 2018 Jan]; [about 3 screens]. Available from: https://www.cmpa-acpm.ca/en/advice-publications/browse-articles/2012/protecting-children-reporting-child-abuse

43. CMPA: empowering better health care [Internet]. Ottawa (ON): Canadian Medical Protective Association. Elder abuse and neglect: balancing intervention and patients' right to confidentiality; 2016 Dec [cited 2018 Jan]; [about 2 screens]. Available from: https://www.cmpa-acpm.ca/en/advice-publications/browse-articles/2016/

elder-abuse-and-neglect-balancing-intervention-and-patients-right-to-confidentiality

44. Canadian Centre for Elder Law. A practical guide to elder abuse and neglect law in Canada. Vancouver (BC): British Columbia Law Institute, University of British Columbia; 2011.

45. CMPA: empowering better health care [Internet]. Ottawa (ON): Canadian Medical Protective Association. Fitness to drive: when do physicians have a duty to report?; 2015 Dec [cited 2018 Jan]; [about 3 screens]. Available from: https://www.cmpa-acpm .ca/en/advice-publications/browse-articles/2015/fitness-to-drive-when-do-physicians-have-a-duty-to-report

46. Toms v Foster, 1994 CanLII 517 (ONCA).

47. Wilberg KR. Report to the Minister of Justice and Solicitor General: Public inquiry into the death of Megan Alyssa Wolitski. Edmonton (AB): Government of Alberta; 2017.

48. Redelmeier DA, Yarnell CJ, Thiruchelvam D, et al. Physicians' warnings for unfit drivers and the risk of trauma from road crashes. N Engl J Med. 2012;367(13): 1228–36. PMID: 23013074.

49. Redelmeier DA, Yarnell CJ, Tibshirani RJ. Physicians' warnings for unfit drivers and risk of road crashes. N Engl J Med. 2013;368(1):87–8. PMID: 23281992.

50. Canadian Medical Association. CMA driver's guide: determining medical fitness to operate motor vehicles. 9th ed. Ottawa (ON): CMA; 2017.

51. Byszewski A. The driving and dementia toolkit. 3rd ed. Ottawa (ON): The Regional Geriatric Program of Eastern Ontario/The Champlain Dementia Network; 2009.

52. Aeronautics Act, R.S.C. 1985, c. A-2.

53. Railway Safety Act, R.S.C. 1985, c. 32 (4th Supp.).

54. Merchant Seamen Compensation Act, R.S.C. 1985, c. M-6.

55. Canadian Medical Protective Association. Medical-legal handbook for physicians in Canada. Version 8.2. Ottawa (ON): CMPA; 2016. Available from: https:// www.cmpa-acpm.ca/static-assets/pdf/ advice-and-publications/handbooks/ com_16_MLH_for_physicians-e.pdf

56. College of Physicians and Surgeons of Ontario. Third party reports [Internet]. Toronto (ON): CPSO; 2002 Nov [updated 2009 Nov, 2012 May, 2018 May, cited 2018 Jan]. Available from: https://www. cpso.on.ca/policies-publications/policy/ third-party-reports

57. Martin AF. The adoption of mandatory gunshot wound reporting legislation in Canada: a decade of tension in lawmaking at the intersection of law enforcement and public health. MJLH. 2016;9:173.

58. May JP, Hemenway D, Hall A. Do criminals go to the hospital when they are shot? Inj Prev. 2002;8(3):236–8. PMID: 12226123.

59. May JP, Hemenway D, Oen R, et al. Medical care solicitation by criminals with gunshot wound injuries: a survey of Washington, DC, jail detainees. J Trauma. 2000;48(1):130–2. PMID: 10647578.

60. CDC. Medical examiners' and coroners' handbook on death registration and fetal death reporting. Hyattsville (MD): Centers for Disease Control and Prevention; 2003.

61. Bourke J, Wessely S. Confidentiality. BMJ. 2008;336(7649):888–91. PMID: 18420695.

62. Lenzer J. Doctors outraged at Patriot Act's potential to seize medical records. BMJ. 2006;332(7533):69. PMID: 16410565.

63. R v Vice Media Canada Inc, SCC 53, Supreme Court of Canada, 2018.

64. Smith v Jones. [1999] 1 SCR 455.

65. O'Shaughnessy RJ, Glancy GD, Bradford JM. Canadian landmark case, Smith v Jones, Supreme Court of Canada: confidentiality and privilege suffer another blow. J Am Acad Psychiatry Law. 1999;27(4): 614–20. PMID: 10638788.

66. Mills MJ, Sullivan G, Eth S. Protecting third parties: a decade after Tarasoff. Am J Psychiatry. 1987;144(1):68–74. PMID: 3799843.

67. Tarasoff v Regents of University of California, 529 P.2d 553 (Cal. 1974).

68. Tarasoff v Regents of University of California, 551 P.2d 334 (Cal. 1976).

69. Johnson R, Persad G, Sisti D. The Tarasoff rule: the implications of interstate variation and gaps in professional training. J Am Acad Psychiatry Law. 2014;42(4):469–77. PMID: 25492073.

70. Glancy GD, Regehr C, Bryant AG. Confidentiality in crisis: Part II: Confidentiality of treatment records. Can J Psychiatry. 1998;43(10):1006–11. PMID: 9868565.

71. Chaimowitz G, Glancy G. The duty to protect. Ottawa (ON): Canadian Psychiatric Association; 2011.

72. CMPA: empowering better health care [Internet]. Ottawa (ON): Canadian Medical Protective Association. When to disclose confidential information; 2015 Mar [cited 2018 Jan]; [about 3 screens]. Available from: https://www.cmpa-acpm.ca/en/advice-publications/browse-articles/2015/when-to-disclose-confidential-information

Chapter 8

1. Starson v Swayze. 2003 SCC 32, [2003] 1 SCR 772.

2. Appelbaum PS, Gutheil TG. Clinical handbook of psychiatry & the law. 4th ed. Philadelphia (PA): Wolters Kluwer/Lippincott Williams & Wilkins; 2007.

3. Gilmour JM. Legal capacity and decision-making. In: Erdman J, Gruben V, Nelson E, editors. Canadian health law and policy. 5th ed. Toronto (ON): LexisNexis Canada; 2017. p. 351–74.

4. Wong JG, Clare IC, Gunn MJ, et al. Capacity to make health care decisions: its importance in clinical practice. Psychol Med. 1999;29(2):437–46. PMID: 10218935.

5. Grisso T, Appelbaum PS. Assessing competence to consent to treatment: a guide for physicians and other health professionals. New York: Oxford University Press; 1998.

6. Beauchamp TL, Childress JF. Principles of biomedical ethics. 5th ed. New York: Oxford University Press; 2001.

7. Gilmour JM. Retrenchment not reform: using law and policy to restrict the entitlement of women with disabilities to social assistance. In: Gavigan S, Chunn D. The legal tender of gender: law, welfare, and the regulation of women's poverty. Oxford: Hart Publishing; 2010. p. 189–216.

8. Cassell EJ, Leon AC, Kaufman SG. Preliminary evidence of impaired thinking in sick patients. Ann Intern Med. 2001;134(12):1120-3. PMID: 11412052.

9. Raymont V, Bingley W, Buchanan A, et al. Prevalence of mental incapacity in medical inpatients and associated risk factors: cross-sectional study. Lancet. 2004;364(9443):1421–7. PMID: 15488217.

10. Sessums LL, Zembrzuska H, Jackson JL. Does this patient have medical decision-making capacity? JAMA. 2011;306(4):420–7. PMID: 21791691.

11. Howell J. ACP Journal Club. Review: several instruments are accurate for evaluating patient capacity for medical treatment decision-making. Ann Intern Med. 2011;155(10):JC5–12. PMID: 22084359.

12. Marson DC, McInturff B, Hawkins L, et al. Consistency of physician judgments of capacity to consent in mild Alzheimer's disease. J Am Geriatr Soc. 1997;45(4):453–7. PMID: 9100714.

13. Gunn M. The meaning of incapacity. Med Law Rev. 1994;2(1):8–29. PMID: 11656866.

14. Etchells E, Darzins P, Silberfeld M, et al. Assessment of patient capacity to consent to treatment. J Gen Intern Med. 1999;14(1): 27–34. PMID: 9893088.

15. Joint Centre for Bioethics. Aid to capacity evaluation [Internet]. Toronto (ON): University of Toronto Joint Centre for Bioethics; 2008. Available from: http://jcb.utoronto.ca/tools/documents/ace.pdf

16. D. Wendler and A. Rid, Systematic review: the effect on surrogates of making treatment decisions for others, Ann Intern Med, 154 (2011): 336–46.

17. K. Marx, The18th Brumaire of Louis Napoleon (1852); In: The Collected Works of Marx and Engels, Vol 11 (New York, International Publishers, 1979): 103.

18. J. Weeks, P. Catalano, A. Cronin, M. Finkelman, J. Mack, N. Keating, and D. Schrag, Patients' expectations about effects of chemotherapy for advanced cancer, New Engl J Med, 367 (2012); 1616–25. DOI:10.1056/NEJMoa124410 "Code" is the code word for CPR (Cardio-Pulmonary Resuscitation) which is called and, hopefully, performed when a patient suffers a cardiac arrest. CPR will generally be performed on a patient unless a "No CODE" order is written on the patient's chart.

19. Sawatzky v Riverview Health Centre Inc., [1998] 167 DLR (4th) 359, 362 (MBQB).

20. Zeytinoglu M. Talking it out: helping our patients live better while dying. Ann Intern Med. 2011;154(12):830–2. DOI: 10.7326/0003-4819-154-12-201106210-00011

21. Fleming v Reid and Gallagher, [1991] 48 OAC 46 (ONCA).

22. Government of Alberta. Fact sheet: the Mental Health Act and the Adult Guardianship and Trusteeship Act. Edmonton (AB): Government of Alberta; 2009.

23. Appelbaum PS. Almost a revolution: mental health law and the limits of change. New York: Oxford University Press; 1994.

24. Williams AR, Caplan AL. Thomas Szasz: rebel with a questionable cause. Lancet. 2012;380(9851):1378–9. PMID: 23091833.

25. Bennion E. A right to remain psychotic? A new standard for involuntary treatment in light of current science. Loyola Los Angel Law Rev. 2013;47:251.

26. Brean J. Professor Starson's landmark case established legal right to refuse medication, but he's still fighting his own battle. National Post [Internet]. 2013 Feb 4;News:[about 4 screens]. Available from: https://nationalpost.com/news/canada/ professor-starsons-landmark-case-established-legal-right-to-refuse-medication-but-hes-still-fighting-his-own-battle

27. Sheehan S. Is there no place on earth for me? New York: Houghton Mifflin; 1982.

28. Braslow JT, Messac L. Medicalization and demedicalization: a gravely disabled homeless man with psychiatric illness. N Engl J Med. 2018;379(20):1885–8. PMID: 30428298.

29. Appelbaum PS. The right to refuse treatment with antipsychotic medications: retrospect and prospect. Am J Psychiatry. 1988;145(4):413–9. PMID: 3279829.

30. Hewak N. The ethical, medical, and legal implications of the forcible treatment provisions of the Criminal Code. Health Law Can. 1995;15(4):107–16. PMID: 10143461.

31. Orr F, Watson D, King-Smith A. Alberta's community treatment order legislation and implementation: the first 18 months in review. Health Law Rev. 2012;20(2):5.

32. C.L. Tait, Ethical programming: Towards a community-centred approach to mental health and addiction programming in aboriginal communities, Pimatisiwin: A Journal of Aboriginal and Indigenous Community Health, 6 (2008): 29–60.

33. Byrick K, Walker-Renshaw B. A practical guide to mental health and the law in Ontario. Toronto (ON): Ontario Hospital Association; 2016.

34. Alberta Health Services. Summary sheet: consent to treatment/procedures: minors/ mature minors [Internet]. Edmonton (AB): AHS; 2010. Available from: https://www.albertahealthservices.ca/assets/about/ policies/ahs-clp-consent-summary-sheet-minors-mature-minors.pdf

35. Jackson MK, Burns KK, Richter MS. Confidentiality and treatment decisions of minor clients: a health professional's dilemma & policy makers challenge. SpringerPlus. 2014;3(1):320. DOI: 10.1186/2193-1801-3-320

36. Alderson P. Children's consent to surgery. Buckingham (UK): Open University Press; 1993.

37. CMPA: empowering better health care [Internet]. Ottawa (ON): Canadian Medical Protective Association. Can a child provide consent?; 2014 Mar [updated 2016 Jun, cited 2018 Feb]; [about 3 screens]. Available from: https://www.cmpa-acpm.ca/en/ advice-publications/browse-articles/2014/ can-a-child-provide-consent

38. Gillick v West Norfolk and Wisbech Area Health Authority, 1 AC 112, 187(D) (HL 1986).

39. Guichon J, Mitchell I. Free and informed choice in medical treatment: making it safe to choose for Jehovah's Witnesses. BJOG. 2009;116(11):1540. PMID: 19769763.

40. Re L.D.K.: Children's Aid Society of Metropolitan Toronto v K and K, [1985] 48 RFL 2d 164 (ONCJ).

41. Gabor JY. The role of children in decision-making and consent to cancer treatment. UTMJ. 2003;80(3):203–7.

42. Robb N. Ruling on Jehovah's Witness teen in New Brunswick may have "settled the law" for MDs. CMAJ. 1994;151(5):625–8. PMID: 8069805.

43. Region 2 Hospital Corp. v Walker, [1994] NBJ 242 (NBCA).

44. Woolley S. Children of Jehovah's Witnesses and adolescent Jehovah's Witnesses: what are their rights? Arch Dis Child. 2005;90(7):715–9. PMID: 15970615.

45. B.H. v Alberta (Director of Child Welfare), 2002 ABQB 371, [2002] AJ No. 518 (ABCQB).

46. Guichon J, Mitchell I. Medical emergencies in children of orthodox Jehovah's Witness families: three recent legal cases, ethical issues and proposals for management. Paediatr Child Health. 2007;12(5):386. PMID: 19030394.

47. AC v Manitoba (Director of Child and Family Services), 2009 SCC 30, [2009] 2 SCR 181.

48. Blackwell T. Makayla Sault's parents say they have no regrets over girl's decision to opt for holistic cancer treatment. National Post [Internet]. 2014 June 6, updated 2015 Jan 24;News:[about 7 screens]. Available from: https://nationalpost.com/news/canada/makayla-saults-parents-say-they-have-no-regrets-over-girls-decision-to-opt-for-holistic-cancer-treatment

49. Warnica R. Makayla Sault went to controversial Florida clinic for "counselling," not medical treatment: mother. National Post [Internet]. 2015 Feb 27 [cited 2018 Feb];News:[about 4 screens]. Available from: http://nationalpost.com/news/canada/makayla-sault-went-to-controversial-florida-clinic-for-counselling-not-medical-treatment-mother

50. McLaren L. Makayla Sault: whose rights are served when a little girl dies? Globe and Mail [Internet]. 2015 Jan 21, updated 2018 May 12;Parenting:[about 3 screens]. Available from: https://www.theglobeandmail.com/life/parenting/whose-rights-are-served-when-a-little-girl-dies/article22562573/

51. Hébert PC. Good medicine: the art of ethical care in Canada. Toronto (ON): Doubleday Canada; 2016.

52. Galloway G. Ontario First Nations girl taken off chemotherapy has died. Globe and Mail [Internet]. 2015 Jan 19, updated 2018 May 12;Health:[about 3 screens]. Available from: https://www.theglobeandmail.com/life/health-and-fitness/health/health-care-must-do-better-at-respecting-aboriginal-patients-journal-urges/article22517597/

53. Casey L. Makayla Sault's parents speak out about daughter's death. CBC [Internet]. 2015 Feb 26, updated 2015 Mar 3;Indigenous:[about 4 screens]. Available from: https://www.cbc.ca/news/indigenous/makayla-sault-s-parents-speak-out-about-daughter-s-death-1.2973938

54. Hamilton Health Sciences Corp. v D.H. 2014 ONCJ 603.

55. Mitchell I, Guichon JR, Wong S. Caring for children, focusing on children. [Erratum appears in Paediatr Child Health. 2015 Nov-Dec;20(8):466-7. PMID: 26744561.] Paediatr Child Health. 2015;20(6):293–5. PMID: 26435666.

56. Jarvis D, Byrick K, de Wit M. Update: recent case regarding parent refusing chemotherapy for First Nations child in favour of traditional medicines: what are the implications for health care providers? [Internet]. CanLII Connects; 2015 [cited 22 Mar 2018]. Available from: http://canliiconnects.org/en/commentaries/37105

Chapter 9

1. Attributed to Balint M by Norell J, letter. The importance of the generalist. Br J Gen Pract. 1992;42(363):442–3. PMC1372245.

2. Canadian Medical Association. CMA code of ethics. Ottawa (ON): CMA; 2004. Available from: https://www.cma.ca/En/Pages/code-of-ethics.aspx

3. Brewin T. Primum non nocere? Lancet. 1994;344(8935):1487–8. PMID: 7968126.

4. Webb B. A patient who changed my practice: the zero option. BMJ. 1995;310:1380. DOI: 10.1136/bmj.310.6991.1380

5. Balint M. The doctor, his patient and the illness. Revised ed. Madison (CT): International Universities Press; 1988. p. 231.

6. Rosenbaum L. The paternalism preference: choosing unshared decision making. N Engl J Med. 2015;373(7):589–92. DOI:10.1056/NEJMp1508418

7. Feinberg J. Freedom and fulfillment: philosophical essays. Princeton (NJ): Princeton University Press, 1992. The child's right to an open future. p. 89.

8. Kodama D, Yanagawa B, Chung J, et al. "Is there a doctor on board?": Practical recommendations for managing in-flight medical emergencies. CMAJ. 2018;190(8):E217–22. DOI: 10.1503/cmaj.170601

9. Smits JM. The Good Samaritan in European private law: on the perils of principles without a programme and a programme for the future [inaugural lecture]. Maastricht: Maastricht University; 2000. Available from: https://works.bepress.com/jan_smits/8/

10. Davies C, Shaul RZ. Physicians' legal duty of care and legal right to refuse to work during a pandemic. CMAJ. 2010;182(2):167–70. DOI: 10.1503/cmaj.091628

11. Crits et al. v Sylvester et al., [1956] OR 132, 143 (ONCA), aff'd [1956] SCR 991.

12. Emanuel EJ. The lessons of SARS. Ann Intern Med. 2003;139(7):589–91. PMID: 14530230.

13. Caplan A. Time to mandate influenza vaccination in health-care workers. Lancet. 2011;378(9788):310–11. PMID: 21789789.

14. Vancouver General Hospital v McDaniel, [1934] 4 DLR 593, 597 (PC); Wilson v Swanson, [1956] 5 DLR 2d 113, 120 (SCC). For a story of "overtreatment" see Warraich HJ. Opinion: the cancer of optimism. New York Times. 2013 May 5;SR9.

15. Bolam v Friern Hospital Management Committee, 2 All ER 118, 122 (QBD 1957).

16. Ter Neuzen v Korn, [1995] 3 SCR 674. Per La Forest, Sopinka, Gonthier, Cory, McLachlin and Iacobucci.

17. Yang Y, Larochelle M, Haffajee R. Managing increasing liability risks related to opioid prescribing. Am J Med. 2017;130(3):249–50. DOI: 10.1016/j.amjmed.2016.08.041

18. Wahl J, Le Clair K, Himel S. The geriatric patient. In: Bloom H, Bay M, editors. A practical guide to mental health, capacity, and consent law of Ontario. Toronto (ON): Carswell; 1996. p. 343–77.

19. Woman who swallowed anti-freeze dies after refusing treatment. Daily Mail [Internet]. 2008 Oct 17;News:[about 4 screens]. Available from: https://www.dailymail.co.uk/news/article-1078439/Woman-swallowed-anti-freeze-dies-refusing-treatment-doctors-feared-assault-claim-saved-her.html

20. Wolff J. Dementia, death and advance directives. Health Econ Policy Law. 2012;7(4):499–506. DOI:10.1017/S1744133112000278

21. Ganzini L, Lee M. Psychiatry and assisted suicide in the United States. N Engl J Med. 1997;336(25):1824–6. DOI: 10.1056/NEJM199706193362511

22. Pochard F, Robin M, Kannas S. Letter to the editor. N Engl J Med. 1998;338:261–2. PMID: 9441236.

23. Grant J. Liability in patient suicide. Curr Psychol. 2004;3(11):80–2.

24. College of Physicians and Surgeons of Alberta. CPSA reprimands doctor for failing to attend a patient in the emergency department. Messenger. 2016 May;224.

25. Muzina D. What physicians can do to prevent suicide. Cleve Clin J Med. 2004;71(3):242–50. PMID: 15055247.

26. Sheridan K. Is it a crime to avoid vaccines? People who refuse are being punished with jail and job loss. Newsweek [Internet]. 2017 Dec 5;Tech and Science:[about 3 screens]. Available from: https://www.newsweek.com/sending-parents-jail-refusing-vaccinate-doesnt-work-say-experts-730439

27. Caulfield T. Stop those naturopaths who spread anti-vaxxer myths. Globe and Mail [Internet]. 2017 Jun 24;Opinion:[about 3 screens]. Available from: https://www.theglobeandmail.com/opinion/stop-those-naturopaths-who-spread-anti-vaxxer-myths/article35444890/

28. Caulfield T. The vaccination picture. Toronto (ON): Penguin Books; 2017.

29. Truth and Reconciliation Commission of Canada. Honouring the truth, reconciling for the future: summary of the final report of the Truth and Reconciliation Commission of Canada. Ottawa (ON): Truth and Reconciliation Commission of Canada; 2015.

30. Gilbert R, Fluke J, O'Donnell M, et al. Child maltreatment: variation in trends and policies in six developed countries. Lancet. 2012;379(9817):758–72. DOI: 10.1016/S0140-6736(11)61087-8

31. Wissow L. Child abuse and neglect. N Engl J Med. 1995;332(21):1425–31. DOI: 10.1056/NEJM199505253322107

32. Picard E. Legal liability of doctors and hospitals in Canada. 2nd ed. Toronto (ON): Carswell; 1984. p. 47.

33. Civil Code of Quebec, S.Q. 1991, c. 64, a. 13.

34. Quoted in Schroeder P. Female genital mutilation: a form of child abuse. N Engl J Med. 1994;331(11):739–40. DOI: 10.1056/NEJM199409153311111

35. B. (R.) v CAS of Metropolitan Toronto, [1995] 1 SCR 315.

36. Wilson J. Letting them die: parents refuse medical help for children in the name of Christ. The Guardian [Internet]. 2016 April 13;News:[about 7 screens]. Available from: https://www.theguardian.com/us-news/2016/apr/13/followers-of-christ-idaho-religious-sect-child-mortality-refusing-medical-help

37. Sandstrom A. Most states allow religious exemptions from child abuse and neglect laws [Internet]. Fact Tank, Pew Research Center; 2016 Aug 12. Available from: http://www.pewresearch.org/fact-tank/2016/08/12/most-states-allow-religious-exemptions-from-child-abuse-and-neglect-laws/

38. Superintendent of Family and Child Service v RD and SD, [1983] 42 BCLR 173 (BCSC).

39. Chambers JD. A practical treatise on the jurisdiction of the High Court of Chancery over the persons and property of infants. London: Saunders and Benning; 1847. p. 175.

40. Carter J quoted in Picard, op. cit.: 49.

41. Minister of Social Services v F & L Paulette, [1991] Saskatchewan Provincial Court, Sask. D. 1568–605 (Prov. Ct.; unreported).

42. E. (Mrs.) v Eve, [1986] 2 SCR 388.

43. Lovinsky D, Gagne J. Legal representation of children in Canada. Ottawa (ON): Department of Justice Canada; 2015. 3: Legal representation of children in Canada: parens patriae jurisdiction. Available from: https://www.justice.gc.ca/eng/rp-pr/other-autre/lrc-rje/p3.html

44. Grekul J. Sterilization in Alberta, 1928 to 1972: gender matters. Can Rev Sociol. 2008;45(3):247–66. PMID: 19579351.

45. Cairney R. "Democracy was never intended for degenerates": Alberta's flirtation with eugenics comes back to haunt it. CMAJ. 1996;155(6):789–92. PMID: 8823227.

46. Samson A. Eugenics in the community: gendered professions and eugenic sterilization in Alberta, 1928–1972. Can Bull Med Hist. 2014;31(1):143–63. PMID: 24909022.

47. Park DC, Radford JP. From the case files: reconstructing a history of involuntary sterilisation. Disabil Soc. 1998;13(3):317–42. PMID: 11660707.

48. Lantos JD. Ethics for the pediatrician: the evolving ethics of cochlear implants in children. Pediatr Rev. 2012;33(7):323–6. DOI: 10.1542/pir.33-7-323.

49. Adapted from Gunther D, Diekama D. Attenuating growth in children with profound developmental disability. Arch Pediatr Adolesc Med. 2006;160(10):1013–17. DOI: 10.1001/archpedi.160.10.1013

50. Solomon A. Far from the tree: parents, children, and the search for identity. New York: Scribner; 2012.

51. Liao LM, Creighton SM. Requests for cosmetic genitoplasty: how should healthcare providers respond? BMJ. 2007;334(7603):1090–2. DOI: 10.1136/bmj.39206.422269.BE

52. Toubia N. Female circumcision as a public health issue. N Engl J Med. 1994; 331(11):712–16. DOI: 10.1056/NEJM199409153311106; Black J, Debelle G. Female genital mutilation in Britain. BMJ. 1995;310(6994):1590–2. PMID: 7787654; Gallard C. Female genital mutilation in France. BMJ. 1995;310(6994):1592–3. PMID: 7787655.

53. Arora KS, Jacobs AJ. Female genital alteration: a compromise solution. J Med Ethics. 2016;42(3):148–54. DOI:10.1136/medethics-2014-102375

54. Nurcombe B, Partlett D. Child mental health and the law. New York: The Free Press; 1994. p. 119–21.

Chapter 10

1. Saundby R. Medical ethics: a guide to professional conduct. 2nd ed. London: Charles Griffin & Co.; 1907. p. 2.

2. Pellegrino E. Medical professionalism: can it, should it survive? J Am Board Fam Pract. 2000;13(2):147–9. PMID:10764200.

3. Hafferty F. Professionalism: the next wave. N Engl J Med. 2006;355(20):2151–2. DOI: 10.1056/NEJMe068217

4. Proposed language may be found in the Uniform Apology Act. CMPA: empowering better health care [Internet]. Ottawa (ON): Canadian Medical Protective Association. Apology legislation in Canada: what it means for physicians; 2008 Sept [revised 2013 Apr]; [about 2 screens]. Available from: https://www.cmpa-acpm.ca/en/advice-publications/browse-articles/2008/apology-legislation-in-canada-what-it-means-for-physicians

5. Huntington B, Kuhn N. Communication gaffes: a root cause of malpractice claims. Proc (Bayl Univ Med Cent). 2003;16(2): 157–61. PMID: 16278732.

6. Medical Professionalism Project. Medical professionalism in the new millennium: a physician charter. Lancet. 2002;359(9305):520–2. DOI: 10.1016/S0140-6736(02)07684-5; Simultaneously published in Ann Intern Med. 2002;136(3):243–6. PMID:11827500.

7. Cassel C, Hood V, Bauer W. A physician charter: the 10th anniversary. Ann Intern Med. 2012;157(4):290–1. DOI: 10.7326/0003-4819-157-4-201208210-00012

8. Frank J, editor. The CanMEDS 2005 physician competency framework: better standards, better physicians, better care [Internet]. Ottawa (ON): Royal College of Physicians and Surgeons of Canada; 2005 [cited 2016 Dec 1]. Available from: http://www.royalcollege.ca/portal/page/portal/rc/common/documents/canmeds/resources/publications/framework_full_e.pdf

9. Frankfurt H. The reasons of love. Princeton (NJ): Princeton University Press; 2004. ft. 5, p. 20.

10. Peabody F. The care of the patient. JAMA. 1927;88(12):877–82. DOI: 10.1001/jama.1927.02680380001001

11. Schneider C. The practice of autonomy: patients, doctors, and medical decisions. New York (NY): Oxford University Press; 1998. p. 227.

12. Riskin A, Erez A, Foulk TA, et al. The impact of rudeness on medical team performance: a randomized trial. Pediatrics. 2015;136(3):487 95. DOI: 10.1542/peds.2015-1385

13. Bar-David S. Trust your canary: every leader's guide to taming workplace incivility. Toronto (ON): Fairleigh Press; 2015.

14. Health Force Ontario. Implementing interprofessional care in Ontario: final report of the Interprofessional Care Strategic Implementation Committee. Ontario: Government of Ontario; 2010. Available from: http://www.healthforceontario.ca/en/Home

15. Lill M, Wilkinson T. Judging a book by its cover: descriptive survey of patients' preferences for doctors' appearance and mode of address. BMJ. 2005;331(7531):1524–7. PMID: 16373739.

16. Rehman S, Nietert P, Cope D, et al. What to wear today? Effect of doctor's attire on the trust and confidence of patients. Am J Med. 2005;118(11):1279–86. DOI: 10.1016/j.amjmed.2005.04.026

17. Reddy R. Slippers and a white coat? Hawai'i physician attire study. Hawaii Med J. 2009;68(11):284–5. PMID: 20034257.

18. Chung H, Lee H, Chang DS, Kim HS, et al. Doctor's attire influences perceived empathy in the patient-doctor relationship,

Patient Educ Couns. 2012;89(3):387–91. DOI: 10.1016/j.pec.2012.02.017

19. Cohen M, Jeanmonod D, Stankewicz H, et al. An observational study of patients' attitudes to tattoos and piercings on their physicians: the ART study. Emerg Med J. 2018;35(9):538–43. DOI: 10.1136/emermed-2017-206887

20. Ambady N, LaPlante D, Nguyen T, Rosenthal R, et al., Surgeons' tone of voice: a clue to malpractice history. Surgery. 2002;132(1):5–9. PubMed PMID: 12110787.

21. Editorial: evidence-based handshakes. Lancet. 2007;370 (9581):2. DOI: 10.1016/S0140-6736(07)61021-6

22. Cruess R, Cruess S, Johnston S. Professionalism and medicine's social contract. J Bone Joint Surg Am. 2000;82-A(8):1189–94. PMID: 10954108.

23. Canadian Medical Protective Association. Medical-legal handbook for physicians in Canada. Version 8.2. Ottawa (ON): CMPA; 2016. Available from: https://www.cmpa-acpm.ca/static-assets/pdf/advice-and-publications/handbooks/com_16_MLH_for_physicians-e.pdf

24. Norberg v Wynrib, [1992] 2 SCR 226.

25. Fickweiler F, Fickweiler W, Urbach E. Interactions between physicians and the pharmaceutical industry generally and sales representatives specifically and their association with physicians' attitudes and prescribing habits: a systematic review. BMJ Open. 2017;7(9):e016408. https://bmjopen.bmj.com/content/7/9/e016408

26. Institute of Medicine. Conflict of interest in medical research, education, and practice. Washington (DC): National Academies Press; 2009.

27. College of Physicians and Surgeons of Ontario v R Devgan (2003). https://www.casewatch.net/foreign/devgan/devgan.pdf

28. Griffin MR, Stein CM, Ray W. Postmarketing surveillance for drug safety: surely we can do better. Clin Pharmacol Ther. 2004;75 (6):491–4. DOI: 10.1016/j.clpt.2004.01.017

29. Hill KP, Ross J, Egilman D, et al. The ADVANTAGE seeding trial: a review of internal documents. Ann Intern Med. 2008;149(4):251–8. PMID: 18711155; see also: Sox H, Rennie D. "Seeding" trials: just say "no." Ann Intern Med. 2008;149(4):279–80. PMID: 18711161.

30. Campbell EG. Doctors and drug companies—scrutinizing influential relationships. N Engl J Med. 2007;357 (18): 1796–7. DOI: 10.1056/NEJMp078141

31. Adapted from Morreim EH. Conflicts of interest for physician entrepreneurs. In: Spece R, Shimm D, Buchanan A, editors. Conflicts of interest in clinical practice and research. New York (NY): Oxford University Press; 1996. p. 251–85.

32. The Centers for Medicare and Medical Services (CMS.gov) keeps track of monies and other benefits made to doctors. CMS [Internet]. Baltimore (MD): US Centers for Medicare and Medicaid Services. Open payments data in context; 2016 Nov 28; [about 2 screens]. Available from: https://www.cms.gov/OpenPayments/About/Open-Payments-Data-in-Context.html

33. Ornstein C. Public disclosure of payments to physicians from industry. JAMA. 2017;317(17):1749–50. DOI: 10.1001/jama.2017.2613

34. ProPublica's Dollars for Docs program keeps track of how industry provides money and other gifts to doctors. Such enrichment may be partly behind the epidemic of opioid related deaths. Dollars for doctors [Internet]. New York (NY): ProPublica; 2018. Available from: https://www.propublica.org/series/dollars-for-docs

35. Such enrichment may be partly behind the epidemic of opioid-related deaths. In the 1990s doctors were reassured by the educational efforts of pharmaceutical companies that patients would not get addicted to prescription painkillers. This has, of course, proven not to be the case, resulting in the overdose deaths of tens of thousands of persons per year. See the NIH website: https://www.drugabuse.gov/drugs-abuse/opioids/opioid-overdose-crisis

36. Canadian Medical Association. Guidelines for physicians in interactions with industry. Ottawa (ON): CMA; 2007. Available from: http://policybase.cma.ca/dbtw-wpd/Policypdf/PD08-01.pdf

37. "Drugs are the third leading cause of death after heart disease and cancer." Gøtzsche P. Deadly medicines and organised crime: how big pharma has corrupted healthcare. London: Radcliffe Publishing; 2013. p. 1.

38. Augustine N, Madhavan G, Nass SJ, editors. Making medicines affordable: a national imperative. A consensus study report of the National Academies of Sciences, Engineering, and Medicine. Washington (DC): National Academies Press; 2018. DOI: 10.17226/24946

39. Mack J. Pharma promotional spending in 2013. Pharma Marketing News. 2014;13(5):1–6.

40. Goel R. Doctors are under the influence of pharma drugs. Huffington Post [Internet]. 2013 Apr 2, updated 2013 Jun 2;The Blog:[about 3 screens]. Available from: https://www.huffingtonpost.ca/ritika-goel/doctors-pharma-drugs_b_2994867.html

41. Brennan T, Rothman D, Blank L, et al. Health industry practices that create conflicts of interest: a policy proposal for academic medical centers. JAMA. 2006;295(4):429–33. DOI: 10.1001/jama.295.4.429

42. Greenway T, Ross J. US drug marketing: how does promotion correspond with health value? BMJ. 2017;357:j1855. DOI: 10.1136/bmj.j1855

43. Lexchin J. The relation between promotional spending on drugs and their therapeutic gain: a cohort analysis. CMAJ Open. 2017;5(3):E724-E728. DOI: 10.9778/cmajo.20170089

44. Steinbrook R. Physicians, industry payments for food and beverages, and drug prescribing. JAMA. 2017;317(17):1754. DOI:10.1001/jama.2017.2477

45. Rosenbloom S. Boundary transgressions in therapeutic relationships [master's thesis]. Petersburg (VA): Virginia State University; 2003. p. 2–3.

46. Norberg v Wynrib, [1992] 2 SCR 226.

47. Hall K. Sexualization of the doctor–patient relationship: is it ever ethically permissible? Fam Pract. 2001;18(5):511–15. https://doi.org/10.1093/fampra/18.5.511.

48. CMA. The patient–physician relationship and the sexual abuse of patients. CMAJ. 1994;150(11):1884A–F. PMID: 8199968; see also, the CMPA: empowering better health care [Internet]. Ottawa (ON): Canadian Medical Protective Association. Maintaining appropriate boundaries; [about 1 screen]. Available from: https://www.cmpa-acpm.ca/serve/docs/ela/goodpracticesguide/pages/professionalism/

Respecting_boundaries/maintaining_appropriate_boundaries-e.html. This is increasingly recognized as an important issue by professional insurers, such as the CMPA: www.cmpa-acpm.ca/en/advice-publications/browse-articles/2014/recognizing-boundary-issue

49. Spence S. Patients bearing gifts: are there strings attached? BMJ. 2005;331(7531):1527–9. DOI: 10.1136/bmj.331.7531.1527

50. Caddell A, Hazelton L. Accepting gifts from patients. Can Fam Physician. 2013;59(12):1259–60. PMID: 24336530.

51. Hilfiker D. Not all of us are saints. Toronto (ON): Hill and Wang; 1994. p. 198–9.

52. Turner psychiatrist ordered to pay $10,000. CBC News [Internet]. 2006 March 31; Newfoundland and Labrador:[about 2 screens]. Available from: www.cbc.ca/canada/newfoundland-labrador/story/2006/03/31/nf-doucet-decision-20060331.html

53. Aravind VK, Krishnaram VD, Thasneem Z. Boundary crossings and violations in clinical settings. Indian J Psychol Med. 2012; 34(1): 21–24. DOI: 10.4103/0253-7176.96151

54. Gutheil T, Gabbard G. Misuses and misunderstandings of boundary theory in clinical and regulatory settings. Am J Psychiatry. 1998;155(3):409–14. DOI: 10.1176/ajp.155.3.409

55. Norberg v Wynrib, [1992] 2 SCR 226.

56. Lagu T, Metayer K, Moran M, et al. Website characteristics and physician reviews on commercial physician-rating websites. JAMA. 2017;317(7):766–8. DOI: 10.1001/jama.2016.18553

57. Rothenfluh F, Schulz PJ. Physician rating websites: what aspects are important to identify a good doctor, and are patients capable of assessing them? A mixed-methods approach including physicians' and health care consumers' perspectives. J Med Internet Res. 2017;19(5):e127. DOI: 10.2196/jmir.6875

58. Daskivich TJ, Houman J, Fuller G, et al. Online physician ratings fail to predict actual performance on measures of quality, value, and peer review. J Am Med Inform Assoc. 2018;25(4):401–7. DOI: 10.1093/jamia/ocx083

59. CMPA: empowering better health care [Internet]. Ottawa (ON): Canadian Medical Protective Association. Online physician reviews: what's to be done?; 2014 Sept [revised 2016 May]; [about 3 screens]. Available from: https://www.cmpa-acpm.ca/en/advice-publications/browse-articles/2014/online-physician-reviews-what-s-to-be-done

60. Jewell D. I do not love thee, Mr Fell: techniques for dealing with "heartsink" patients. BMJ. 1988;297(6647):498–9. PMID: 3139174.

61. Zlomislic D, Mendleson R, Cribb R, et al. Bad doctors who cross the border can hide their dirty secrets: we dug them up. Toronto Star. 2018 May 1;A1 and ff. Available from: http://projects.thestar.com/doctor-discipline/index.html

62. Collier R. Professionalism: the privilege and burden of self-regulation. CMAJ. 2012;184(14):1559–60. DOI: 10.1503/cmaj.109-4286

63. Horsley T, Lockyer J, Cogo E, et al. National programmes for validating physician competence and fitness for practice: a scoping review. BMJ Open. 2016;6(4):e010368. DOI: 10.1136/bmjopen-2015-010368

64. See, for example: 1. Medical Board of Australia. Medical practitioners' ongoing fitness and competence to practice: report. North Sydney: Medical Board of Australia; 2016. "The Medical Board of Australia (the Board), in partnership with the Australian Health Practitioner Regulation Agency is currently considering whether the introduction of revalidation of medical practitioners is needed as a more proactive step to contribute to the 'protection of the public'." 2. General Medical Council. Guidance for doctors: requirements for revalidation and maintaining your licence. Manchester: GMC; 2010. "Every doctor that is licensed to practice, whether working in the NHS or in private hospitals, must go through revalidation every five years." Available from: https://www.gmc-uk.org/-/media/registration-and-licensing/guidance_for_doctors_requirements_for_revalidation_and_maintaining_your_licence.pdf.

65. Canadian Medical Protective Association. Physicians and blood borne viral infections: understanding and managing the risks. Ottawa (ON): CMPA; 2010.

66. Bailey TB, Jefferies CSG. Physicians with health conditions: law and policy reform to protect the public and physician-patients.

Edmonton (AB): Health and Law Institute; 2012. Available from: http://cpsa.ca/wp-content/uploads/2015/06/Physicians_with_Health_Conditions_Complete1.pdf

67. Teasdale GM, Council of the Society of British Neurological Surgeons. Learning from Bristol: report of the public inquiry into children's heart surgery at Bristol Royal Infirmary 1984–1995. Br J Neurosurg. 2002;16(3):211–16. PMID: 12201391.

68. Dyer C. UK introduces far reaching law to protect whistleblowers. BMJ. 1999;319(7201):7. PMID: 10390434.

69. Sinclair M. The report of the Manitoba Pediatric Cardiac Surgery Inquest: inquiry into twelve deaths at the Winnipeg Health Sciences Centre in 1994. Winnipeg (MB): Provincial Court of Manitoba; 2000.

70. Beerstecher HJ. Whistleblowing: a word of warning from an unreasonable man. BMJ. 2017;358:j4205. DOI: 10.1136/bmj.j4205

71. Winslow D. Treating the enemy. Ann Intern Med. 2007;147(4):278–9. PMID: 17709761.

72. With thanks to Saporta A, Gibson BE at the University of Toronto for permission to use this case. Ethics of self-referral for profit: case example of a physician-owned physiotherapy clinic. Physiother Can. 2007;59(4):266–71. DOI: 10.3138/ptc.59.4.266

Chapter 11

1. Chretien KC. Should I be "friends" with my patients on social networking web sites? Am Fam Physician. 2011;84(1):105, 108. PubMed PMID: 21766761.

2. Evans M. DocMikeEvans YouTube channel [Internet]. [cited 2018 Feb]. Available from: https://www.youtube.com/user/DocMikeEvans

3. ACOG Committee on Professional Liability. Committee Opinion No. 622: Professional use of digital and social media. Obstet Gynecol. 2015;125(2):516-20. DOI: 10.1097/01.AOG.0000460783.32467.bf

4. Shore R, Halsey J, Shah K, et al. Report of the AMA Council on Ethical and Judicial Affairs: professionalism in the use of social media. J Clin Ethics. 2011;22(2):165–72. PubMed PMID: 21837888.

5. The College of Physicians and Surgeons of Ontario. Social media: appropriate use by physicians [Internet]. Toronto (ON): CPSO; 2012 [cited 2017 Oct 20].

Available from: https://www.cpso.on.ca/Policies-Publications/Positions-Initiatives/Social-Media-Appropriate-Use-by-Physicians#toc1

6. The College of Physicians and Surgeons of Ontario. FAQs: Appropriate use of social media by physicians [Internet]. Toronto (ON): CPSO; 2013 May [cited 2017 Oct 20]. Available from: http://www.cpso.on.ca/uploadedFiles/policies/positions/Social-Media-FAQ.pdf

7. College of Physicians and Surgeons of Alberta. Social media: what physicians need to know [Internet]. Edmonton (AB): CPSA; 2015 [cited 2017 Oct 20]. Available from: http://www.cpsa.ca/wp-content/uploads/2015/08/Social-Media-Advice-Document.pdf

8. CMPA: empowering better health care [Internet]. Ottawa (ON): Canadian Medical Protective Association. Social media: the opportunities, the realities; 2014 Oct [cited 2017 Oct 20]; [about 4 screens]. Available from: https://www.cmpa-acpm.ca/en/advice-publications/browse-articles/2014/social-media-the-opportunities-the-realities

9. Canadian Medical Association. Social media and Canadian physicians: issues and rules of engagement [Internet]. Ottawa (ON): CMA; 2011 [cited 2017 Oct 30]. Available from: https://www.cma.ca/Assets/assets-library/document/en/advocacy/CMA_Policy_Social_Media_Canadian_Physicians_Rules_Engagement_PD12-03-e.pdf.

10. College of Physicians and Surgeons of Alberta. Social media: what physicians need to know [Internet]. Edmonton (AB): CPSA; 2015 [cited 2018 Feb]. Available from: http://www.cpsa.ca/wp-content/uploads/2015/08/Social-Media-Advice-Document.pdf

11. Modahl M, Tompsett L, Moorhead T. Doctors, patients & social media. Waltham (MA): QuantiaMD, CareContinuum Alliance; 2011.

12. Bosslet GT, Torke AM, Hickman SE, et al. The patient-doctor relationship and online social networks: results of a national survey. J Gen Intern Med. 2011;26(10):1168–74. PubMed PMID: 21706268.

13. Desai DG, Ndukwu JO, Mitchell JP. Social media in health care: how close is too close? Health Care Manager. 2015;34(3):225–33. PubMed PMID: 26217998.

14. Pare M. Boundary issues, in CanMEDS physician health guide: a practical handbook for physician health and well-being. Eds. Puddester D, Flynn L, and Cohen J. Ottawa (ON): The Royal College of Physicians and Surgeons of Canada; 2009. p. 76-7.

15. CMPA: empowering better health care [Internet]. Ottawa (ON): Canadian Medical Protective Association. Respecting boundaries; [cited 2017 Oct 20]; [about 1 screen]. Available from: https://www.cmpa-acpm.ca/serve/docs/ela/goodpracticesguide/pages/professionalism/Respecting_boundaries/maintaining_appropriate_boundaries-e.html

16. Chretien KC, Tuck MG. Online professionalism: a synthetic review. Int Rev Psychiatry. 2015;27(2):106–17. PubMed PMID: 25804627.

17. Chretien KC, Farnan JM, Greysen SR, et al. To friend or not to friend? Social networking and faculty perceptions of online professionalism. Acad Med. 2011;86(12):1545–50. PubMed PMID: 22030752.

18. Brown J. How to master electronic communication with patients. Med Econ. 2013;90(7):60–2, 64–7. PubMed PMID: 24066458.

19. Chretien KC, Greysen SR, Chretien J-P, et al. Online posting of unprofessional content by medical students. JAMA. 2009;302(12):1309–15.

20. Greysen SR, Kind T, Chretien KC. Online professionalism and the mirror of social media. J Gen Intern Med. 2010;25(11):1227–9. PubMed PMID: 20632121.

21. Greysen SR, Chretien KC, Kind T, et al. Physician violations of online professionalism and disciplinary actions: a national survey of state medical boards. JAMA. 2012;307(11):1141–2. PubMed PMID: 22436951.

22. Bosslet GT. Commentary: the good, the bad, and the ugly of social media. Acad Emerg Med. 2011;18(11):1221–2. PubMed PMID: 22092907.

23. Rosen J. The web means the end of forgetting. New York Times Magazine. 2010 July 21: p. 25.

24. O'Hanlon S, Shannon B. Comments further to: privacy, professionalism and Facebook: a dilemma for young doctors. Med Educ. 2011;45(2):209. PubMed PMID: 21208267.

25. Grauschopf S. A complete guide to Facebook's privacy settings: how (and why!) to control who sees your Facebook posts [Internet]. New York: The Balance; 2016 [updated 2018 Aug 29, cited 2017 Oct 26]. Available from: https://www.thebalance.com/understanding-facebook-s-privacy-levels-892796

26. Luckerson V. Make your Facebook profile more private in 6 easy steps. Time [Internet]. 2016 Jan 5;Tech:[about 8 screens]. Available from: http://time.com/4166749/facebook-privacy-settings-guide/

27. Zheleva E, Terzi E, Getoor L. Privacy in social networks. Synthesis Lectures on Data Mining and Knowledge Discovery. 2012;3(1):1–85.

28. Aghasian E, Garg S, Gao L, et al. Scoring users' privacy disclosure across multiple online social networks. IEEE Access. 2017;5:13118–30. DOI: 10.1109/ACCESS.2017.2720187

29. Aljohani M, Nisbet A, Blincoe K. A survey of social media users' privacy settings & information disclosure. In: Johnstone M, editor. Proceedings of the 14th Australian Information Security Management Conference, 2016 Dec 5–6, Edith Cowan University, Perth, Western Australia. Perth: Security Research Institute, Edith Cowan University; 2016. p. 67–75. Available from: https://kblincoe.github.io/publications/2016_SECAU_Social_Media.pdf

30. Solon O. You are Facebook's product, not customer. Wired UK [Internet]. 2011 Sept 21;Technology:[about 2 screens]. Available from: https://www.wired.co.uk/article/doug-rushkoff-hello-etsy

31. Ovide S. Google and Facebook divide up your eyeballs. Bloomberg [Internet]. 2016 Nov 21 [cited 2017 Oct 27];Gadfly. Available from: https://www.bloomberg.com/gadfly/articles/2016-11-21/google-and-facebook-divide-up-your-advertising-viewing

32. Lanchester J. You are the product. London Review of Books. 2017 Aug 17;39(16):3–10. Available from: https://www.lrb.co.uk/v39/n16/john-lanchester/you-are-the-product

33. Wu T. The attention merchants. New York: Random House; 2016.

34. Meyer R. The Cambridge Analytica scandal, in 3 paragraphs. The Atlantic [Internet]. 2018 Mar 20;Technology:[about 3 screens]. Available from: https://www.theatlantic.

com/technology/archive/2018/03/the-cam-bridge-analytica-scandal-in-three-para-graphs/556046/

35. Wikipedia [Internet]. Wikimedia Foundation, Inc.; 2018. Facebook-Cambridge Analytica data scandal; 2018 [updated 2018 Nov 29, cited 2018 May 19]; [about 3 screens]. Available from: https://en.wikipedia.org/wiki/Facebook%E2%80%93Cambridge_Analytica_data_scandal

36. Facebook [Internet]. Menlo Park (CA): Facebook, Inc.; 2018. Data policy; revised 2018 Apr 19 [cited 2017 Oct 28]; [about 14 screens]. Available from: https://www.facebook.com/policy.php

37. Schneier B. Data and Goliath: the hidden battles to collect your data and control your world. New York: WW Norton & Company; 2015.

38. Facebook is "deliberately killing privacy," says Schneier 2010 [cited 2017 Nov 24, 2017]. Available from: https://www.information-age.com/facebook-is-deliberately-killing-privacy-says-schneier-1290603/

39. Nazem N. Can my doctor be my Facebook friend? BBC News [Internet]. 2013 Nov 22 [cited 2017 Oct 25];Health[about 3 screens]. Available from: http://www.bbc.com/news/health-24850051

40. CPSO. Social media offers benefits, risks. CPSO Dialogue. 2013;9(2):30–2.

41. Devi S. Facebook friend request from a patient? Lancet. 2011;377(9772):1141–2. PubMed PMID: 21465700.

42. Volpe R, Blackall G, Green M, et al. Googling a patient. Hastings Cent Rep. 2013;43(5):14–15. PubMed PMID: 24224192.

43. Yu S, Wilkerson RG. Facebook: a last resort for patient contact. Am J Emerg Med. 2017;35(9):1375–6. DOI: 10.1016/j.ajem.2017.03.045

44. Warner J. Anything you post can and will be used against you: the legal dos and don'ts of social media. Super Lawyers: a special advertising supplement to the New York Times. 2017:8–11. Available from: https://www.superlawyers.com/united-states/article/anything-you-post-can-and-will-be-used-against-you/8783055d-aa01-405e-b825-99867be32fd8.html

45. Chretien KC, Kind T. Social media and clinical care: ethical, professional, and social implications. Circulation. 2013;127(13):1413–21. PubMed PMID: 23547180.

46. Doctor sued for posting breast augmentation photos. Kansas City Star [Internet]. 2012 August 13;Local:[about 1 screen]. Available from: https://www.kansascity.com/news/local/article306966/Doctor-sued-for-posting-breast-augmentation-photos.html

47. CMPA: empowering better health care [Internet]. Ottawa (ON): Canadian Medical Protective Association. Using clinical photography and video for educational purposes; 2011 Mar [cited 2017 Oct 15]; [about 3 screens]. Available from: https://www.cmpa-acpm.ca/en/advice-publications/browse-articles/2011/using-clinical-photography-and-video-for-educational-purposes

48. Devon KM. A piece of my mind. Status update: whose photo is that? JAMA. 2013;309(18):1901–2. PubMed PMID: 23652521.

49. Valencia N, Fernandez B, Deaton J. Photos of drinking, grinning air mission doctors cause uproar. CNN [Internet]. 2010 Feb 3 [cited 2017 Nov 6];World:[about 2 screens]. Available from: http://www.cnn.com/2010/WORLD/americas/01/29/haiti.puerto.rico.doctors/index.html

50. Ventola CL. Social media and health care professionals: benefits, risks, and best practices. Pharm Ther. 2014;39(7):491–520. PMID: 25083128.

51. Carone DA. The limitation of blogging about patients [Internet]. Nashua (NH): KevinMD; 2011 Oct 18 [cited 2017 Nov 7]; [about 1 screen]. Available from: http://www.kevinmd.com/blog/2011/10/limitation-blogging-patients.html

52. Patterson K. Talk to me like my father: frontline medicine in Afghanistan. Mother Jones. 2007 July/August.

53. Freeman A. Doctor's gory tale angers soldier's family. Globe and Mail [Internet]. 2007 August 4, updated 2018 Apr 26;News:[about 3 screens]. Available from: https://www.theglobeandmail.com/news/national/doctors-gory-tale-angers-soldiers-family/article690429/

54. College of Physicians and Surgeons of British Columbia. Disciplinary report on Dr. Kevin Patterson [Internet]. Vancouver (BC):

CPSBC; 2009 Jan 27 [cited 2018 May 22]. Available from: https://www.cpsbc.ca/files/disciplinary-actions/Dr_Kevin_Lee_Patterson_090127_f.pdf

55. B.C. doctor disciplined for writing about soldier's death. CBC News [Internet]. 2009 Jan 27 [cited 2018 May 22];British Columbia:[about 2 screens]. Available from: http://www.cbc.ca/news/canada/british-columbia/b-c-doctor-disciplined-for-writing-about-soldier-s-death-1.790277

56. Gibson E. Publication of case reports: is consent required? Paediatr Child Health. 2008;13(8):666–7. PubMed PMID: PMC2606070.

57. Ofri D. Doctor-writers: what are the ethics? Huffington Post [Internet]. 2010 Jul 5 [updated 2011 May 25, cited 2017 Oct]:[about 2 screens]. Available from: https://www.huffingtonpost.com/danielle-ofri-md-phd/doctor-writers-what-are-t_b_563664.html

58. Osipov R. Healing narrative: ethics and writing about patients. Virtual Mentor. 2011;13(7):420.

59. Reisman A. Should doctors write about patients? The benefits—and ethical pitfalls—of telling true stories as a physician. The Atlantic [Internet]. 2015 Feb 18;Health:[about 4 screens]. Available from: https://www.theatlantic.com/health/archive/2015/02/should-doctors-write-about-their-patients/385296/

Chapter 12

1. The reaction, or foreign conservatism. Blackwood's Edinburgh Magazine. 1849 May;65(303):537. Available from: https://babel.hathitrust.org/cgi/pt?id=chi.26398629;view=1up;seq=545

2. Hilfiker D. Facing our mistakes. N Engl J Med. 1984;310(2):118–22. DOI: 10.1056/NEJM198401123100211. The original classic paper on self-disclosure of harmful error. "Medicine has no place for its mistakes," Hilfiker wrote. How times have changed—at least for some.

3. Davies J, Hébert PC, Hoffman C. Canadian patient safety dictionary. Ottawa (ON): RCPSC; 2003. p. 26–8.

4. Lord Denning, "We must not condemn as negligence that which is only a misadventure." Quoted in Picard E, Robertson G. Legal liability of doctors and hospitals in Canada. 3rd ed. Toronto (ON): Carswell Thomson Canada; 1996. p. 212.

5. The quotation in Box 12.3 is taken from Mahon v Osborne, 2 KB 14, 31 (CA 1939).

6. Baker GR, Norton PG, Flintoft V, et al. The Canadian adverse events study: the incidence of adverse events among hospital patients in Canada. CMAJ. 2004;170(11):1678–86; PMID: 15159366; Wilson R, Runciman W, Gibberd R, et al. The quality in Australian health care study. Med J Aust. 1995;163(9):458–71. PMID: 7476634; An organisation with a memory. London: UK Department of Health; 2000. Available from: www.doh.gov.uk; Gawande A, Thomas E, Zinner M, et al. The incidence and nature of surgical adverse events in Colorado and Utah in 1992. Surgery. 1999;126(1):66–75. DOI: 10.1067/msy.1999.98664

7. Institute of Medicine. To err is human: building a safer health system. Washington (DC): National Academy Press; 1999.

8. Institute of Medicine. Crossing the quality chasm: a new health system for the 21st century. Washington (DC): National Academy Press; 2001.

9. Arriaga A, Bader A, Wong J, et al. Simulation-based trial of surgical-crisis checklists. N Engl J Med. 2013;368(3):246–53. DOI: 10.1056/NEJMsa1204720

10. See, for example, Camiré E, Moyen E, Stelfox T. Medication errors in critical care: risk factors, prevention and disclosure. CMAJ. 2009;180(9):936–43. DOI: 10.1503/cmaj.080869

11. Klein G. Sources of power: how people make decisions. Cambridge (MA): MIT Press; 1998.

12. Vicente K. The human factor: revolutionizing the way we live with technology. Toronto (ON): Vintage Canada Books; 2004.

13. "Managing test results effectively is vital to quality patient care." College of Physicians and Surgeons of Ontario. Test results management. Toronto (ON): CPSO; 2011. (Policy 11-1.) Available from: https://www.cpso.on.ca/Policies-Publications/Policy/Test-Results-Management

14. Shobridge v Thomas, [1999] BCJ No. 1747 (BCSC).

15. Brown S, Lehman C, Truog R, et al. Stepping out further from the shadows: disclosure of harmful radiologic errors to

patients. Radiology. 2012;262(2):381–6. DOI: 10.1148/radiol.11110829

16. Balint M. The doctor, his patient and the illness. Rev ed. Madison (CT): International Universities Press; 1988. p. 69–80.

17. Braun v Vaughan, [2000] MJ No. 63 (MBCA).

18. Garvey C, Connolly S. Radiology reporting: where does the radiologist's duty end? Lancet. 2006;367(9508):444. DOI: 10.1016/S0140-6736(06)68145-2

19. Berlin L. Using an automated coding and review process to communicate critical radiologic findings: one way to skin a cat. AJR Am J Roentgenol. 2005;185(4):840–3. DOI: 10.2214/AJR.05.0651. The author has written extensively and eloquently on error in radiology and the scope of the radiologist's duty to disclose mistakes to patients. See: Berlin L. Malpractice issues in radiology. 3rd ed. Leesburg (VA): ARRS; 2009.

20. Wu A. Medical error: the second victim. The doctor who makes the mistake needs help too. BMJ. 2000;320(7237):726–7. PMID: 10720336.

21. Boyte R. Casey's legacy. Health Aff. 2001;20(2):250–4. PMID: 11260951.

22. Davidoff F. Shame: the elephant in the room. BMJ. 2002;324(7338):623–4. PMID:11895807.

23. Iezzoni L, Rao S, DesRoches C, et al. Survey shows that at least some physicians are not always open or honest with patients. Health Aff. 2012;31(2):383–91. DOI: 10.1377/hlthaff.2010.1137

24. Varjavand N, Bachegowda L, Gracely E, et al. Changes in intern attitudes toward medical error and disclosure. Med Educ. 2012;46(7):668–77. DOI: 10.1111/j.1365-2923.2012.04269.x

25. Gallagher TH, Denham CR, Leape LL, et al. Disclosing unanticipated outcomes to patients: the art and practice. J Patient Saf. 2007;3:158–65. DOI: 10.1097/pts.0b013e3181451606

26. Kleinman A. Presence. Lancet. 2017;389(10088):2466–7. DOI: 10.1016/S0140-6736(17)31620-3

27. Canadian Patient Safety Institute. Canadian disclosure guidelines: being open with patients and families. Edmonton (AB): CPSI; 2011.

28. Kraman S, Hamm G. Risk management: extreme honesty may be the best policy. Ann Intern Med. 1999;131(12):963–7. PMID: 10610649.

29. Kachalia A, Kaufman S, Boothman R, et al. Liability claims and costs before and after implementation of a medical error disclosure program. Ann Intern Med. 2010;153(4);213–21. DOI: 10.7326/0003-4819-153-4-201008170-00002

30. Lazare A. On apology. New York (NY): Oxford University Press; 2004.

31. Castel M. The impact of the Canadian Apology Legislation when determining civil liability in Canadian private international law. Advocates' Quarterly. 2012;39:440–51.

32. Proposed language may be found in the Uniform Apology Act. CMPA: empowering better healthcare. Ottawa (ON): Canadian Medical Protective Association. Apology legislation in Canada: what it means for physicians; 2008 Sept [revised 2013 Apr]; [about 2 screens]. Available from: https://www.cmpa-acpm.ca/en/advice-publications/browse-articles/2008/apology-legislation-in-canada-what-it-means-for-physicians

33. Sorry Works! [Internet]. Glen Carbon (IL): Sorry Works! States with apology laws; [about 1 screen]. Available from: http://sorryworkssite.bondwaresite.com/apology-laws-cms-143

34. Apology Act, 2009, S.O. 2009, c. 3.

35. Alcorn T. Meningitis outbreak reveals gaps in US drug regulation. Lancet. 2012;380(9853):1543–4. Perfect J. Iatrogenic fungal meningitis: tragedy repeated. Ann Intern Med. 2012;157(11):825–6. DOI: 10.7326/0003-4819-157-11-201212040-00558

36. Dudzinski D, Hébert PC, Foglia MB, et al. The disclosure dilemma: large-scale adverse events. N Engl J Med. 2010;363(10):978–86. DOI: 10.1056/NEJMhle1003134

37. Hormone testing: judicial inquiry probes faulty breast cancer tests. CBC News [Internet]. 2008 March 18;In Depth:[about 3 screens]. Available from: https://www.cbc.ca/news2/background/cancer/inquiry.html

38. Cameron MA, Commissioner. Commission of Inquiry on Hormone Receptor Testing [Internet]. St. John's (NL): Commission of Inquiry on Hormone Receptor Testing; 2007. Available from: http://www.cihrt.

nl.ca; http://www.releases.gov.nl.ca/re-leases/2009/health/CameronInquiry.pdf

39. Mustapha v. Culligan of Canada Ltd., 2008 SCC 27, [2008] 2 SCR 114.

40. Healey v. Lakeridge Health Corp., 2011 ONCA 55, [2011] 103 OR 3d 401 (ONCA).

41. Elwy R, Bokhour BG, Maguire EM, et al. Improving healthcare systems' disclosures of large-scale adverse events: a department of veterans affairs leadership, policymaker, research and stakeholder partnership. J Gen Intern Med. 2014;29(Suppl 4):S895–903. DOI: 10.1007/s11606-014-3034-3.

42. Hall J. Horae vacivae, or, essays: some occasionall considerations. London;E.G. for J. Rothwell, at the Sun and Fountaine in Pauls Church-yard; 1646. p. 6. Available from: https://quod.lib.umich.edu/cgi/t/text/text-idx?c=eebo;idno=A86786.0001.001

Chapter 13

1. DeLillo D. Mao II. New York: Viking Penguin; 1991. p. 16.

2. Oxford English Dictionary [CD-ROM]. 2nd ed. Version 3.0. Oxford: Oxford University Press; 2002.

3. Adapted from Iezzoni L. Boundaries. what happens to the disabled poor when insurers draw a line between what's "medically necessary" and devices that can improve quality of life? Health Aff. 1999;18(6):171–6. PMID: 10650700.

4. Iezzoni L. Eliminating health and health care disparities among the growing population of people with disabilities. Health Aff. 2011;30(10):1947–54. DOI: 10.1377/hlthaff.2011.0613

5. Cheng J. Confronting the social determinants of health: obesity, neglect, and inequity. N Engl J Med. 2012;367(21):1976–7. DOI: 10.1056/NEJMp1209420

6. Hilfiker D. Not all of us are saints: a doctor's journey with the poor. Toronto (ON): Macmillan; 1994.

7. Rawls J. Justice as fairness: a restatement. Cambridge (MA): Harvard University Press; 2001. p. 9.

8. Adapted from McIntyre J, quoted in Jackman M. The Canadian Charter as a barrier to unwanted medical treatment of pregnant women in the interests of the foetus. Health Law Can. 1993;14(2):53. PMID: 10131254.

9. Adapted from Council on Ethical and Judicial Affairs, AMA. Ethical considerations in the allocation of organs and other scarce medical resources among patients. Arch Intern Med. 1995;155(1):40. PMID: 7802518.

10. Alexander S. They decide who lives, who dies. Life Magazine. 1962 Nov 9;102ff.

11. Eggers P. Medicare's end stage renal disease program. Health Care Financ Rev. 2000;22(1):55–60. PMID: 25372768.

12. Baker R. Visibility and the just allocation of health care: a study of age-rationing in the British NHS. Health Care Anal. 1993;1(2):139–50. DOI: 10.1007/BF02197107

13. Clarke K, Gray D, Keating N, et al. Do women with acute myocardial infarction receive the same treatment as men? BMJ. 1994;309(6954):563–6. PMID: 7916228.

14. Kaul P, Chang W, Westerhout C, et al. Differences in admission rates and outcomes between men and women presenting to emergency departments with coronary syndromes. CMAJ. 2007;177(10):1193–9. DOI: 10.1503/cmaj.060711

15. Udell J, Koh M, Qiu F, et al. Outcomes of women and men with acute coronary syndrome treated with and without percutaneous coronary revascularization. J Am Heart Assoc. 2017,6(1).e004319. DOI: 10.1161/JAHA.116.004319

16. Borkhoff C, Hawker G, Kreder H, et al. The effect of patients' sex on physicians' recommendations for total knee arthroplasty. CMAJ. 2008;178(6):681–7. DOI: 10.1503/cmaj.071168

17. Aristotle. Nicomachean ethics. Ostwald M, translator. New York: Bobbs-Merrill Publishers; 1962. Book V.

18. American Physiological Society. Women's heart disease tied to small blood vessels. ScienceDaily [Internet]. 2011 Oct 14;Health & Medicine:[about 2 screens]. Available from: www.sciencedaily.com/releases/2011/10/111014095622.htm

19. Williams RI, Fraser AG, West RR. Gender differences in management after acute myocardial infarction: not 'sexism' but a reflection of age at presentation. J Public Health. 2004; 26(3):259–63. DOI: 10.1093/pubmed/fdh159

20. Royal College of Surgeons of England. Access all ages: assessing the impact of ages on access to surgical treatment. London: RCSENG; 2012. Available from: http://www.rcseng.ac.uk/publications/docs/access-all-ages

21. Miller D, Jahnigan D, Gorbien M, et al. CPR: How useful? Attitudes and knowledge of an elderly population. Arch Intern Med. 1992;152(3):578–82. PMID: 1546921.

22. Mariotto A, De Leo D, Buono MD, et al. Will elderly patients stand aside for younger patients in the queue for cardiac services? Lancet. 1999;354(9177):467–70. ISSN: 0140-6736. PMID: 10465171.

23. Howe E. Mixed agency in military medicine: ethical rules in conflict. In: Beam T, Sparacino L, Pellegrino E, et al., editors. Military medical ethics. Vol 1. Washington DC: Office of the Surgeon General; 2003. p. 339–43.

24. Earle CC, Landrum MB, Souza JM, et al. Aggressiveness of cancer care near the end of life: is it a quality-of-care issue? J Clin Oncol. 2008;26(23):3860–6. DOI: 10.1200/JCO.2007.15.8253

25. Wennberg J. Tracking medicine. 2010, New York: Oxford University Press; 2010. Understanding supply-sensitive care; p. 130.

26. Katz S, Jagsi R, Morrow M. Reducing overtreatment of cancer with precision medicine: just what the doctor ordered. JAMA. 2018;319(11):1091–2. DOI: 10.1001/jama.2018.0018

27. La Puma J. Managed care ethics. New York (NY): Hatherleigh Press; 1998.

28. Ubel P. Pricing life: why it's time for health care rationing. Cambridge (MA): First MIT Press; 2001.

29. Brook RH. Assessing the appropriateness of care: its time has come. JAMA. 2009;302(9):997–8. DOI: 10.1001/jama.2009.1279

30. Laine C. High-value testing begins with a few simple questions. Ann Intern Med. 2012;156(2):162–3. DOI: 10.7326/0003-4819-156-2-201201170-00016

31. Gawande A. Overkill. The New Yorker [Internet]. 2015 May 11;Annals of Health Care:[about 28 screens]. Available from: https://www.newyorker.com/magazine/2015/05/11/overkill-atul-gawande

32. Choosing Wisely [Internet]. Philadelphia (PA): ABIM Foundation; 2018. Available from: http://www.choosingwisely.org

33. Brody H. From an ethics of rationing to an ethics of waste avoidance. N Engl J Med. 2012;366(21):1949–51. DOI: 10.1056/NEJMp1203365

34. Choosing Wisely Canada. We've told patients to ask us, but what do WE need to ask

ourselves?. Choosing Wisely Canada; 2018. Available from: https://choosingwiselycanada.org/event/jan2018talk/

35. Harari YN. Sapiens: a brief history of humankind. Toronto (ON): McClelland & Stewart; 2014.

36. Sandel M. What money can't buy: the moral limits of markets. New York: Farrar, Straus and Giroux; 2012.

37. Martin D, Miller AP, Quesnel-Vallée A, et al. Canada's universal health-care system: achieving its potential. Lancet. 2018;391(10131):1718–35. DOI: 10.1016/S0140-6736(18)30181-8

38. Martin D. Better now: six big ideas to improve health care for all Canadians. Toronto (ON): Penguin Random House; 2017.

39. Canada Health Act. Wikipedia. Available from: https://en.wikipedia.org/wiki/Canada_Health_Act

40. Canada Health Act, R.S.C. 1985, c. C-6.

41. Canada.ca. Ottawa (ON): Government of Canada; 2018. Canada's health care system; 2016 Aug 22; [about 4 screens]. Available from: http://www.canada.ca/en/health-canada/services/canada-health-care-system.html

42. Eliminating Code Gridlock in Canada's Health Care System: 2015 Wait Time Alliance Report Card. Available from: http://www.waittimealliance.ca/wta-reports/2015-wta-report-card/

43. Chaoulli v Quebec (Attorney General), 2005 SCC 35, [2005] 1 SCR 791.

44. Yeo M, Lucock C. Quality v. equality: the divided court in Chaoulli v. Québec. Health Law J. 2006;14:129–50. PMID: 17563960.

45. Schroeder S, Cantor J. On squeezing balloons. Cost control fails again. N Engl J Med. 1991;325(15):1099–100. DOI: 10.1056/NEJM199110103251510

46. Flood C, Zimmerman M. Judicious choices: health care resource decisions and the Supreme Court of Canada. In: Downie J, Gibson E, editors. Health law at the Supreme Court of Canada. Toronto (ON): Irwin Law; 2007. p. 54.

47. National Institute for Health and Care Excellence [Internet]. London: NICE; 2018. Available from: https://www.nice.org.uk

48. Cochrane UK [Internet]. London: The Cochrane Collaboration; 2018. About us;

[about 2 screens]. Available from: http://uk.cochrane.org/about-us

49. Eddy D. Clinical decision making: from theory to practice: practice policies: what are they? JAMA. 1990;263(6):877–80. PMID:2296151.

50. Ransohoff D, Pignone M, Sox H. How to decide whether a clinical practice guideline is trustworthy. JAMA. 2013;309(2):139–40. DOI: 10.1001/jama.2012.156703

51. Oshima Lee E, Emanuel EJ. Shared decision making to improve care and reduce costs. N Engl J Med. 2013;368(1):6–8. DOI: 10.1056/NEJMp1209500

52. Hummel E, Ubel P. Cost and clinical practice guidelines: can two wrongs make it right? Virtual Mentor. 2004;6(12):558–60. Available from: http://virtualmmentor.ama-assn.org/2004/12/pfor1-0412.html.

53. Kredo T, Bernhardsson S, Machingaidze S, et al. Guide to clinical practice guidelines: the current state of play. Int J Qual Health Care. 2016;28(1):122–8. DOI: 10.1093/intqhc/mzv115

54. Daniels, N. Just health. New York (NY): Cambridge University Press; 2008. How can we meet health needs fairly when we can't meet them all? Accountability for reasonable resource allocation. p. 103–39.

55. Biller-Andorno N, Lee TH. Ethical physician incentives: from carrots and sticks to shared purpose. N Engl J Med. 2013;368(11):980–2. DOI: 10.1056/NEJMp1300373

56. Wennberg J. Tracking medicine: a researcher's quest to understand health care. New York: Oxford University Press; 2010. p. 10.

57. Kassirer J. Managed care and the morality of the marketplace. N Engl J Med. 1995;333(1):50–2. DOI: 10.1056/NEJM199507063330110

58. Hopkins D. Disease eradication. N Engl J Med. 2013;368(1):54–63. DOI: 10.1056/NEJMra1200391

59. Caulfield T. The vaccination picture. Toronto (ON): Penguin Books; 2017.

60. See: US Department of Health and Human Services, US Department of Homeland Security. 'Updated interim planning guidance on allocating and targeting pandemic influenza vaccine. Washington (DC): US Department of Health and Human Services, US Department of Homeland Security; 2018. p. 5. Available from: https://www.cdc.gov/flu/pandemic-resources/national-strategy/planning-guidance/index.html

61. Henry B, Gadient S, on behalf of the Canadian Pandemic Influenza Preparedness (CPIP) Task Group. Canada's pandemic vaccine strategy. CCDR. 2017;43(7/8):164–7. Available from: https://www.canada.ca/content/dam/phac-aspc/migration/phac-aspc/publicat/ccdr-rmtc/17vol43/dr-rm43-7-8/assets/pdf/17vol43_7_8-ar-05-eng.pdf

62. UNOS [Internet]. Richmond (VA): United Network for Organ Sharing; 2018. Available from: www.unos.org

63. Benjamin M, Cohen C, Grochowski E. What transplantation can teach us about health care reform. N Engl J Med. 1994;330(12):858–60. DOI: 10.1056/NEJM199403243301211

64. Daniels N. Four unsolved rationing problems. A challenge. Hastings Cent Rep. 1994;24(4):27–9. PMID: 7960702.

65. Radcliffe Richards J. The ethics of transplants: why careless thought costs lives. Oxford: Oxford University Press; 2012.

66. Truog RD. The ethics of organ donation by living donors. N Engl J Med. 2005;353(5):444–6. DOI: 10.1056/NEJMp058155

67. Everybody can save a life. Matching Donors [Internet]. Canton (MA): MatchingDonors; 2003–2018. Available from: http://matchingdonors.com/life/index.cfm

68. Steinbrook R. Public solicitation of organ donors. N Engl J Med. 2005;353(5):441–4. DOI: 10.1056/NEJMp058151

69. Couri T, Cotter TG, Chen D, et al. Use of hepatitis C positive organs: patient attitudes in urban Chicago. Am J Nephrol 2019; 49:32–40 doi.org/10.1159/000495263

70. Denner J. Paving the path toward porcine organs for transplantation. New Engl J Med. 2017, 377 (19): 1892–3. DOI: 10.1056/NEJMcibr1710853

71. Singer P. Ethics in the real world: 82 brief essays on things that matter. Princeton (NJ): Princeton University Press; 2016.

72. Farmer P, Yong Kim J, Kleinman A, et al. Reimagining global health: an introduction. Los Angeles (CA): University of California Press; 2013.

Chapter 14

1. Reference re Assisted Human Reproduction Act, 2010 SCC 61, [2010] 3 SCR 457.

2. Templeton A, Grimes DA. A request for abortion. N Engl J Med. 2011;365(23):2198–204. DOI: 10.1056/NEJMcp1103639

3. On this point, and many other points in this chapter, the authors are extremely grateful for the close critical reading by Dr Rhonda Zwingerman.

4. Thomas WD. The Badgley report on the abortion law. CMAJ. 1977;116(9):966. PMID: 858113.

5. Badgley R. Report of the committee on the operation of the abortion law. Ottawa (ON): Department of Justice; 1977.

6. R v Morgentaler, [1988] 44 DLR (4th) 385, 402 (SCC).

7. Browne A, Sullivan B. Abortion in Canada. Camb Q Healthc Ethics. 2005;14(3):287–91. PMID: 16028541.

8. Abortion Rights Coalition of Canada. Statistics: abortion in Canada [Internet]. Vancouver (BC): Abortion Rights Coalition of Canada; January 30, 2019.. Available from: http://www.arcc-cdac.ca/backrounders/statistics-abortion-in-canada.pdf

9. Dunn S, Cook R. Medical abortion in Canada: behind the times. CMAJ. 2014;186(1):13–14. DOI: 10.1503/cmaj.131320

10. Gruben V. Regulating reproduction. In: Erdman J, Gruben V, Nelson E, editors. Canadian health law and policy. 5th ed. Toronto (ON): LexisNexis Canada; 2017. p. 399–428.

11. Sedgh G, Henshaw S, Singh S, et al. Induced abortion: estimated rates and trends worldwide. Lancet. 2007;370(9595):1338–45. DOI: 10.1016/S0140-6736(07)61575-X

12. R v Morgentaler, [1988] 1 SCR 30.

13. Grisez G, Boyle J, Finnis J, et al. "Every marital act ought to be open to new life": toward a clearer understanding. The Thomist. 1988;52(3):365–426.

14. Weir M, Evans M, Coughlin K. Ethical decision making in the resuscitation of extremely premature infants: the health care professional's perspective. J Obstet Gynaecol Can. 2011;33(1):49–56. DOI: 10.1016/S1701-2163(16)34773-9

15. Harris L. Divisions, new and old: conscience and religious freedom at HHS. N Engl J Med. 2018;378(15):1369–71. DOI: 10.1056/NEJMp1801154

16. Thomson JJ. A defense of abortion. Phil and Public Affairs. 1971; 1(1)47–66. https://www.jstor.org/stable/2265091

17. Lee P, George R. The wrong of abortion. In: Cohen AI, Wellman CH, editors. Contemporary debates in applied ethics. Malden (MA): Blackwell Publishing; 2005. p. 13-26.

18. Roe v Wade, 410 US 113 (1973). Roe v Wade, (No. 70-18) 314 F. Supp. 1217 (US 1973), aff'd in part and rev'd in part.

19. Igo S. The known citizen: a history of privacy in modern America. Cambridge (MA): Harvard University Press; 2018. p. 158–9.

20. Guttmacher Institute [Internet]. New York: Guttmacher Institute; 2018. An overview of abortion laws; 2018 Feb 1; [about 5 screens]. Available from: https://www.guttmacher.org/state-policy/explore/overview-abortion-laws

21. Greene M, Ecker J. Abortion, health and the law. N Engl J Med. 2004;350(2):184–6. DOI: 10.1056/NEJMsb035739

22. I Stand With Planned Parenthood [Internet]. Planned Parenthood Federation of America Inc. and Planned Parenthood Action Fund, Inc.; 2018. "Defund" defined; [about 4 screens]. Available from: https://www.istandwithpp.org/defund-defined

23. Carlsen A, Ngu A, Simon S. What it takes to get an abortion in the most restrictive U.S. state. New York Times [Internet]. 2018 July 20;U.S.:[about 6 screens]. Available from: https://www.nytimes.com/interactive/2018/07/20/us/mississippi-abortion-restrictions.html

24. Herskovitz J. Floor tiles, water fountains, clinic doors weigh on Texas abortion case. Reuters [Internet]. 2016 Feb 28;Supreme Court:[about 2 screens]. Available from: https://www.reuters.com/article/us-usa-court-abortion-clinics-id USKCN0W10HT

25. R v Morgentaler, [1988] 1 SCR 30.

26. Tremblay v Daigle, [1989] 2 SCR 530.

27. Kent CA. Medical ethics: the state of the law. Toronto (ON): LexisNexis Canada; 2005.

28. Dickens BM, Cook, RJ. The scope and limits of conscientious objection. Int J Gynaecol Obstet. 2000;71(1):71–7. PMID: 11044548.

29. College of Physicians and Surgeons of Ontario. Effective referral [Internet]. Toronto (ON): CPSO; 2016. Available from: https://www.cpso.on.ca/CPSO/media/documents/Policies/Policy-Items/PAD-Effective-Referral-FactSheet.pdf

30. Breen K, Cordner S, Thomson C. Good medical practice: professionalism, ethics and law. 4th ed. Kingston (AU): Australia Medical Council; 2016. p. 483.

31. Charo RA. The partial death of abortion rights. N Engl J Med. 2007;356(21):2125–8. DOI: 10.1056/NEJMp078055

32. Rodgers S, Downie J. Abortion: ensuring access. CMAJ. 2006;175(1):9. DOI: 10.1503/cmaj.060548

33. Shawn Winsor, personal communication, 2017.

34. Rudrappa S. India outlawed commercial surrogacy: clinics are finding loopholes. The Conversation [Internet]. 2017 Oct 23 [cited 2018 Jan 29];Politics:[about 4 screens]. Available from: http://theconversation.com/india-outlawed-commercial-surrogacy-clinics-are-finding-loopholes-81784

35. Castro RJ. Mitochondrial replacement therapy: the UK and US regulatory landscapes. J Law Biosci. 2016;3(3):726–35. DOI: 10.1093/jlb/lsw051

36. Fraga, J. After IVF, some struggle with what to do with leftover embryos. NPR [Internet]. 2016 Aug 20;Treatments:[about 3 screens]. Available from: https://www.npr.org/sections/health-shots/2016/08/20/489232868/after-ivf-some-struggle-with-what-to-do-with-leftover-embryos

37. Rivard G, Hunter J. The law of assisted human reproduction. Toronto (ON): LexisNexis Canada; 2005.

38. Reference re Assisted Human Reproduction Act, 2010 SCC 61, [2010] 3 SCR 457.

39. Ikemoto L. ART use among neighbours: commercialization concerns in Canada and the U.S., in the global context. In: Lemmens T, Martin AF, Lee IB, Milne C, editors. Regulating creation: the law, ethics, and policy of assisted human reproduction. Toronto (ON): University of Toronto Press; 2017. p. 253–73.

40. Ethics Committee of the American Society for Reproductive Medicine. Preconception gender selection for nonmedical reasons. Fertil Steril. 2004;82 Suppl 1:S232-5. DOI: 10.1016/j.fertnstert.2004.05.013

41. Ethics Committee of the American Society for Reproductive Medicine. Financial compensation of oocyte donors: an Ethics Committee opinion. Fertil Steril. 2016;106(7):e15-e19. DOI: 10.1016/j.fertnstert.2016.09.040

42. Blackwell T. Illegal purchase of sperm, eggs and surrogacy services leads to 27 charges against Canadian fertility company and CEO. National Post [Internet]. 2013 Feb 15;News:[about 6 screens]. Available from: https://nationalpost.com/news/illegal-purchase-of-sperm-eggs-and-surrogacy-services-leads-to-27-charges-against-canadian-fertility-company-and-ceo

43. James S, Chilvers R, Havemann D, et al. Avoiding legal pitfalls in surrogacy arrangements. Reprod Biomed Online. 2010;21(7):862–7. DOI: 10.1016/j.rbmo.2010.06.037

44. Sensible Surrogacy is one of many private sites devoted to helping arrange surrogate pregnancy. "We seek out the best, most successful IVF clinics and service providers worldwide. We negotiate the lowest prices on behalf of our clients. And we provide the guidance to ensure that our clients have the best chance at success." For more info, visit: Sensible Surrogacy [Internet]. Las Vegas (NV): Sensible Surrogacy; 2018. Available from: https://www.sensiblesurrogacy.com

45. Sarah Cohen, personal communication, 2018 January 19.

46. Food and Drugs Act, R.S.C. 1985, c. F-27.

47. See HFEA statement on Donor Conceived Register. 2018 April 17. Available from: https://www.hfea.gov.uk/about-us/news-and-press-releases/2018-news-and-press-releases/hfea-statement-on-donor-conceived-register/

48. Pratten v BC (Attorney General), 2011 BCSC 656, [2011] 22 BCLR (5th) 307 (BCSC).

49. Zomorodi S. Should s. 7 Charter rights impose positive state obligations in the context of donor anonymity? Reg Offenses and Compliance Newsletter. 2011;40:1–5.

50. Gruben V. A number but no name: is there a constitutional right to know one's sperm donor in Canadian law? In: Lemmens T, Martin AF, Lee IB, Milne C, editors. Regulating creation: the law, ethics, and policy of assisted human reproduction. Toronto

(ON): University of Toronto Press; 2017. p. 145–77.

51. Gurmankin AD, Caplan AL, Braverman AM. Screening practices and beliefs of ART programs. Fertil Steril. 2005;83(1):61–7. DOI: 10.1016/j.fertnstert.2004.06.048

52. Light AD, Obedin-Maliver J, Sevelius JM, et al. Transgender men who experienced pregnancy after female-to-male gender transitioning. Obstet Gynecol. 2014;124(6):1120–7. DOI: 10.1097/AOG.0000000000000540

53. Potter v Korn, [1995] BCCHRD No. 20.

54. Korn v Potter, [1996] BCJ No. 692 (BCSC).

55. Ethics Committee of the American Society for Reproductive Medicine. Access to fertility treatment by gays, lesbians, and unmarried persons. Fertil Steril. 2009;92(4):1190–3. DOI: 10.1016/j.fertnstert.2009.07.977

56. Ethics Committee of the American Society for Reproductive Medicine. Child-rearing and the provision of fertility services. Fertil Steril. 2009;92(3):864–7. DOI: 10.1016/j.fertnstert.2009.07.978

57. Boorse C. On the distinction between disease and illness. In: Cohen M, Nagel T, Scanlon T, editors. Medicine and moral philosophy. Princeton (NJ): Princeton University Press; 1981. p. 3–48.

58. Cameron v Nova Scotia (Attorney General), [1999] NSJ No. 297 para 170 (NSCA).

59. Marvel S, Tarasoff L, Epstein R, et al. Listening to LGBTQ people on assisted human reproduction: access to reproductive material, services, and facilities. In: Lemmens T, Martin AF, Lee IB, Milne C, editors. Regulating creation: the law, ethics, and policy of assisted human reproduction. Toronto (ON): University of Toronto Press; 2017. p. 325–58.

60. Flood C, Thomas B. Regulatory failure: the case of the private-for-profit IVF sector. In: Lemmens T, Martin AF, Lee IB, Milne C, editors. Regulating creation: the law, ethics, and policy of assisted human reproduction. Toronto (ON): University of Toronto Press; 2017. p. 359–88.

61. Claiborne A, English R, Kahn J, editors. Committee on the Ethical and Social Policy Considerations of Novel Techniques for Prevention of Maternal Transmission of Mitochondrial DNA Diseases; Board on Health Sciences Policy; Institute of Medicine; National Academies of Sciences, Engineering and Medicine. Mitochondrial replacement techniques: ethical, social, and policy considerations. Consensus study report. Washington (DC): National Academy of the Sciences; 2016.

62. Annas GJ. Assisted reproduction: Canada's Supreme Court and the "global baby." N Engl J Med. 2011;365(5):459–63. DOI: 10.1056/NEJMhle1101361

63. NGA Law [Internet]. Nr Salisbury: Natalie Gamble Associates; 2014. Single parent surrogacy: remedial order goes to Parliament; 2017 Nov 29; [about 2 screens]. Available from: http://www.nataliegambleassociates.co.uk/blog/2017/11/29/single-parent-surrogacy-remedial-order-goes-to-parliament

64. All Families Are Equal Act (Parentage and Related Registrations Statute Law Amendment), 2016, S.O. 2016, c. 23–Bill 28.

65. Drummond S. Fruitful diversity: revisiting the enforceability of gestational carriage contracts. In: Lemmens T, Martin AF, Lee IB, Milne C, editors. Regulating creation: the law, ethics, and policy of assisted human reproduction. Toronto (ON): University of Toronto Press, 2017. p. 274–324.

66. Tolstoy LN. Anna Karenina. Edmonds R, translator. Harmondsworth (UK): Penguin Books; 1969.

67. Jordan K. Fertility law, assisted reproduction and alternative family building. In: Wilson J. Wilson on children and the law. Toronto (ON): LexisNexis Canada; 2017.

68. Edmiston J. Woman wins couple's embryo tug of war. National Post. 2018 Aug 2; A1, 10.

69. Slack J. Stem cells: a very short introduction. Oxford: Oxford University Press; 2012.

70. Ptaszek LM, Mansour M, Ruskin JN, et al. Towards regenerative therapy for cardiac disease. Lancet. 2012;379(9819):933–42. DOI: 10.1016/S0140-6736(12)60075-0

71. Bolli R, Chugh AR, D'Amario D, et al. Cardiac stem cells in patients with ischaemic cardiomyopathy (SCIPIO): initial results of a randomized phase 1 trial. Lancet. 2011;378(9806):1847–57. DOI: 10.1016/S0140-6736(11)61590-0

72. Goff ZD, Kichura AB, Chibnall JT, et al. A survey of unregulated direct-to-consumer treatment centers providing stem cells for

patients with heart failure. JAMA Intern Med. 2017;177(9):1387–8. DOI: 10.1001/jamainternmed.2017.2988

73. Marks PW, Witten CM, Califf RM. Clarifying stem-cell therapy's benefits and risks. N Engl J Med. 2017;376(11):1007–9. DOI: 10.1056/NEJMp1613723

74. Jameson J, Longo D. Precision medicine: personalized, problematic, and promising. N Engl J Med. 2015;372(23):2229–34. DOI: 10.1056/NEJMsb1503104

75. Charo RA, Sipp D. Rejuvenating regenerative medicine regulation. N Engl J Med. 2018;378(6):504–5. DOI: 10.1056/NEJMp1715736

76. Laidlaw S. Battle lines being drawn for new war over stem cells. Toronto Star [Internet]. 2007 Aug 25;Insight:[about 4 screens]. Available from: https://www.thestar.com/news/insight/2007/08/25/battle_lines_being_drawn_for_new_war_over_stem_cells.html

77. Cavaliere G. A 14-day limit for bioethics: the debate over human embryo research. BMC Med Ethics. 2017;18(1):38. DOI: 10.1186/s12910-017-0198-5

78. Ethics Committee of the American Society for Reproductive Medicine. Financial compensation of oocyte donors. Fertil Steril. 2007;88(2):305–9. DOI: 10.1016/j.fertnstert.2007.01.104

Chapter 15

1. Beckett S. Waiting for Godot. New York: Grove Press, 1954.

2. Rodriguez v British Columbia (Attorney General), [1993] 3 SCR 519.

3. Terminally ill woman wins right to refuse treatment. CBC [Internet]. 1992 Feb 13 [updated 2018 April 8];Digital Archives:[video]. Available from: http://www.cbc.ca/player/play/1757272257

4. Nancy B. v Hotel-Dieu de Quebec, [1992] 86 DLR 4th 385 (QCCS).

5. Hussain JA, Flemming K, Murtagh FE, et al. Patient and health care professional decision-making to commence and withdraw from renal dialysis: a systematic review of qualitative research. Clin J Am Soc Nephrol. 2015;10(7):1201–15. PMID: 25943310.

6. Murphy E, Germain MJ, Cairns H, et al. International variation in classification of dialysis withdrawal: a systematic review.

Nephrol Dial Transplant. 2014;29(3):625–35. PMID: 24293659.

7. Aggarwal Y, Baharani J. End-of-life decision making: withdrawing from dialysis: a 12-year retrospective single centre experience from the UK. BMJ Support Palliat Care. 2014;4(4):368–76. PMID: 24844585.

8. Birmele B, Francois M, Pengloan J, et al. Death after withdrawal from dialysis: the most common cause of death in a French dialysis population. Nephrol Dial Transplant. 2004;19(3):686-91. PMID: 14767027.

9. Murtagh FEM, Spagnolo AG, Panocchia N, et al. Conservative (non dialytic) management of end-stage renal disease and withdrawal of dialysis. Prog Palliat Care. 2009;17(4):179–85. DOI: 10.1179/096992609X12455871937143

10. Davison SN, Torgunrud C. The creation of an advance care planning process for patients with ESRD. Am J Kidney Dis. 2007;49(1):27–36. PMID: 17185143.

11. United States Renal Data System. 2017 USRDS annual data report: Epidemiology of kidney disease in the United States [Internet]. Bethesda (MD): National Institutes of Health, National Institute of Diabetes and Digestive and Kidney Diseases; 2017 [cited 2018 Jun 28]. Available from: https://www.usrds.org/2017/view/Default.aspx

12. Turgeon AF, Lauzier F, Simard JF, et al. Mortality associated with withdrawal of life-sustaining therapy for patients with severe traumatic brain injury: a Canadian multicentre cohort study. CMAJ. 2011;183(14):1581–8. PMID: 21876014.

13. Baumrucker SJ, Sheldon JE, Morris GM, et al. Withdrawing treatment for the "wrong" reasons. Am J Hosp Palliat Med. 2007;24(6):509–14. PMID: 18182638.

14. Rodgers C, Field HL, Kunkel EJ. Countertransference issues in termination of life support in acute quadriplegia. Psychosomatics. 1995;36(3):305–9. PMID: 7638319.

15. von Gunten CF, Ferris FD, Emanuel LL. The patient–physician relationship. Ensuring competency in end-of-life care: communication and relational skills. JAMA. 2000;284(23):3051–7. PMID: 11122596.

16. Crawley LM, Marshall PA, Lo B, et al. End-of-Life Care Consensus Panel. Strategies for culturally effective end-of-life care. Ann

Intern Med. 2002;136(9):673–9. PMID: 11992303.

17. Gilmour JM. Legal capacity and decision-making. In: Erdman J, Gruben V, Nelson E, editors. Canadian health law and policy. 5th ed. Toronto (ON): LexisNexis Canada; 2017. p. 351–74.

18. Perkins HS. Controlling death: the false promise of advance directives. Ann Intern Med. 2007;147(1):51–7. PMID: 17606961.

19. Breslin J. Think carefully about advance requests for medical assistance in dying [Internet]. CMAJ Blogs; 2016 August 4; [about 4 screens]. Available from: https://cmajblogs.com/think-carefully-about-advance-requests-for-medical-assistance-in-dying/

20. Silveira MJ, Kim SY, Langa KM. Advance directives and outcomes of surrogate decision making before death. N Engl J Med. 2010;362(13):1211-8. PMID: 20357283.

21. Smith AK, Williams BA, Lo B. Discussing overall prognosis with the very elderly. N Engl J Med. 2011;365(23):2149–51. PMID: 22150033.

22. Goold SD, Williams B, Arnold RM. Conflicts regarding decisions to limit treatment: a differential diagnosis. JAMA. 2000;283(7):909–14. PMID: 10685716.

23. Pence GE. Medical ethics: accounts of ground-breaking cases. 5th ed. New York (NY): McGraw-Hill; 2008.

24. Jin (next friend of) v Calgary Health Region, 2007 ABQB 593.

25. Lunau K. The story behind a vegetative patient's shocking recovery. MacLean's [Internet]. 2015 Dec 31;Health:[about 9 screens]. Available from: https://www.macleans.ca/society/health/the-story-behind-a-vegetative-patients-shocking-recovery/

26. Carter v Canada (Attorney General), 2012 BCSC 886.

27. Waite M, Taylor D. Case Summary: Rasouli v Cuthbertson 2013. 2018 March 12. Available from: https://www.cba.org/Sections/Health-Law/Resources/Resources/2013/Case-Summary-em-Rasouli-v-Cuthbertson-em

28. Cuthbertson v Rasouli, 2013 SCC 53, [2013] 3 SCR 341.

29. Hawryluck L, Baker AJ, Faith A, et al. The future of decision-making in critical care after Cuthbertson v Rasouli. Can J Anaesth. 2014;61(10):951-8. PMID: 25164242.

30. Waite MA. End of life and critical care decisions: legal and ethical considerations [Internet]. Ottawa (ON): Canadian Bar Association; 2009 May 22 [cited 2018 Mar 12]. Available from: http://www.cba.org/cba/cle/pdf/Michael_Waite_paper.pdf

31. Boyle T. Hassan Rasouli to move out of Sunnybrook after long end-of-life court battle. Toronto Star [Internet]. 2013 Dec 31;Health & Wellness:[about 4 screens]. Available from: https://www.thestar.com/life/health_wellness/2013/12/31/hassan_rasouli_to_move_out_of_sunnybrook_after_long_endoflife_court_battle.html

32. Barbulov v Cirone, 2009 CanLII 15889 (ONSC).

33. Child and Family Services of Central Manitoba v Lavallee et al, 1997 CanLII 3742 (MBCA).

34. I.H.V. (Re), 2008 ABQB 250.

35. Children's Aid Society of Ottawa-Carleton v M.C., 2008 CanLII 49154 (ONSC).

36. Jin (next friend of) v Calgary Health Region, 2007 ABQB 593.

37. Golubchuk v Salvation Army Grace General Hospital et al, 2008 MBQB 49.

38. Sawatzky v Riverview Health Centre Inc., [1998] 133 Man.R. 2d 41 (MBQB).

39. Doctors offer to treat dying Winnipeg man after colleagues refuse. CBC News [Internet]. 2008 Jun 18 [cited 2018 April 11];Manitoba:[about 3 screens]. Available from: http://www.cbc.ca/news/canada/manitoba/doctors-offer-to-treat-dying-winnipeg-man-after-colleagues-refuse-1.759160

40. Dean MM, Cellarius V, Henry B, et al. Librach Canadian Society of Palliative Care Physicians Taskforce SL. Framework for continuous palliative sedation therapy in Canada. J Palliat Med. 2012;15(8):870–9. PMID: 22747192.

41. Billings JA. Double effect: a useful rule that alone cannot justify hastening death. J Med Ethics. 2011;37(7):437-40. PMID: 21478423.

Chapter 16

1. Law Reform Commission of Canada. Euthanasia, aiding suicide, and cessation of treatment. Ottawa (ON): Law Reform Commission of Canada; 1983.

2. Who owns my life? The story of Sue Rodriguez. CBC Radio [Internet]. 2016 Jun 11 [cited 2018 April 8];Rewind:[audio, 53 mins]. Available from: http://www.cbc.ca/

radio/rewind/who-owns-my-life-the-story-of-sue-rodriguez-1.3621902

3. Emanuel EJ, Onwuteaka-Philipsen BD, Urwin JW, et al. Attitudes and practices of euthanasia and physician-assisted suicide in the United States, Canada, and Europe. JAMA. 2016;316(1):79-90. PMID: 27380345.

4. Doctor-assisted suicide supported by majority of Canadians in new poll. CBC News [Internet]. 2014 Oct 8 [cited 2018 March 27];Health:[about 2 screens]. Available from: http://www.cbc.ca/news/health/doctor-assisted-suicide-supported-by-majority-of-canadians-in-new-poll-1.2792762

5. Morrow A. Majority of Canadians approve of assisted suicide: poll. Globe and Mail [Internet]. 2013 October 11, updated 2018 May 11;News:[about 2 screens]. Available from: https://www.theglobeandmail.com/news/national/majority-of-canadians-approve-of-assisted-suicide-poll/article14819642/

6. Browne A, Russell JS. Physician-assisted death in Canada. Camb Q Healthc Ethics. 2016;25(3):377-83. PMID: 27348822.

7. Li M, Watt S, Escaf M, et al. Medical assistance in dying: implementing a hospital-based program in Canada. N Engl J Med. 2017;376(21):2082-8. PMID: 28538128.

8. Keown J. A Right to Voluntary Euthanasia? Confusion in Canada in Carter. Notre Dame J Law Ethics Public Policy. 2014;28(1):1-45.

9. Keown J. Euthanasia in the Netherlands: sliding down the slippery slope? Notre Dame J Law Ethics Public Policy. 1995;9(2):407 at 32.

10. Fitzpatrick K. Should the law on assisted dying be changed? No. BMJ. 2011;342:d1883. PMID: 21511803.

11. Hizo-Abes P, Siegel L, Schreier G. Exploring attitudes toward physician-assisted death in patients with life-limiting illnesses with varying experiences of palliative care: a pilot study. BMC Palliat Care. 2018;17(1):56. PMID: 29618364.

12. Oczkowski SJW, Ball I, Saleh C, et al. The provision of medical assistance in dying: protocol for a scoping review. BMJ Open. 2017;7(8):e017888. PMID: 28801443.

13. Gandsman A. Paradox of choice and the illusion of autonomy: the construction of ethical subjects in right-to-die activism. Death Stud. 2018;42(5):329-35. PMID: 29279002.

14. An Act to amend the Criminal Code and to make related amendments to other Acts (medical assistance in dying), S.C. 2016, c. 3.

15. Downie J. End of life law and policy. In: Erdman J, Gruben V, Nelson E, editors. Canadian health law and policy. 5th ed. Toronto (ON): LexisNexis Canada; 2017. p. 453–77.

16. Cheyfitz K. Suicide machine, part 1: Kevorkian rushes to fulfill his clients' desire to die. Detroit Free Press. 1997 March 3.

17. Death with Dignity Act [Internet]. Salem (OR): Oregon Health Authority. Frequently asked questions; [revised 2018 Aug 1, cited 2018 May 17]; [about 6 screens]. Available from: http://www.oregon.gov/oha/PH/PROVIDERPARTNERRESOURCES/EVALUATIONRESEARCH/DEATHWITHDIGNITYACT/Pages/faqs.aspx#prescription

18. Tegel S. Colombia just legalized euthanasia. Here's why that's a big deal. Global Post [Internet]. 2015 Apr 19;Health:[about 4 screens]. Available from: https://www.pri.org/stories/2015-04-29/colombia-just-legalized-euthanasia-heres-why-thats-big-deal

19. Mendoza-Villa JM, Herrera-Morales LA. Reflections on euthanasia in Colombia. Colomb J Anesthesiol. 2016;44(4):324-9. DOI: 10.1016/j.rcae.2016.06.007.

20. Rodriguez v British Columbia (Attorney General), [1993] 3 SCR 519.

21. Sue Rodriguez and the right to die debate [Internet]. CBC Digital Archives [cited 2018 March 23]. Available from: http://www.cbc.ca/archives/topic/sue-rodriguez-and-the-right-to-die-debate

22. Select Committee on Dying with Dignity. Dying with dignity: report. Quebec (QC): National Assembly of Quebec; 2012.

23. Act Respecting End-of-Life Care, R.S.Q. 2014, c. S-32.0001.

24. Todd D. The story at the heart of Friday's Supreme Court ruling on assisted suicide. Vancouver Sun [Internet]. 2015 Feb 4;News:[about 7 screens]. Available from: https://vancouversun.com/news/staff-blogs/b-c-woman-chooses-a-dignified-death-in-switzerland

25. Carter v Canada (Attorney General), 2012 BCSC 886.

26. Inside Gloria Taylor's battle for the right to die. CBC News [Internet]. 2012 Oct

12;Canada:[about 5 screens]. Available from: https://www.cbc.ca/news/canada/inside-gloria-taylor-s-battle-for-the-right-to-die-1.1186092

27. Carter v Canada (Attorney General), 2015 SCC 5, [2015] 1 SCR 331.

28. Gilmour JM. Legal capacity and decision-making. In: Erdman J, Gruben V, Nelson E, editors. Canadian health law and policy. 5th ed. Toronto (ON): LexisNexis Canada; 2017. p. 351–74.

29. Bolt EE, Flens EQ, Pasman HR, et al. Physician-assisted dying for children is conceivable for most Dutch paediatricians, irrespective of the patient's age or competence to decide. Acta Paediatr. 2017;106(4):668-75. PMID: 27727473.

30. Friedel M. Does the Belgian law legalising euthanasia for minors really address the needs of life-limited children? Int J Palliat Nurs. 2014;20(6):265-7. PMID: 25040860.

31. Samuel H. Belgium authorized euthanasia of a terminally ill nine and 11-year-old in youngest cases worldwide. The Telegraph [Internet]. 2018 Aug 7;News:[about 4 screens]. Available from: https://www.telegraph.co.uk/news/2018/08/07/belgium-authorised-euthanasia-terminally-nine-11-year-old-youngest/

32. Andrew S. Where is euthanasia legal? Three terminally ill minors choose to die in Belgium, new report finds. Newsweek [Internet]. 2018 Aug 7;Health:[about 2 screens]. Available from: https://www.newsweek.com/child-euthanasia-legal-belgium-three-minors-died-1061587

33. Malette v Shulman, [1990] 72 OR 2d. 417 (ONCA).

34. Fleming v Reid and Gallagher, [1991] 48 OAC 46 (ONCA).

35. Breslin J. Think carefully about advance requests for medical assistance in dying [Internet]. CMAJ Blogs; 2016 August 4; [about 4 screens]. Available from: https://cmajblogs.com/think-carefully-about-advance-requests-for-medical-assistance-in-dying/

36. de Boer ME, Hertogh CM, Droes RM, et al. Advance directives in dementia: issues of validity and effectiveness. Int Psychogeriatr. 2010;22(2):201–8. PMID: 19664311.

37. Menzel PT, Chandler-Cramer MC. Advance directives, dementia, and withholding food and water by mouth. Hastings Cent Rep. 2014;44(3):23–37. PMID: 24821250.

38. van Delden JJ. The unfeasibility of requests for euthanasia in advance directives. J Med Ethics. 2004;30(5):447–51; discussion 51–2. PMID: 15467074.

39. Auckland C. Protecting me from my directive: ensuring appropriate safeguards for advance directives in dementia. Med Law Rev. 2018;26(1):73–97. PMID: 28981694.

40. Hertogh CM, de Boer ME, Droes RM, et al. Would we rather lose our life than lose our self? Lessons from the Dutch debate on euthanasia for patients with dementia. Am J Bioeth. 2007;7(4):48–56. PMID: 17454999.

41. Schuklenk U, van de Vathorst S. Treatment-resistant major depressive disorder and assisted dying. J Med Ethics. 2015;41(8):577–83. PMID: 25935906.

42. Vandenberghe J. Physician-assisted suicide and psychiatric illness. N Engl J Med. 2018;378(10):885–7. PMID: 29514019.

43. Deschepper R, Distelmans W, Bilsen J. Requests for euthanasia/physician-assisted suicide on the basis of mental suffering: vulnerable patients or vulnerable physicians? JAMA Psychiatry. 2014;71(6):617–8. PMID: 24759890.

44. Dembo J, Smith D. Assisted dying for patients with psychiatric disorders. CMAJ. 2016;188(14):1036. DOI: 10.1503/cmaj.1150120. PMID: PMC5047825.

45. Vandenberghe J. Euthanasia in patients with intolerable suffering due to an irremediable psychiatric illness. In: MacKellar C, Gastmans C, Jones DA, editors. Euthanasia and assisted suicide: lessons from Belgium. Cambridge (UK): Cambridge University Press; 2017. p. 133–49. (Cambridge Bioethics and Law; 42).

46. Miller FG, Appelbaum PS. Physician-assisted death for psychiatric patients: misguided public policy. N Engl J Med. 2018;378(10):883-5. PMID: 29514026.

47. Owens D, Horrocks J, House A. Fatal and non-fatal repetition of self-harm. Systematic review. Br J Psychiatry. 2002;181:193-9. PMID: 12204922.

48. Canada (Attorney General) v E.F., 2016 ABCA 155.

49. New challenge to assisted-death law could expose Ottawa's gamble as flawed. Globe and Mail [Internet]. 2016 June 28,

updated 2018 May 16; Editorial:[about 1 screen]. Available from: https://www.theglobeandmail.com/opinion/editorials/new-challenge-to-assisted-death-law-could-expose-ottawas-gamble-as-flawed/article30653265/

50. Lamb v Canada (Attorney General), 2017 BCSC 1802.

51. Grant K. Medically assisted death allows couple married almost 73 years to die together. Globe and Mail [Internet]. 2018 Apr 1;Canada:[about 9 screens]. Available from: https://www.theglobeandmail.com/canada/article-medically-assisted-death-allows-couple-married-almost-73-years-to-die/

52. Wright DK, Fishman JR, Karsoho H, et al. Physicians and euthanasia: a Canadian print-media discourse analysis of physician perspectives. CMAJ Open. 2015;3(2):E134-9. PMID: 26389090.

53. College of Family Physicians of Canada. ePanel #2: Physician assisted suicide and euthanasia [Internet]. Mississauga (ON): CFPC; 2015. Available from: http://www.cfpc.ca/uploadedFiles/Health_Policy/_PDFs/ePanel_psa_results_EN.pdf

54. College of Physicians and Surgeons of Ontario. Medical assistance in dying: frequently asked questions [Internet]. Toronto (ON): CPSO; [cited 2018 Apr]. Available from: http://www.cpso.on.ca/cpso/media/documents/policies/policy-items/medical-assistance-in-dying-faq.pdf

55. Fine S. Christian doctors challenge Ontario's assisted-death referral requirement. Globe and Mail [Internet]. 2016 Jun 22 [updated 2018 May 16];News:[about 3 screens]. Available from: https://www.theglobeandmail.com/news/national/christian-doctors-challenge-ontarios-assisted-death-referral-policy/article30552327/

56. Centre for Effective Practice. Medical assistance in dying (MAID): Ontario [Internet]. Toronto (ON): Centre for Effective Practice; revised 2017. Available from: https://cep.health/clinical-products/medical-assistance-in-dying/

57. Abortion Rights Coalition of Canada. Position paper #8: problems with hospital access to abortion [Internet]. Vancouver (BC): Abortion Rights Coalition of Canada; 2017 [cited 2018 May 19]. Available from: http://www.arcc-cdac.ca/postionpapers/08-Hospital-Access-Problems.PDF

58. Canadian Institute for Health Information. Statistics on abortion [Internet]. Ottawa (ON): CIHI; 2014 [cited 2018 May 19]. Available from: https://www.cihi.ca/en/ta_10_alldatatables20120417_en.pdf

59. Tonelli MR. Terminal sedation. N Engl J Med. 1998;338(17):1230; author reply -1. PMID: 9556397.

Chapter 17

1. Macklin R. Against relativism: cultural diversity and the search for ethical universals in medicine. Oxford: Oxford University Press; 1999. p. 37.

2. Sanders L. Every patient tells a story: medical mysteries and the art of diagnosis. New York: Random House; 2009.

3. Hudson KL. Genomics, health care, and society. N Engl J Med. 2011;365(11):1033–41. DOI: 10.1056/NEJMra1010517

4. Ginsberg G, Willard H. The foundations of genomic and personalized medicine. In: Ginsberg G, Willard H, editors. Essentials of genomic and personalized medicine. San Diego (CA): Elsevier; 2010. p. 1–10. Available from: http://www.sciencedirect.com/science/book/9780123749345

5. Feero WG. Introducing "Genomics and Precision Health." JAMA. 2017;317(18):1843. DOI: 10.1001/jama.2016.20625

6. Cardarella S, Johnson BE. The impact of genomic changes on treatment of lung cancer. Am J Respir Crit Care Med. 2013;188(7):770–75. DOI: 10.1164/rccm.201305-0843PP

7. Bradbury PA, Tu D, Seymour L, et al. Economic analysis: randomized placebo-controlled clinical trial of erlotinib in advanced non–small cell lung cancer. J Natl Cancer Inst. 2010;102(5):298-306. DOI: 10.1093/jnci/djp518

8. Reis A, Hornblower B, Robb B, et al. CRISPR/CaS9 & targeted genome editing: new era in molecular biology. Ipswich (MA): New England BioLabs; 2014 [cited 2018 Oct 22]. Available from: https://www.neb.com/tools-and-resources/feature-articles/crispr-cas9-and-targeted-genome-editing-a-new-era-in-molecular-biology

9. Rodriguez E. Ethical issues in genome editing using CRISPR/Cas9 system. J Clin Res Bioeth. 2016;7(2):266. DOI:10.4172/2155-9627.1000266

10. Brokowski C, Adli M. CRISPR ethics: moral considerations for applications of a powerful tool. J Mol Biol. 2018;431(1):88–101. DOI: 10.1016/j.jmb.2018.05.044

11. Genome editing [Internet]. Bethesda (MD): National Human Genome Research Institute; 2017 Aug 3. Available from: https://www.genome.gov/27569222/genome-editing/

12. Fisher C, Harrington McCarthy E. Ethics in prevention science involving genetic testing. Prev Sci. 2013;14(3):310–8. DOI: 10.1007/s11121-012-0318-x

13. Palmor M, Fiester A. Incidental findings of nonparentage: a case for universal nondisclosure. Pediatrics. 2014;134(1):163–8. DOI: 10.1542/peds.2013-4182

14. Thanks to Dr Richard Wells for pointing this out.

15. Kalia SS, Adelman K, Bale SJ, et al. Recommendations for reporting of secondary findings in clinical exome and genome sequencing, 2016 update (ACMG SF v2.0): a policy statement of the American College of Medical Genetics and Genomics. Genet Med. 2017;19(2):249–55. DOI: 10.1038/gim.2016.190

16. Burke W, Evans BJ, Jarvik GP. Return of results: ethical and legal distinctions between research and clinical care. Am J Med Genet Part C Semin Med Genet. 2014;166C(1):105–11. DOI: 10.1002/ajmg.c.31393

17. Weiner C. Anticipate and communicate: ethical management of incidental and secondary findings in the clinical, research, and direct-to-consumer contexts. (December 2013 report of the Presidential Commission for the Study of Bioethical Issues.) Am J Epidemiol. 2014;180(6):562-4. DOI: 10.1093/aje/kwu217

18. Berlin L. To telephone or not to telephone: how high is the standard? Malpractice issues in radiology. 3rd ed. Leesburg (VA): American Roentgen Ray Society; 2009. p. 91–5.

19. Adapted from Leung WC, Mariman E, van der Wouden JC, et al. Ethical debate: Results of genetic testing: when confidentiality conflicts with a duty to warn relatives.

BMJ. 2000;321(7274):1464–6. PMID: 11110744.

20. Houchens N, Dhaliwal G, Askari F, et al. Clinical problem-solving. The essential element. N Engl J Med. 2013;368(14):1345–51. DOI: 10.1056/NEJMcps1203173

21. UNESCO. International declaration on human genetic data [Internet]. Paris: UNESCO; 2003. Available from: http://portal.unesco.org/en/ev.php-URL_ID=17720&URL_DO=DO_TOPIC&URL_SECTION=201.html

22. Lucassen A, Parker M. Confidentiality and sharing genetic information with relatives. Lancet. 2010;375(9725):1507–9. DOI: 10.1016/S0140-6736(10)60173-0

23. Manolio T. Genomewide association studies and assessment of the risk of disease. N Engl J Med. 2010;363(2):166–76. DOI: 10.1056/NEJMra0905980

24. May T. Sociogenetic risks: ancestry DNA testing, third-party identity, and protection of privacy. N Engl J Med. 2018;379(5):410–11. DOI: 10.1056/NEJMp1805870

25. Coupland R, Martin S, Dutli MT. Protecting everybody's genetic data. Lancet. 2005;365(9473):1754–6. DOI: 10.1016/S0140-6736(05)66563-4

26. Havasupai Tribe of Havasupai Reservation v Arizona Board of Regents, 204 P.3d 1063 (Ariz. App. Div. 1 2008).

27. Canadian Institutes of Health Research, Natural Sciences and Engineering Research Council of Canada, Social Sciences and Humanities Research Council of Canada. Tri-council policy statement: ethical conduct for research involving humans. Ottawa (ON): Interagency Secretariat on Research Ethics; 2010. p. 107.

28. Tait CL. Ethical programming: towards a community-centred approach to mental health and addiction programming in Aboriginal communities. Pimatisiwin: J Aboriginal Indigenous Commun Health. 2008;6(1):51.

29. Hudson K. Genomics, health care, and society. N Engl J Med. 2011;365(11):1033–41. DOI: 10.1056/NEJMra1010517

30. Sen A. Identity and violence: the illusion of destiny. New York: W W Norton; 2006.

31. Landstreet P. A world of sociology, part 1: the basic concepts. 2010. Unpublished manuscript.

32. Tucker CM, Marsiske M, Rice KG, et al. Patient-centered culturally sensitive health

care: model testing and refinement. Health Psychol. 2011;30(3):342–350. DOI: 10.1037/a0022967

33. College of Nurses of Ontario. Culturally sensitive care. Toronto (ON): CNO; 2009. Pub. No. 41040.

34. Registered Nurses' Association of Ontario. Embracing cultural diversity in health care: developing cultural competence. Toronto (ON): RNAO; 2007.

35. Adapted from Epner D, Baile W. Patient-centered care: the key to cultural competence. Ann Oncol. 2012;23 Suppl 3:iii33–iii42. DOI: 10.1093/annonc/mds086

36. Landry J. Delivering culturally sensitive care to LGBTQI patients. J Nurse Pract. 2017;13(5):342-7. DOI: 10.1016/j.nurpra.2016.12.015

37. Gay and Lesbian Medical Association. Guidelines for the care of lesbian, gay, bisexual, and transgender patients [Internet]. San Francisco (CA): GLMA; 2006. Available from: http://www.glma.org/index/cfm?fuseaction=Page.viewPage&pageID=1025&grandparentsID=534&parentID=940&nodeID=1

38. The World Professional Association for Transgender Health. Standards of care for the health of transsexual, transgender, and gender nonconforming people [Internet]. 7th version. East Dundee (IL): WPATH; 2011. Available from: www.wpath.org

39. Fraser Health Authority. Providing diversity competent care to people of the Sikh faith: a handbook for health care providers. British Columbia: Diversity Services, Fraser Health Authority; 2013.

40. Indigenous Physician's Association of Canada, Association of Faculties of Medicine of Canada. First Nations, Inuit, Métis health: core competencies [Internet]. Ottawa (ON): IPAC, AFMC; 2009. Available from: http://www.ipac-amac.ca/wp-content/uploads/2018/08/02-IPAC-RCPSC-CME-DOC.pdf

41. Eiser A, Ellis G. Cultural competence and the African American experience with health care: the case for specific content in cross-cultural education. Acad Med. 2007; 82(2):176–83. DOI: 10.1097/ACM.0b013e31802d92ea

42. Amris S, Blaauw M, Danielsen L, et al. Medical physical examination of alleged torture victims: a practical guide to the Istanbul Protocol for medical doctors. Copenhagen: International Rehabilitation Council for Torture Victims; 2009. Available from: www.irct.org

43. Dr Wendell Block, personal communication.

44. Forrest D, Hutton F. Guidelines for the examination of survivors of torture [Internet]. 2nd ed. London: Medical Foundation for the Care of Victims of Torture; 2002. Available from: https://www.freedomfromtorture.org/sites/default/files/documents/Forrest%2C guidelines%2C2002.pdf

45. Fadiman A. The spirit catches you and you fall down: a Hmong child, her American doctors, and the collision of cultures. New York: Noonday Press, Farrar, Straus and Giroux; 1997.

46. Fox M. Lia Lee dies: life went on around her, redefining care. New York Times [Internet]. 2012 Sept 14;US:[about 8 screens]. Available from: https://www.nytimes.com/2012/09/15/us/life-went-on-around-her-redefining-care-by-bridging-a-divide.html

47. Padela A, Punekar B. Emergency medical practice: advancing cultural competence and reducing healthcare disparities. Acad Emerg Med. 2009;16(1):69–75. DOI: 10.1111/j.1553-2712.2008.00305.x

48. This list is adapted from Kleinman A, in Fadiman A. op. cit.: 260–1.

49. Oram J, Murphy P. Diagnosis of death. Contin Educ Anaesth Crit Care Pain. DOI.org/10.1093/bjaceaccp/mkr008.

50. Wijdicks EFM. Deliberating death in the summer of 1968. N Engl J Med. 2018;379(5):412–5. DOI: 10.1056/NEJMp1802952

51. "Policies may include specific accommodations, such as the continuation of artificial respiration under certain circumstances, as well as guidance on limits to accommodation." New York State Department of Health. Guidelines for determining brain death. Albany (NY): New York State Department of Health; 2005 Dec. p. 2–3.

52. Olick R, Braun E, Potash J. Accommodating religious and moral objections to neurological death. J Clin Ethics. 2009;20(2):183–91. PMID: 19554827.

53. Goffin P. Woman to be taken off life support: judge. Toronto Star. 2018 June 27:GT4.

54. Bugge J. Brain death and its implications for management of the potential organ donor. Acta Anaesthesiol Scand. 2009;53(10):1239–50. DOI: 10.1111/j.1399-6576.2009.02064.x

55. "Ultimately, the heart stops in brain death . . . despite full cardiovascular support, 97% of . . . brain-dead bodies developed asystole in a week." Wijdicks EFM, Atkinson JLD. Pathophysiologic responses to brain death. In: Wijdicks EFM, editor. Brain death. Philadelphia (PA): Lippincott Williams & Wilkins; 2001. p. 35.

56. Powner D, Bernstein I. Extended somatic support for pregnant women after brain death. Crit Care Med. 2003;31(4):1241–9. DOI: 10.1097/01.CCM.0000059643.45027.96

57. Brett A, Jersild P. "Inappropriate" treatment near the end of life: conflict between religious convictions and clinical judgment. Arch Intern Med. 2003;163(14):1645–9. DOI: 10.1001/archinte.163.14.1645

58. Marx K, Engels F. Marx/Engels selected works. Moscow: Progress Publishers; 1969. Third thesis on Feuerbach. p. 1.

59. Tait CL. Ethical programming: towards a community-centred approach to mental health and addiction programming in Aboriginal communities. Pimatisiwin: J Aboriginal Indigenous Commun Health. 2008;6(1):29–60.

60. Kleinman A. Moral experience and ethical reflection: can ethnography reconcile them? A quandary for the "new bioethics." Daedalus. 1999:128(4):70. *JSTOR*, www.jstor.org/stable/20027589.

61. Harris, S., The moral landscape: how science can determine human values. New York: Free Press; 2010. p. 2.

62. Suing, J. Sorry to burst your bubble: memes are actually good for democracy; political memes offer an opportunity to stimulate a more in-depth discussion on matters they set forth. [Internet] 2017 Feb 9 [about 6 screens]. Available from: https://www.huffingtonpost.com/entry/sorry-to-burst-your-bubble-memes-are-actually-good_us_589c1306e4b061551b3e0793

63. Laframboise K. Former Jehovah's Witness says blood transfusion after childbirth saved her life. CBC News [Internet]. 2017 Nov 15;Montreal:[about 3 screens]. Available from: http://www.cbc.ca/news/canada/montreal/jehovah-witness-blood-transfusion-woman-speaks-out-1.4404193

64. Rosenberg AR, Starks H, Unguru Y, et al. Truth telling in the setting of cultural differences and incurable pediatric illness. JAMA Pediatr. 2017;171(11):1113–9. DOI: 10.1001/jamapediatrics.2017.2568

65. Thanks to Dr Mary Rose MacDonald for making this point.

Chapter 18

1. Chalmers I. What do I want from health research and researchers when I am a patient? BMJ, 1995;310(6990):1315–18. PMID: 7773050.

2. Porter R. The greatest benefit to mankind: a medical history of humanity. New York: WW Norton & Company; 1999.

3. Lifton RJ. The Nazi doctors: medical killing and the psychology of genocide. New York: Basic Books; 1988, Updated 2000.

4. Gaw A. Exposing unethical human research: the transatlantic correspondence of Beecher and Pappworth. Ann Intern Med. 2012;156(2):150–5. DOI: 10.7326/0003-4819-156-2-201201170-00012

5. Nix E. Tuskegee experiment: the infamous syphilis study. 2017 May 16. Available from: https://www.history.com/news/the-infamous-40-year-tuskegee-study

6. MK-ULTRAViolence: or, how McGill pioneered psychological torture. 2012 September 6. Available from: https://www.mcgilldaily.com/2012/09/mk-ultraviolence/

7. Freedman B. Equipoise and the ethics of clinical research. N Engl J Med. 1987;317(3):141–5. DOI: 10.1056/NEJM198707163170304

8. Lo B. A parallel universe of clinical trials. N Engl J Med. 2018;379(2):101–3. DOI: 10.1056/NEJMp1804552

9. Sacristán JA, Aguarón A, Avendaño-Solá C, et al,. Patient involvement in clinical research: why, when, and how. Patient Prefer Adherence. 2016;10:631–40. DOI: 10.2147/PPA.S104259

10. Goldacre B. Bad pharma: how drug companies mislead doctors and harm patients. Toronto: McClelland and Stewart; 2012. p. 186.

11. ICMJE. Recommendations for the conduct, reporting, editing, and publication of scholarly work in medical journals. [Internet] 2018 Dec. Available from: http://www.icmje.org/icmje-recommendations.pdf

12. Roxby P. Northwick Park drug trial disaster: could it happen again? BBC News, 2013

May 24. Available from: http://www.bbc.com/news/health-22556736

13. Matharu H. The troubled history of clinical drug trials. The Independent. 2016 Jan 15. Available from: https://www.independent.co.uk/life-style/health-and-families/health-news/the-drug-trials-that-went-wrong-a6814696.html

14. In this chapter we will only look at the ethics of RCTs—there are, of course, many other types of research such as qualitative studies, that we cannot, for reasons of space, consider.

15. Goldacre B. Bad Pharma. Toronto: McClelland and Stewart; 2012. p. 130.

16. Ibid. p. 168–70.

17. Burton JL, Wells M. The Alder Hey affair: Implications for pathology practice. J Clin Path. 2001;54(11):820–3. PMID: 11684712.

18. Skloot R. The immortal life of Henrietta Lacks. New York: Crown Publishers; 2010.

19. Cheung C, Martin B, Asa S, Defining diagnostic tissue in the era of personalized medicine. CMAJ. 2013;185(2):135–9. DOI: 10.1503/cmaj.120565

20. Moore v Regents of the University of California, 793 P.2d 479 (Cal. 1990).

21. Caulfield T. Who owns your tissue: you'd be surprised. Globe and Mail. 2014 Jun 20. Updated 2017 Dec 11.

22. Washington University v William J. Catalona. 06-2286 (2007). Court of Appeals for the Eighth Circuit.

23. Limbaugh J. Catalona v Washington University (2006), as quoted in Schmidt, C. Tissue banks trigger worry about ownership issues. JNCI: Journal of the National Cancer Institute. 2006;98(17):1174–5. Available from: https://doi.org/10.1093/jnci/djj380

24. Dickens B. Living tissue and organ donors and property law: more on Moore. J. Contemp. Health L. & Pol'y 1992;8(1):73–86.

25. Adapted from Mello M and Wolf L. The Havasupai Indian tribe case: lessons for research involving stored biologic samples. N Engl J Med. 2010;363(3):204–7. DOI: 10.1056/NEJMp1005203

26. Emerson C, Singer PA, Upshur R. Access and use of human tissues from the developing world: ethical challenges and a way forward using a tissue trust. BMC Med Ethics. 2011;12(2). DOI: 10.1186/1472-6939-12-2

27. Burns J. British council bars doctor who linked vaccine with autism. NY Times. 2010 May 24. Available from: http://www.nytimes.com/2010/05/25/health/policy/25autism.html

28. Koski, G., Kennedy, L., Tobin, M., et al. Accreditation of clinical research sites: moving forward. N Engl J Med. 2018;379(5):405–7. DOI: 10.1056/NEJMp1806934

29. Goldacre B. Bad pharma: how drug companies mislead doctors and harm patients. Toronto: Random House Canada; 2012.

30. Gutmann A., Safeguarding children: pediatric research on medical countermeasures, N Engl J Med. 2013;368(13):1171–3. DOI: 10.1056/NEJMp1302093

31. Gelinas L, Largent EA, Cohen IG, et al. A framework for ethical payment to research participants. February 22, 2018. N Engl J Med 2018;378(8):766-771. DOI: 10.1056/NEJMsb1710591

32. Walter JK, Burke JF, Davis MM. Research participation by low-income and racial/ethnic minority groups: how payment may change the balance. Clin Transl Sci. 2013;6(5):363–71. DOI: 10.1111/cts.12084

33. Kass N, Pronovost P, Sugarman J, et al. Controversy and quality improvement: lingering questions about ethics, oversight, and patient safety oversight. Jt Comm J Qual Patient Saf. 2008;34(6):349–53. PMID: 18595381.

34. Kim JU, Oleribe O, Njie R, Taylor-Robinson SD. A time for new north–south relationships in global health. Int J Gen Med. 2017;10:401–8. DOI: 10.2147/IJGM.S146475

35. A collection of US Regulations for Drug Studies, the Code of Federal Regulations, and European Directives on Good Clinical Practice is usefully found in one book: Selected regulations & guidance for drug studies. Philadelphia: Clinical Research Resources; 2012.

36. Silberman G, Kahn K. Burdens on research imposed by institutional review boards: the state of the evidence and its implications for regulatory reform. Milbank Q, 2011;89(4):599–627. DOI: 10.1111/j.1468-0009.2011.00644.x

37. Ormond K. Medical ethics for the genome world. J Mol Diagn. 2008; 10(5):377–82. DOI: 10.2353/jmoldx.2008.070162

38. Lavery J, Grady C, Wahl E, and Emanuel E, (eds.). Ethical issues in international

biomedical research: a casebook. Oxford (UK): Oxford University Press; 2007. p. 192–4.

39. Editorial. Strengthening clinical research in India. The Lancet. 2007;369(9569):1233. DOI: 10.1016/S0140-6736(07)60568-6

40. Kharawala S, Dalal J. Challenges in conducting psychiatry studies in India. Perspect Clin Res. 2011;2(1):8–12. DOI: 10.4103/2229-3485.76284

41. Glickman S, McHutchison J, Peterson E, et al. Ethical and scientific implications of the globalization of clinical research. N Engl J Med. 2009;360(8):816–23. DOI: 10.1056/NEJMsb0803929

42. Canadian Institutes of Health Research Natural Sciences and Engineering Research Council of Canada Social Sciences and Humanities Research Council of Canada. Tri-council policy statement: ethical conduct for research involving humans. 2014. Available from: http://www.pre.ethics.gc.ca/pdf/eng/tcps2-2014/TCPS_2_FINAL_Web.pdf

43. Indian Council of Medical Research. National ethical guidelines for biomedical and health research involving human participants. Available from: https://icmr.nic.in/guidelines/ICMR_Ethical_Guidelines_2017.pdf

44. UK Medical Research Council. Good research practice: principles and guidelines. 2011. Available from: https://mrc.ukri.org/publications/browse/good-research-practice-principles-and-guidelines/

45. Australian National Health and Medical Research Council. Australian code for the responsible conduct of research. Updated 2018. Available from: https://www.nhmrc.gov.au/research/responsible-conduct-research-0

46. National Institute of Health. Ethical guidelines and regulations. Available from: https://humansubjects.nih.gov/ethical-guidelines-regulations

47. US FDA regulations relating to good clinical practice and clinical trials. Available from: https://www.fda.gov/scienceresearch/specialtopics/runningclinicaltrials/ucm155713.htm–FDA Regulations

48. The Global Forum on Bioethics in Research. http://www.gfbr.global/about-the-gfbr/

49. WHO. Standards and operational guidance for ethics review of health-related research with human participants. 2011.

Available from: http://apps.who.int/iris/bitstream/handle/10665/44783/9789241502948_eng.pdf;jsessionid=999BCEDF3E157C-DAFE34CAB94F290E09?sequence=1

Conclusion

1. Popper K. In search of a better world: lectures and essays from thirty years. 1st ed. London: Routledge; 1995. p. 1.

2. Jha V, Robinson A. Religion and medical professionalism: moving beyond social and cultural nuances. J Grad Med Educ. 2016;8(2):271-3. DOI: 10.4300/JGME-D-16-00104.1

3. American College of Physicians. Ethics manual. 6th ed. [Internet]. 2012 Jan. Available from: https://www.acponline.org/clinical-information/ethics-and-professionalism/acp-ethics-manual-sixth-edition-a-comprehensive-medical-ethics-resource

4. Jin P. The physician charter on medical professionalism from the Chinese perspective: a comparative analysis. J Med Ethics. 2015;41(7):511–4. DOI: 10.1136/medethics-2014-102318

5. Wang X, Shih J, Kuo FJ, et al. A scoping review of medical professionalism research published in the Chinese language. BMC Med Educ. 2016;16(1):300. DOI: 10.1186/s12909-016-0818-7

6. Abdel-Razig S, Ibrahim H, Alameri H, et al. Creating a framework for medical professionalism: an initial consensus statement from an Arab nation. J Grad Med Educ. 2016; 8(2):165–72. DOI: 10.4300/JGME-D-15-00310.1

7. Gellner E. Thought and change. Chicago (IL): Midway Reprints, University of Chicago Press; 1964.

8. Miller D. Critical rationalism: a restatement and defence. Chicago (IL): Open Court; 1994.

9. Ostrom E. Governing the commons. Cambridge (UK): Cambridge University Press; 2015.

10. Global Fund overview [Internet]. Geneva: The Global Fund to Fight AIDS, Tuberculosis and Malaria; 2018. Available from: https://www.theglobalfund.org/en/overview/

11. Gourevitch PA, Lake DA, Stein JG. The credibility of transnational NGOs: when virtue is not enough. Cambridge (UK): Cambridge University Press; 2012.

12. Kristof N. Why 2017 was the best year in human history. New York Times. 2018 Jan 6;Sunday Review.

13. Rosenthal DI, Verghese A. Meaning and the nature of physicians' work. N Engl J Med. 2016;375(19):1813–5. DOI: 10.1056/NEJMp1609055

14. Wright A, Katz I. Beyond burnout: redesigning care to restore meaning and sanity for physicians. N Engl J Med. 2018;378(4):309–11. PMID: 29365301.

15. Muir Gray, JA. The resourceful patient. Oxford: Rosetta Press; 2002.

16. McKinlay J, Marceau L. When there is no doctor: reasons for the disappearance of primary care physicians in the US during the early 21st century. Soc Sci Med. 2008;67(10):1481–91. DOI: 10.1016/j.socscimed.2008.06.034

17. Zuger A. Dissatisfaction with medical practice. N Engl J Med. 2004;350(1):69–75. DOI: 10.1056/NEJMsr031703

18. World Health Organization. Attacks on health care [Internet]. Available from: https://www.who.int/emergencies/attacks-on-health-care/en/

19. Gebien D, as told to Laidlaw K. Disgraced. Toronto Life [Internet]. 2017 Mar 28;City:[about 18 screens]. Available from: http://torontolife.com/city/crime/doctor-perfect-life-got-hooked-fentanyl/

20. Wallach R. Stuck in despair. Hopkins Medicine [Internet]. 2016. Available from: https://www.hopkinsmedicine.org/news/publications/hopkins_medicine_magazine/features/spring-summer-2016/stuck-in-despair

21. Russell BJ. Physicians and substance abuse [Internet]. Ottawa (ON): Royal College of Physicians and Surgeons of Canada. Available from: http://royalcollege.ca/rcsite/bioethics/cases/section-3/physicians-substance-abuse-e

22. Edwards N, Kornacki MJ, Silversin J. Unhappy doctors: what are the causes and what can be done? BMJ. 2002;324(7341):835. PMID: 11934779.

23. Mokluk A. Hallway health care. Toronto Life. 2018 May;44–8.

24. Dickens C. Hard times. Peterborough (ON): Broadview Press; 1996.

25. Adams J, Mounib EL, Pai A, et al. Healthcare 2015: win-win or lose-lose? Somers (NY): IBM Institute for Business Value; 2006.

26. Roberts LW, Hammond KAG, Geppert CM, et al. The positive role of professionalism and ethics training in medical education: a comparison of medical student and resident perspectives. Acad Psychiatry. 2004;28(3):170. PMID: 15507551.

27. LeBlanc C, Heyworth J. Emergency physicians:" burned out" or" fired up"? CJEM. 2007;9(2):121. DOI: 10.1017/S1481803500014913

28. Sandars J. The use of reflection in medical education: AMEE Guide No. 44. Med Teach. 2009;31(8):685–95. PMID: 19811204.

29. Horowitz CR, Suchman AL, Branch WT, et al. What do doctors find meaningful about their work? Ann Intern Med. 2003;138(9):772–5. PMID: 12729445.

30. Weinstein M. Out of the straitjacket. N Engl J Med. 2018;378(9):793–5. PMID: 29490178.

31. Porter R. The greatest benefit to mankind: a medical history of humanity (the Norton history of science). New York: WW Norton & Company; 1999.

32. Alderson P. Children's consent to surgery. Buckingham (UK): Open University Press; 1993.

33. Balint M. The doctor, his patient and the illness. Madison (CT): Harvester Int; 1988.

34. Beauchamp T, Childress J. Principles of biomedical ethics. 7th ed. New York: Oxford University Press; 2013.

35. Berger J, Mohr J. A fortunate man. New York: Pantheon Books; 1967.

36. Breen KJ, Cordner SM, Thomson CJH. Good medical practice: professionalism, ethics, and the law. 4th ed. Kingston (AU): Australian Medical Council Ltd; 2016.

37. Gawande A. Being mortal: medicine and what matters at the end. Toronto (ON): Anchor Books; 2014.

38. Gottlieb A. The dream of enlightenment: the rise of modern philosophy. New York (NY): Norton and Company; 2016.

39. Ingelfinger F. Arrogance. N Engl J Med. 1980;303(26):1507–11. DOI: 10.1056/NEJM198012253032604

40. Jameson L. The empathy exams: essays. Minneapolis (MN): Graywolf Press; 2014.

41. British Medical Association. Medical ethics today: the BMA's handbook of ethics and law. London: John Wiley & Sons; 2012.

42. Verghese A. Cutting for stone. Toronto (ON):Vintage Books Canada; 2010.

42. Williams J. Medical ethics manual. 3rd ed. Ferney-Voltaire Cedex (FR): World Medical Association; 2015.

Index

abortion, 16, 83, 254–62; barriers to, 260; conscience and, 261–2; history of, 256–7; medical, 257; second- and third-term, 258
"above all, do no harm," 7
abuse: child, 122–3, 166; elder, 123, 174; sexual, 188; spousal, 34, 35–6
accessibility: abortion, 260, 262; assisted reproductive technology and, 266–7, 268; *Canada Health Act* and, 243; healthcare and, 235–6
accountability: errors and, 217–18, 222
"accountability for reasonableness," 247
actionability, medical, 322
Act Respecting End of Life Care, An, 301
administration: *Canada Health Act* and, 243
advance directives, 138, 139, 140, 141, 281–4; assisted dying and, 304, 307–9; consent and, 98; dementia and, 163; tattooed, 58
adverse events, 215–16; cause of, 217–18; "large-scale," 225–8; preventable/unpreventable, 215; rates of, 216–17; *see also* errors
advertising: direct-to-consumer (DTC), 253; social media and, 202–3
advice: ethics and, 41
Aeronautics Act, 124
Affordable Care Act, 184
age: consent and, 146; discrimination and, 235; majority, 146
"agent," 139
"aid in dying," 298
Alberta: driving safety in, 124; eugenics in, 170
Alberta Health Services, 120
Aljohani M, 203
All Families Are Equal Act, 270
allocation: costs and, 240–2; criteria for, 234; decisions on, 244–7; discrimination and, 235–9; guidelines for, 245–7; justice and, 247–51; principles of, 248–9; resources and, 242–5
altruism, 19, 25; research and, 355
Alzheimer's disease: truthtelling and, 87; *see also* dementia
American College of Genetics and Genomics, 322
American Society for Reproductive Medicine, 274
amniocentesis, 255–6
amyotrophic lateral sclerosis (ALS), 300
Androgen Insensitivity Syndrome, 87, 88
anonymity: "collusion of", 219; photography and, 207, 210
anorexia nervosa, 43–6
anosognosia, 142, 144

antibiotics, 2–4
antipsychotics, 81–2; refusal of, 57, 144–5
apologies: liability and, 224–5; professionalism and, 177
"Apology Acts," 224
appearance, physicians', 180
Appelbaum P, 143
appreciation: capacity and, 135, 137, 142, 144
"appropriate therapeutic distance," 198
Aristotle, 18, 236
"arm": clinical trial and, 345, 346–7
Arndt v Smith, 83
assisted decision-making, 141–2
assisted dying, 293, 294, 296–318; administration of, 298, 299, 300; advance directives and, 304, 307–9; children and, 304, 305–7; conscience issues and, 313–17; eligibility for, 303; mental illness and, 304–5, 310–13; v palliative sedation, 292; safeguards for, 304; in various jurisdictions, 299–300; *see also* medical assistance in dying (MAID)
Assisted Human Reproductive Act, 263–5, 269
assisted reproduction technology (ART), 254, 262–75; commercialization of, 264–5; cost of, 265; federal agency for, 266, 269; funding of, 268–9; guidelines for, 263; prohibitions on, 264–5; stem cells and, 273; values and, 266–7
"assisted suicide," 298
attitude, professional, 180–1
"attorney for personal care," 139
Australia: duty to refer in 261
autonomy, 5, 6, 38, 40–1; assisted dying and, 296; beneficence and, 153; capacity and, 93, 149; consent and, 85; justice and, 239; legal articulation of, 72; limits to, 66; meaning of, 53–4; patient-based care and, 50–68; as patient's preference, 54–6; v protection, 131, 145; "relational," 26; reversible factors in, 64–6; right to refuse and, 142–3

Balint M, 151, 219
Barbulov v Cirone, 292
battery, 61, 72
Beecher HK, 340
Belgium: assisted dying in, 299, 300, 310–11, 312; child's assisted dying in, 306; physician support for assisted dying in, 315
beneficence, 5, 6, 38, 40–1; justice and, 239; nonmaleficence and, 151–74; principles of, 151–6
benevolence, 47

"best interests of the patient," 235
best-interests standard: children and, 165
bias: allocation and, 235–6; cultural, 329
"Big Pharma," 183–6
Bill C-14, 302–4; challenge to, 312–13
bioethics, feminist, 25, 26, 28, 29
biologic agents: cost of, 244, 253
birth control, 146; emergency, 257
birthing, 254–60, 262–72
"birth mother," 270
births: reporting of, 126
Blackburn S, 1
Blackwood's Edinburgh Magazine, 214
Block W, 330
blogs, 209
blood cells: stem cells and, 272
blood transfusion, 56–8, 147, 167
body art, 180
Bok S, 88
bone marrow: donation of, 170; stem cells and, 272
boundaries: professional, 186–91; social media and, 197–200
"brain dead," 333–4
breast hormone assay inquiry, 225–6
Breslin J, 308–9
bricolage, 30
British Columbia: driving safety in, 123; eugenics in, 170
British Columbia Civil Liberties Association (BCCLA), 301, 302
British Columbia Court of Appeal, 302

Calgary Health Region, 288
California Supreme Court, 128
Cameron ED, 341
Canada: abortion in, 256–7, 260, 262; assisted reproductive technology in, 263–5; compensation for error in, 222; disclosure in, 121–9; duty to warn in, 128–9; healthcare system in, 242–4; informed consent in, 74–83; pharmaceutical industry in, 185; privacy in, 111; recordings in, 119; right to refuse in, 145
Canada Health Act, 243
Canadian HIV/AIDS Legal Network, 122
Canadian Medical Association, 124, 185, 187, 314, 316; Code of Ethics, 129
Canadian Medical Protective Association, 125, 193
Canadian Paediatrics Society, 305–6
Canadian Psychiatric Association, 115
cancer: truthtelling and, 86–7
"CanMEDS" (Canadian Medical Education Directions for Specialists), 178
Canterbury v Spence, 73–4
capability theory, 23–4, 25, 28, 29

capacity, 131–50; assessment of, 134–6; autonomy and, 53, 149; children and, 145–9; consent and, 136–7; informed choice and, 89, 92–3, 102; mental illness and, 134, 136, 142–5; as term, 132; see also incapacity
cardiopulmonary resuscitation (CPR), 58, 288; see also No CPR; Do not resuscitate
Cardozo B, 69
Carter K, 301–2
Carter v Canada, 289, 293, 302
casuistry, 25, 26–8
"categorical imperative," 20
causation: test of, 80–1
central problem: identifying, 39–40
Centre for Effective Practice, 316
Chalmers I, 340
Chaoulli v Quebec, 243–4
chaperones, 329–30
Charter of Rights and Freedoms: abortion and, 256, 260, 266, 268; assisted dying and, 300, 301, 302, 312
Child and Family Services of Central Manitoba v Lavellee et al, 292
children: abuse and neglect of, 122–3, 166; assisted dying and, 304, 305–7; assumed capacity and, 146; best-interests standard and, 165; competency and, 133; consent and, 102; disclosure and, 335–8; experimental treatment and, 169; as martyrs, 167; parental refusal of care and, 165–9; parental request for treatment and, 169–73; research and, 351–2; right to refuse and, 145–9; "saviour," 273, 274; views of, 165, 172
child welfare authorities, 166, 168
Children's Aid Society of Ottawa-Carleton v M.C., 292
China: privacy in, 111
choices: foolish, 60–2; good, 58–60; "informed," 78; reproductive, 254–75; self-destructive, 62–4
"Choosing Wisely" initiative, 240–2
Christian Science, 169
Ciarlariello v Schacter, 100
"circle of care," 35–6
circumcision: female, 172; male, 170
circumstances: importance of, 34–7; informed consent and, 80, 97–105
class action lawsuits, 226
clinical trials, 344–5, 346–7; equipoise and, 342–4; new drug, 183–4, 185–6; see also research
cloning, 264
co-decision-maker, 142
cochlear implants, 171, 338–9
Cockerham H, 50

codes of ethics, 129, 151
coercion: informed consent and, 94, 95
cogito ergo sum, 54
cognitive impairment: assisted dying and, 307–9
Cohen S, 265
College of Family Physicians of Canada, 315, 316
College of Physicians and Surgeons of Ontario, 315
"collusion of anonymity," 219
Colombia: assisted dying in, 300
commercialization: assisted reproductive technology and, 264–5, 275, 268–72; stem cells and, 273; tissue samples and, 348–9
communication, *xvi–xviii*; cross-cultural, 331–2, 336–7; electronic, 115–17; "facilitative," 223; unexpected findings and, 220–1
community: research and, 350
"community treatment orders," 145
compassion, 19
compensation: disclosure and, 222; large-scale adverse effects and, 226–7; research and 352
competency: autonomy and, 53, 57; as functional capacities, 133; informed choice and, 92–3; maintenance of, 191; presumption of, 133; as term, 132
comprehension: capacity and, 135, 137; informed choice and, 89, 91–2
comprehensiveness: *Canada Health Act* and, 243
compromises: clinical decisions and, 239
computerization, *xvii–xviii*; confidentiality and, 108, 115–17; errors and, 218
confidentiality, 108–30; children and, 146; commitment to, 114; after death, 209–10; duty to warn and, 128; justifications for, 111–12; limits to, 121–9; as outdated, 109; patient, 36; v privacy, 108–9; social media and, 198; trust and, 110–15
conflict: cross-cultural, 333–5; ethical principles and, 39, 40–1; patient and professionals, 2–3; patient's family and, 290–2, 293, substitute decision maker and, 284–6, 289
conflicts of interest, 181–6; research and, 349, 352
conscientious objection: abortion and, 261–2; assisted dying and, 313–17
consent: age of, 146; assisted dying and, 308, 309; capacity and, 136–7; choice and, 78; end-of-life decisions and, 289, 290–2; exceptions to, 97–8; excised tissue and, 347–8; genetic testing and, 325, 326; implied and express, 70–1; informed consent, 72–4; major cases on, 292; medical, 69–71; oral, 69–71; as permission, 85; photography and, 207, 208–9; refusal of, 106; research and, 340–1, 344–50, 351; simple, 69–71; tiered, 349; types of, 71; voluntary, 340; waiver of, 98–9;

withdrawal of, 100–1; written, 71, 89, 207, 208, 209; *see also* informed consent
Consent and Capacity Board (CCB), 139, 141, 290–1
consequence, unintended, 321
consequentialism, 18, 21–3, 27
continuous palliative sedation therapy (CPST), 292–3
contraception: children and, 146; "emergency," 257
coordination: multiple specialties and, 220–1
costs: allocation and, 240–2; assisted reproduction technology (ART), 265; biologic agents, 244, 253; drug, 244–5, 253; genomics, 320
courts: medical evidence and, 115; substitute decision-maker and, 141; *see also* law; lawsuits; specific cases/courts
cover-up: errors and, 218
crime: reporting past/future, 127–8
Criminal Code: assisted dying in, 301, 302; sexual assault in, 115; suicide in, 300
CRISPR (Clustered Regularly Interspaced Short Palindromic Repeats), 319–22; non-therapeutic purposes of, 321
CRISPR-associated (Cas9) genes, 321
"critical rationalism," 29–30, 358
"crossings," boundary, 186–7
"cultural navigators," 334–5
culturally sensitive healthcare, 328–9, 336–7
culture: death and, 332–5; disclosure and, 335–8; ethics and, *xx–xxi*; 34, 327–38; gap in, 327–8, 332; idea of, 327; interpretation of illness and, 331–2; overlap of, 328; refusal of treatment and, 166–7; research and, 358–9; respect for, 336; truthtelling and, 87
curriculum: hidden, 10–12; medical, *xvi–xviii*
custody: assisted reproductive technology and, 270

dangers: assessment of, 161–2
Daniels N, 246–7
data collection: social media and, 202–3
Dawson S, 168
Deaf community, 338
death: allowing, 276–81; brain, 333–4; culture and, 332–5; medical assistance in, 296–318; "reasonably foreseeable," 303, 310, 312–13; "suspicious," 126; *see also* assisted dying; end of life
deception: disclosure and, 337–8; errors and, 218–19; physicians and, 86–8; "protective," 87–8
decisions: allocation, 244–7; assisted, 142–3; autonomy and, 53; competent, 281–4; emotions and, 9–10; end-of-life, 276–95;

ethical management and, 41–2; foolish,
60–2; good, 58–60; self-destructive, 62–4;
shared, 105; unilateral end-of-life, 289–92;
withdrawal of treatment, 284–6; *see also*
substitute decision-makers
Declaration of Helsinki, *xxi,* 340
de-identification, 118
delegation: informed consent and, 72–4, 75, 77
DeLillo D, 230
dementia: advance directives and, 163; assisted
dying and, 307–9
deontology, 18, 20–1
depression, "treatment-resistant," 310
Descartes R, 54
"designer babies," 321
developing countries: medical missions to, 207–8;
research in, 354–6
diagnosis, "differential," 30
dialysis, 90, 91–2, 278
Dickens C, 360
digital technology, *xvii–xviii;* confidentiality and,
108, 115–17; errors and, 218
dilemmas: "existential," 36–7; managing, 33–4
"Diogenes syndrome," 64
diphtheria, 248
disability: capacity and, 138; competency and,
133; mental, 138
disclosure: adequate and truthful, 89, 90–2;
compensation and, 222; concept of, 78; delay
in, 226; discretionary/mandatory, 121–7;
errors and, 218–19, 220–4; genomics and,
322–5, 335–7; informed choice and, 89,
90–2; limits on, 101–5; patient privacy and,
36; patients and, 13–14; physician-based v
patient-based, 74; as proportionate duty, 223;
risks and, 72–4; scope of, 80, 91; suggestions
for, 103; timing of, 223; truthtelling and,
85–9; *see also* reporting
discretionary therapy: children and, 165–6
discrimination, 234–9; assisted reproductive
technology and, 267–8, 269
disease: communicable, 121–2; inheritable, 325;
see also illness; specific diseases
distributive justice, 239–42, 247; meanings
of, 231–3
diversity: ethics and, *xx–xxi*
DNA, 320–2
"Dollars for Docs," 184
Do not resuscitate (DNR) order, 67, 138–9; end-
of-life decisions and, 280–1, 282, 283–4, 288;
see also No CPR
"Don't call us, we'll call you," 218
"double effect doctrine, 293
driving: health information and, 123–4
"Driving and Dementia Toolkit," 124

drugs: abortion, 257; consent and, 76, 99–100;
cost benefit analysis of, 245; cost of, 244–5,
253; effects of, 81–2; off-label use of, 82; *see
also* specific drugs
Durrell L, 85
duty: to attend, 156–8; of care, 143, 151, 158;
fiduciary, 85, 181–2; morality and, 20–1; to
offer help, 156; physician's, 157–60; referral
and, 313, 315–16; reporting and, 123, 126,
127; to rescue, 154–6; of social assistance,
158; to warn and protect, 128–9

E (Mrs) v Eve, 169–72
eggs (human): purchase of, 264–5, 275
elderly people, 62–4, 68; abuse and, 123;
competency and, 133; *see also* vulnerable
people
email: guidelines for use of, 117; privacy and,
115–17; security and, 116
embryos, 264; ownership of, 270–1, 273; surplus,
263, 273–4
emergencies: children and, 167; consent and, 351;
duty to respond in, 157–8; informed choice
and, 91, 97–8
emotions: decision-making and, 9–10; ethics and,
24; reason and, 47
empathy, 7–9, 25
employers: health information and, 124–5
"end justifies the means," 21
end of life: decisions on, 276–95; studies of,
278–9
end-stage renal disease (ESRD), 278
entitlement: patients and, 237, 240–1;
transplantation and, 250
"entrustment model," 96
equipoise: clinical trials, and, 342–4, 345
errors: cause of, 217–18; disclosure of, 218–19,
220–4; guidelines for disclosure of, 224;
human, 217–18; management of, 214–29;
medical, 214–22; mistakes and, 215; rates of,
216–17; response to, 221; systemic, 217–18;
see also adverse effects
ethical management process, 33; application of,
43–7; steps in, 37–42
ethics, *xix–xx;* care-based, 26–8; management
of, 33–49; obstacles to, 12–13; preventative,
325–7; professional, 28–30; research and,
340–57; suggested readings on, 361
ethnic minorities: guidelines for treatment of, 328
ethnography, 335
eugenics, 170
European Convention of Human Rights, 269
European Union: duty of social assistance in, 158
euthanasia: voluntary/involuntary/non-
voluntary, 298–9

Eve case, 169–72
experience, physicians', 76
explanation: errors and, 222

Facebook, 197–200, 202; -Cambridge Analytica
    scandal, 202
facilities: assisted dying and, 316–17
Fadiman A, 331–2
fairness, 6–7; justice and, 231–3, 239, 251
fallibilism, 29–30
family: advance directives and, 283; cessation of
    treatment and, 284–6, 289; changing nature
    of, 270–2; death and culture and, 332–5;
    disagreement with, 290–2, 293; disclosure
    and, 335–8; genetic disclosure and, 322–3,
    335–7; guidelines for working with, 286;
    informed consent and, 83–4
fathers: rights of, 260–1
feedback, patient, 192
fee-for-service, 181
feminist bioethics, 25, 26, 28, 29
fetal alcohol syndrome (FAS), 274–5
fetus: status of, 257–60
fiduciary duty, 85, 181–2
fitness: medical practice and, 191–4
Fleming v Reid and Gallagher, 57, 308
food: dementia and, 309; prescribed, 252
Food and Drug Act, 265
force: feeding and, 43–7; use of, 14
"framing effect," 95
Frankfurt H, 9
fraud: healthcare, 126; research, 350
Freedman B, 342
friends, Facebook, 197–200
furor therapeuticus, 154, 156

gametes, 264
Gawande A, 25
Gellner E, 29, 358–9
gender: discrimination and, 235–6
"genital nicking," 172
"gestational carrier," 270
gestational contract, 267
gifts, 189–90; from industry, 183–6
Gillick v West Norfolk, 146
Glasgow Coma Scale, 333
Global Fund to Fight AIDS, Tuberculosis, and
    Malaria, 359
"goals of care," 280
golden rule test, 23
Golubchuk case, 291, 292
good conscience test, 23
Good Samaritan laws, 157–8
Google: data-mining and, 116
"grievous and irremediable medical condition," 303

guardian, 41
guardianship laws, 123
guidelines, clinical, 245–7
gunshot wounds: reporting of, 125–6

Halappanavar S, 16
Hall J, 228
Halls v Mitchell, 121
Hard Times, 360
harm, 7, 151–2; clear, 172–3; errors and, 214;
    negligence and, 216; "zero option" and,
    153–6
Harris S, *xvii*
health, physicians', 193–4
Health Canada, 257
healthcare: aggressive, 238; culturally sensitive,
    328–9, 336–7; inappropriate, 240; "managed,"
    238; patient-based, 50–68; paying for, 242;
    universal, 222; *see also* medicine
Health Care Consent Act, 290, 291
healthcare professionals: liability and, 164; risks
    to, 158–60; *see also* physicians; specific
    specialties
"healthcare representative,"139
healthcare system, 242–4; mutually recognized,
    234
"health custodian," 114
health information: access to, 112–14; actionable,
    322; computerized, 218; control over, 325–7;
    disclosure of, 121–7; employers and, 124–5;
    genetic testing and, 322–5; legislation on,
    111, 113, 128; ownership of, 114, 210–11;
    patient, 108–30; psychiatric, 114–15; research
    and, 352–3; written consent and, 71
health insurance: private, 243–4; public, 242–3
*Heath Insurance Portability and Accountability
    Act (HIPPA)*, 111
"HeLa cells," 347
heteronomy, 53
Hippocrates, 194, 214
Hippocratic Oath, 30–1, 151
HIV status, 122
honesty: apologies and, 224; errors and, 218,
    223, 228
hope: truthtelling and, 104–5
Hopp v Lepp, 74–7, 91
hospices: assisted dying and, 316–17
hospitals: abortion and, 262; assisted dying and,
    316–17
Hughes B, 147
Human Fertilisation and Embryology
    Authority, 266
Human Genome Project, 319
humans: experimentation on, 340
Hume D, 33, 47

humiliation: as suffering, 309
humility, 19
hybrid theories, 18, 23–8

ICH–GCP ("International Conference on
    Harmonization of technical requirements for
    registration of pharmaceuticals for human
    use" – "Good Clinical Practice"), 355–6
identification: genomics and, 325–7; research
    and, 353
I.H.V. (Re), 292
illness: as deviation from normal, 268;
    interpretation of, 331–2; "orphan," 322; *see
    also* disease; mental illness; specific illnesses
immunization, 166, 248–9
impairments, physicians', 193
incapacity, 131–50; causes and prevalence of,
    133–4; recognition of, 134; research and,
    351–2; *see also* capacity
incarceration: psychotic patients and, 143
incidental findings, 322–5; research and, 352
incompetence: assumption of, 133
India: surrogacy in, 262
Indigenous peoples: forced sterilization and, 170;
    genetic testing and, 325–7; guidelines for
    treatment of, 328; refusal of care and, 148–9;
    removal of children and, 166
industry: professionalism and, 183–6
infections, physicians', 193
infertility, 268
"informed choice," 78; elements of, 89–95; opiates
    and, 99–100; requirements of, 92; specific
    circumstances and, 97–105; truthtelling
    and, 85–107
informed consent: delegation and, 77, 78–9;
    legal roots of, 69–84; requirements of, 92; as
    term, 72; *see also* consent
Informed Consent Forms (ICFs): research and, 344
"informed dissent," 85
injustice, 236; *see also* justice
Instagram, 202
Institutional Review Board (IRB), 350
institutions: assisted dying and, 316–17
instructions: advance, 56; prior, 46; *see also*
    advance directives
insurance, health, 242–4
"intended couple," 271
"interests of justice," 115
international aid organizations, 359
Internet: information and, 359; privacy and, 201;
    see also social media
interprofessionalism, 180
interventions: criteria for, 241
interviewing, patient-based, 52
"intransigence," patient, 161

in vitro techniques, 262
"I think, therefore I am," 54
Ireland: law in, 16
IUD, 257

Jehovah's Witnesses, 56, 147, 167
Jin v Calgary Health Region, 292
Jin Z, 287–9
"JJ," 148–9
Jordan K, 271
journals: more rigorous rules and, 344
jurisprudence, *xxii;* informed consent and,
    71–83; North American, 72; *see also* courts;
    law; lawsuits; specific cases/courts
justice, 5, 6–7, 38, 40–1; allocation and, 247–51;
    distributive, 231–3, 239–42, 247; healthcare
    and, 230–53; "interests of," 115; social, 358

Kahneman D, 95
Kant I, 20–1, 27, 53, 274
Kekes J, 29
Kevorkian J, 299
Kleinman A, 332
Kraman S, Hamm G, 222

"labelling": truthtelling and, 102
Lacks H, 347
Lamb v Canada, 310, 312–13
Landstreet P, 327
language: as barrier, 331; competency and, 133
"large-scale adverse effects," 225–8; guidelines
    for, 227
law: abortion, 256–7, 260–2; advance directives
    and, 282; assisted reproductive technology
    and, 268–72; end-of-life decisions and,
    289–92; errors and, 218–19; ethics and,
    16–17; forced feeding and, 45; guardianship,
    123; health information and, 111, 113, 128;
    informed consent and, 69–84; parental
    obligation and, 166; refusal of treatment and,
    276–7; standard of care and, 159; suicide,
    300, 302–3; *see also* courts; specific cases/
    courts/laws
Law Reform Commission Report, 296, 317
lawsuits, 222; class action, 226; wrongful life, 83
Lee P, George R, 259
lesbian, gay, bisexual, transgender, queer
    (LGBTQ+) people: assisted reproductive
    technology and, 267, 269, 270–2; guidelines
    for treatment of, 328
leukemia, 272, 272
Lévi-Strauss C, 30
liability: apologies and, 224–5; errors and,
    218–19; suicide and, 164–5
life: beginning of, 273

LinkedIn, 200
lithium, 344–5
litigation: guidelines and, 246
"living wills," 138, 281–4; advance directive, 281
Luxembourg: assisted dying in, 299, 300
Lyttelton G, 108

McGregor C, 128–9
Macklin R, 319
McKneally M, 96–7
McLachlin B, 131, 144
majority: age of, 146
Malette v Shulman, 56–8, 308
malpractice, 222, 246
"managed care," 238
management of the healthcare system:
    mandatory notifications and, 126
mandatory disclosure, 121–7
Mandatory Gunshot Wounds Reporting Act, 125
mandatory outpatient treatment, 145
manipulation: informed consent and, 94
manners, professional, 178–80
Martin S, 288
Marx K, 335
maturation: intervening in, 171–2
"mature minor doctrine," 146, 147
mature minors: assisted dying and, 305–7
maturity: children and, 145, 146, 147
measles, 248
medical actionability, 322
medical assistance in dying (MAID), 296–318;
    legislation for, 302–4; terminology and,
    298–300; *see also* assisted dying
Medical Officer of Health, 121–2
"Medical Professionalism in the New Millennium:
    A Physician Charter," 177–8, 358
medical records: computerized, 218; written
    consent and, 71; *see also* health information
medicare, 242–3
medications: *see* drugs; specific medications
medicine: legacy of, 340–1; narrative, 9;
    patient-based, *xx, xxi;* "personalized," 320;
    "precision," 320; regenerative, 272; *see also*
    healthcare
memes, 336, 337
mental disability: capacity and, 138
mental illness: assisted dying and, 304–5, 310–13;
    autonomy and, 64; capacity and, 134, 136,
    142–5; denial of, 144; right to refuse
    and, 142–5
Mifegymiso, 257
Mill JS, 21, 42
Miller FG, Appelbaum PS, 311
"mimetics," 336
minimally conscious state, 289

miscommunication: informed consent and, 95–6
mistakes: errors and, 215; *see also* errors
mitochondrial DNA (mtDNA), 320
mitochondrial replacement therapy (MRT),
    262–3, 269
MMSE (Mini-Mental State Examination), 107
"modified objective test," 79–82
"moral monism," 23
Morgentaler H, 256
"morning after pill," 257
mothers: rights of, 260–1
MSF (Médecins Sans Frontières), 359
"mutual aid": research and, 355
"mutual recognition," 234–9

narcotics: loss of, 126; prescription of, 159–60; *see
    also* drugs; opiates; opioid crisis
narrative theory, 24–6, 29
National Institutes of Health, 320
National Security Agency, 111
"navigators," cultural 334–5
Nazis: human experimentation and, 340
"necessaries/necessities of life," 166
negligence, 75, 159–60, 215–16
Netherlands: assisted dying in, 299, 300, 310–11,
    312; child's assisted dying in, 306; physician
    support for assisted dying in, 315
New England Journal of Medicine, 58
Newfoundland and Labrador: large-scale adverse
    effect in 225–6
NICE (National Institute for Health and Care
    Excellence), 244–5
No CPR (cardiopulmonary resuscitation) order,
    138–9, 280–1, 295; *see also* Do not resuscitate
non-disclosure: culture and, 335–8; genomics
    and, 322, 323, 325
non-governmental organizations (NGOs), 359
nonmaleficence, 5, 7, 8, 38, 40–1; beneficence
    and, 151–74; principles of, 151–6; "zero
    option" and, 154
North America: health information disclosure
    in, 121–2
nursing: culturally sensitive competence and, 328
Nussbaum M, 9–10, 23–4, 152

Obermeyer Z, Lee TH, *xviii*
Oken D, 86
Ontario: capacity in, 139; consent in, 290; duty to
    refer in, 261; health information in, 121–2;
    mandatory gunshot reporting in, 125
Ontario Court of Appeal, 56
Open Payments Program, 184
opiates: consent and, 99–100
opioid crisis, 159–60
options: ethical management and, 40–1

organs: purchase of, 249, 250, 251; solicitation of, 251
outcomes research, 245–6
overmedication, 63
overtreatment, 240
ownership: embryos and, 270–2, 273; photography and, 208; tissue samples and, 348
OXFAM, 359

pain, 31–2; consent and, 99–100; palliative sedation and, 293
palliative care, 8; v assisted death, 315
palliative sedation, 292–3
pandemics: vaccines and, 248–9
Pappworth M, 340
parens patriae doctrine, 170
parents: assisted reproductive technology and, 270–2; child's assisted dying and, 306; refusal of care and, 165–9; requests for treatment and, 169–73
Parfit D, 15, 29
paternalism, 73, 58–60; acceptable, 156; deception as, 86, 87–8; defensible, 105; therapeutic privilege and, 104
patients: "best interests" of, 235; as consumers, 51; elderly, 62–4, 68, 123, 133; empathy and, 7–9; errors and, 222–3; ethics and, 6–7; as "friends," 198, 199; incidental findings and, 322–5, 352; increasing power of, 359; "intransigent," 161; just treatment of, 235–9; online privacy of, 205, 206–11; preference of, 54–6, 237; psychotic, 143–4; reckless, 162–5; refusal of treatment and, 276–81; truth and, 86–8; unexpected findings and, 220; use of social media by, 204–6; views of, 153; *see also* vulnerable people
Patriot Act: medical records and, 127
Patterson K, 209–10
Peabody F, 178
Pellegrino E, Thomasma D, 17
Pennsylvania Supreme Court, 78–9
Perkin R, 1–2
permission: consent and, 85; simple consent and, 69, 70–1
persistent vegetative state (PVS), 287–9
Personal Health Information Protection Act (PHIPA), 111
Personal Information Protection and Electronic Documents Act (PIPEDA), 111
"personal/private": social media and, 201–4
"personal/professional": social media and, 200, 204
"personalized medicine," 320
personhood, 257–8
persuasion: v coercion, 94
pharmaceutical industry, 183–6; research and, 343

philosophy: ethics and, 15–32
photography: clinical, 206–9; ownership of, 208; patient privacy and, 206–9; written consent and, 71
Physician Charter, A, 177–8, 358
physician-accelerated death, 298
"physician-assisted dying," 298
"physician-assisted suicide," 299
physicians: abortion and, 258, 261–2; burnout and, 359, 360–1; conscience and, 313–17; impairments of, 193; "reasonable," 73; support for assisted dying among, 314–15; *see also* healthcare professionals
"pillow angel," 171–2
placebos, 104–5, 345–7
point system: transplantation and, 249
Popper K, *xxi*
portability: *Canada Health Act* and, 243
portals, patient, 113
"post-professionalism," 175
power: informed choice and, 85; patients', 359; trainees and, 10–12, 13
Power of Attorney for Personal Care, 139
preceptors: as "friends," 199–200
"precision medicine," 320
pregnancy, 254–60, 339; burden of, 259; "right to," 268
preimplantation genetic diagnosis, 338–9
prescriptions: safety and, 159–60; "special diet" and, 252
President's Commission on Ethical Problems in Medicine, 86–7
preventative ethics, 325–7
prevention science, 322
primum non nocere, 7
Prince v Massachusetts, 167
"principlism," 23
principles, ethical, 2–7, 28–30
privacy, 108–30; breaches of, 116; vii confidentiality, 108–9; genetics and, 324, 325; justifications for, 111–12; limits to, 121–9; meaning of, 110; new risks to, 115–21; photography and, 206–9; research and, 352–3; right to, 111, 112, 260; social media and, 197–200; trust and, 110–15
privacy settings, 198, 200, 202–4
"private/personal": social media and, 201–4
Procrustes, 172
professionalism, 175–96, 358–61; v "doing your job," 180–1; industry and, 183–6; new, 177–81, 194; social media and, 198
"professional/personal": social media and, 200, 204
prognosis: errors in, 287–9
proportionality: justice and, 231–3, 239
protection: *v* autonomy, 131, 145, 149

provinces: assisted dying and, 303; driving safety in, 123–4; mandatory gunshot reporting in, 125; privacy in, 111; *see also* specific provinces
"proxy," 139
prudence, 19
psychedelics, 341
psychiatry: boundaries and, 190; capacity assessment and, 136; confidentiality in, 114–15
"psychic driving," 341
psychotherapy: boundaries and, 187
psychotic patients: right to refuse and, 143–4
public guardian/trustee, 139
publicity test, 23
public opinion polls: transplantation and, 249–50

quality improvement (QI) studies, 354
quality of care, 152
quality-of-life issues, 152, 153
Quebec: age of consent in, 146; assisted dying in, 301; duty of social assistance in, 158
"quickening," 273
Quinlan KA, 287

R v Morgentaler, 256, 257, 261
race: discrimination and, 235
radiologists: unexpected findings and, 220, 323
Railway Safety Act, 124
randomized controlled trial (RCT), 344–5, 346–7; *see also* research
Rasouli H, 289–91
Rasouli v Sunnybrook Health Sciences, 292
RateMD, 191
rating sites, 191–3
"rationalism," critical, 29–30, 358
rationing, 238–9, 244–5; guidelines for, 245–7; rationale for, 247
Rawls J, 21, 234, 247
reason: capacity and, 137; commitment to, 30; emotion and, 47
reasonableness: standard of care and, 216
reasonable person, 74, 79–82; disclosure and, 90; first use of, 78
reasonable physician, 73
"reasonably foreseeable death," 303, 310, 312–13
recklessness, patient, 162–5
recording: guidelines for, 120; legality of, 119; patients', 118–21
records: *see* health information; medical records
referral: assisted dying and, 313, 315–16; conscientious objection and, 261–2; "effective," 313, 315–16
refusal: information sharing and, 36; physician's, 5–6

refusal of care, 56–8, 161–3; children and, 145–9; death and, 276–81; "informed," 58; life-sustaining treatment and, 147; parental, 165–9
"regenerative medicine," 272
registry: ART donors and, 266
regulation: genomics and, 321; professional, 193; research and, 343–4; stem cells and, 273
Reibl v Hughes, 74, 77–82, 90
relativism: cultural, 336–7; moral/cultural, 358–9
religion, 328; death and, 333–4; morality and, 15; refusal of care and, 168
"removing life support," 334
reporting: child abuse and, 122–3, 166; circumstances requiring, 121–7; colleagues' fitness and, 194; elder abuse and, 123; ethical violations and, 188; *see also* disclosure
reproduction, 254–75; new age of, 262–72
requests for treatment: inappropriate, 190–1; parental, 169–73
rescue: limited duty to, 154–6
research: consent and, 340–1, 344–7, 347–50, 351; equipoise and, 342–4, 345; ethics and, 340–57; fraud in, 350; Indigenous peoples and, 325–7; international, 354–6; nonclinical purposes of, 347; online guidelines for, 356; outcomes, 245–6; placebos and, 345–7; purpose of, 341–4; regulation of, 343–4
research ethics board (REB), 345, 350; depth of review and, 354
research participants: information needed by, 344; payment of, 352; privacy of, 352–3
respect for persons, 30; truthtelling and, 87–8
results, missed or overlooked, 218
revalidation, 193
rights: assisted reproductive technology and, 267–8; children of ART and, 265–6; fetal, 254, 257–60; privacy and, 111, 112, 260; security of the person and, 260; women's, 254, 257–60, 260–1
right to refuse, 142–5; children and, 145–9; limits on, 145
risks: disclosure of, 72–4, 75, 77; healthcare professionals and, 158–60; material, 90; minimizing, 80–1
Rodriguez S, 276–7, 296, 300, 301
Rodriguez v British Columbia, 293
Roe v Wade, 260
Roma people, 339
Rosen J, 201
Rosenthal DI, Verghese A, 359

Sacks O, 25
safety: child, 166–7; driving, 123–4; duty of professionals and, 159–60; flying, train, and marine, 124

Salasel P, 290, 291
Salgo v Leland Standford Jr, 72–4
Sault M, 148–9
Saundby R, 175
"saviour child," 273, 274
Sawatsky v Riverview Health Centre, 292
scarcity: resources and, 244
Schloendorff v Society of New York Hospital, 72
Schneider C, 53
"Screen for the Identification of Cognitively
    Impaired Medically at Risk Drivers"
    (SIMARD) test, 124
second opinion, 58
security: email and, 116
security of the person, 260
sedation: consent and, 99–100;
    palliative, 292–3
"seeding," 183
self-determination: assisted dying and, 296
self-disclosure, 193; social media and, 198
self-endangering, 160–5
self-referral, 194–5
self-regulation, professional, 193
Selzer R, 25
Sen A, 23, 33, 152
Sessums LL, 135 10
sex: selection for, 256, 258, 264
sexual assault: confidentiality and, 115
sexual relations: patients and, 187–8
"shared decision-making," 105
Shobridge v Thomas, 218–19
Short Messaging Service (SMS), 118
Siegler M, 109, 129
SIMARD ("Screen for the Identification of
    Cognitively Impaired Medically at Risk
    Drivers") test, 124
Singer P, 22
Skloot R, 347
smallpox, 248
smartphone app, 120
Smith L, 301
Smith v Jones, 115, 127–8
Snowden E, 111
social justice, 358
social media, 197–213; business page and, 200;
    guidelines for, 211, 212
Sophie's Choice, 36–7
"special diets," 252
sperm: purchase of, 264–5
stab wounds: reporting of, 125–6
standard of care: legal, 159; negligence and, 216;
    research and, 342–3, 344
standard practice, 159–60
standards, research, 355–6
Starson v Swayze, 144–5

stem cells, 254, 272–4; embryonic, 272, 273–4;
    induced pluripotent, 272; regulated
    research and treatment using, 273; therapies
    using, 272–4
sterilization: forced, 170; parental request for,
    169–72; surgical, 58–9
stillbirths: reporting of, 126
stories, patients', 9, 24–6
students: power over, 10–12, 13
Styron W, 36
substitute decision-makers (SDM), 41, 82;
    capacity and, 102, 138–42; disagreement
    with, 284–6, 289; emergencies and, 97–8;
    hierarchy of, 140; living will and, 281, 282–3;
    patient's wishes and, 141; refusal of consent
    and, 106
suffering, intolerable, 292–3, 309, 310, 311, 313
suicide, 162–5; "assisted," 298; law and, 300,
    302–3; prevention of, 312; "rational," 163,
    311; survivors of, 311
suicide note, 163, 164
supported decision-maker, 142
Supreme Court (British Columbia), 266, 301
Supreme Court of Canada: abortion and, 256,
    260; assisted dying and, 300, 304, 313, 315;
    blood transfusions and, 147, 167; child
    sterilization and, 170; competency and,
    144; confidentiality and, 127; consent to
    withdrawal of treatment and, 100, 290–1;
    fiduciary duty and, 181; informed consent
    and, 76, 78, 83; palliative sedation and, 293;
    private insurance and, 243–4; refusal of
    treatment and, 277
Supreme Court (Nova Scotia), 268–9
Supreme Court (US), 111
surrogacy, 262–72, 275; gestational/traditional, 267
surrogate contract, 271
"surrogate decision-maker," 139
Switzerland: assisted dying in, 299, 300, 301
syphilis, 341

Tarasoff, 128
tattoo, 58
Taylor G, 301–2
termination, pregnancy: *see* abortion
terminology: assisted dying and, 298–300; end-
    of-life decisions and, 278, 281
Ter Neuzen v Korn, 159
tests: apnea, 333; genetic, 322–5, 325–7;
    guidelines for ordering, 240;
    preimplantation, 262–3; prenatal, 255–6, 258;
    purpose of, 326; *see also* specific tests
text messaging: privacy and, 118
theories: ethical, 15–32; hybrid, 18, 23–8;
    typology of, 18; *see also* specific theories

"Therapeutic Abortion Committee," 256
"therapeutic misconception," 342
"therapeutic nihilism," 7
"therapeutic privilege," 104
therapy, discretionary, 165–6
"third party examiner," 125
Thomsen JJ, 259
tissue: control over, 350; research and, 347–50
Toms v Foster, 123
"toolbox approach," 30
Torres J, 288–9
torture: victims of, 328, 329, 330
trainees: as "friends," 199–200; power over,
    10–12, 13
tranquilizers, 62–4, 68
transplantation, 248, 249–51
"transplant tourism," 249–51
treatment: disproportionate, 155; experimental,
    169; futile/ineffectual, 284; not covered by
    medicare, 243; potentially life-sustaining,
    278, 284–6, 289–92; proportionate, 152;
    "zero," 153–6
Tremblay v Daigle, 261
triage, 238
triazolam, 62–4, 68
trust: confidentiality and, 110–15; ethics
    and, 30–1; informed consent and, 95–7;
    professionalism and, 181–3
trustworthiness, 19
truth: Kant and, 20; utilitarianism and, 21
Truth and Reconciliation Commission, 148
truthtelling: disclosure and, 85–9; importance of,
    88–9; informed choice and, 85–107; limits
    on, 101–5
tubal ligation, 58–9
tuberculosis, 121
Tuskegee Syphilis Study, 341

ultrasound, 255–6
"Ulysses contract," 45–6
unconsciousness, end-of-life, 287–8
underdeveloped countries: missions to, 207–8;
    research in, 354–6
"undue influence," 94
unexpected findings, 220–1, 323
Uniform Apology Act, 224–5
United Kingdom: assisted reproductive
    technology in, 264, 266, 269; recordings in,
    119; "whistle-blowers" in, 194

United States: abortion in, 260, 262; assisted
    dying in, 299–300; assisted reproductive
    technology in, 264; crime reporting in,
    127, 128; informed consent in, 72–4;
    malpractice in, 222; pharmaceutical
    industry in, 184–5; privacy in, 111;
    recordings in, 119; refusal of treatment in,
    168; right to refuse in, 145
universality: *Canada Health Act* and, 243
University of Michigan Health System, 222
unmarried people: assisted reproductive
    technology and, 267
urgency: informed choice and, 91, 97–8
utilitarianism, 21, 28

vaccination, 248–9; refusal of, 166
Vanderberghe J, 311, 312
vasectomy, 59
ventilator: removal of, 333–4
violations, boundary, 186, 187–8
"violinist analogy," 259
virtue theory, 17–20
voluntariness: informed choice and, 89, 93–5
"voluntary euthanasia," 298
vulnerable people, 12; capacity and, 131–2, 133,
    137–9; duty to attend and, 156; patients
    as, 95; refusal of care and, 161–3; *see also*
    patients

Waiting for Godot, 276
wait times, 243
Wait Times Alliance Canada, 243
Walker J, 147
war: medical treatment and, 238
WebMD, 191
Wennberg J, 246, 247
"whistle-blowers," 194
white coat, 180
Whole Genome Sequencing, 322
Williams B, 10
"withdrawal of care," 278
"withdrawal of potentially life-sustaining
    treatment," 278; criteria for, 279, 290–1;
    decisions on, 284–6
"withholding of care," 278; decisions on, 284–6
work: fitness to, 124–5
wrongful life suit, 83

"zero option," 90, 153–6